**Nigel Cawthorne** has written over a hundred books including the *Sex Lives* series, *The World's Greatest Royal Scandals*, *The World's Greatest Political Scandals*, *Sordid Sex Lives*, *Sex Secrets of Old England*, *A Brief History of Robin Hood*, *A Brief Guide to James Bond* and *A Brief Guide to Sherlock Holmes*.

# THE MAMMOTH BOOK OF
# Sex Scandals

Nigel Cawthorne

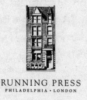

ROBINSON    RUNNING PRESS
PHILADELPHIA · LONDON

Constable & Robinson Ltd
55–56 Russell Square
London WC1B 4HP
www.constablerobinson.com

First published in the UK by Robinson,
an imprint of Constable & Robinson Ltd, 2012

A copy of the British Library Cataloguing in Publication
Data is available from the British Library

UK ISBN: 978-1-78033-538-4 (paperback)
UK ISBN: 978-1-78033-539-1 (ebook)

1 3 5 7 9 10 8 6 4 2

First published in the United States in 2012 by Running Press Book Publishers,
A Member of the Perseus Books Group

Books published by Running Press are available at special discounts for bulk
purchases in the United States by corporations, institutions, and other organizations.
For more information, please contact the Special Markets Department at the
Perseus Books Group, 2300 Chestnut Street, Suite 200, Philadelphia, PA 19103, or
call (800) 810-4145, ext. 5000, or e-mail special.markets@perseusbooks.com.

US ISBN: 978-0-7624-4593-6
US Library of Congress Control Number: 2011939122

9 8 7 6 5 4 3 2 1
Digit on the right indicates the number of this printing

Running Press Book Publishers
2300 Chestnut Street
Philadelphia, PA 19103-4371

Visit us on the web!
www.runningpress.com

Printed and bound in the UK

# Contents

# Introduction

The world is awash with sex scandals. They began when Adam and Eve were thrown out of the Garden of Eden for inappropriate behaviour. And that got press. The story is carried in the Bible, the Torah and the Koran. Thousands of years later, people are still talking about it.

But then history is full of sex scandals. The ancient Egyptians were strong on incest. Wealth was handed down the matriarchal lines. So for a pharaoh to hold on to his money when his wife died, he would marry his daughter, and when she died he would marry his granddaughter/daughter. Later, the Ptolemaic pharaohs married within the immediate family to preserve their Macedonian blood. Cleopatra had married her brother, before she banged Julius Caesar and Mark Antony.

Then there were the Greeks. Well, we all know what the Greeks got up to. The Romans were little better. Julius Caesar swung both ways – his legionaries sang about it as they marched. Tiberius, Caligula and Nero are bywords for sexual excess, though the others, such as Elagabalus, were far worse.

Medieval popes and potentates indulged themselves. Crusaders, courtiers and clerics turned the pages of history blue. After nailing his Ninety-Five Theses to the door of the church in Wittenberg, Martin Luther married a nun. Henry VIII changed history for a bit of the other. His first wife had been a hand-me-down from his brother, while he had already slept with his second wife's sister. Louis XIV, the Sun King, surrounded himself with mistresses who were involved in poisoning and the nude rites of the black mass.

Napoleon only said, "Not tonight, Joséphine," because he had other women to sleep with. Dictators know how to get their way. British prime ministers and the occupants of the White House have hardly been paragons. When they get found out, it is, of course, scandalous. But it is also hilarious. Nothing is funnier than the great and the good being caught with their pants down. Indeed, we've all been there. What do you want to do, laugh or cry?

Sex and scandal have been the stuff of comedy since Aristophanes (450–388 BC). Likewise, the Romans laughed their togas off at a bit of saucy innuendo. Suetonius followed his *Lives of the Twelve Caesars* – which is racy enough – with *Lives of Famous Whores*. Pietro Aretino, Boccaccio, Rabelais, Cervantes, Swift and Voltaire have also raised a laugh with a bit of slap and tickle, often at the expense of those set above them. Musical hall and burlesque used sexual humour as a staple. The "Whitehall farces" put on in the Whitehall Theatre in London between 1950 and 1959, have become synonymous with sexual shenanigans in seat of the British establishment and the *Carry On* films made between 1958 and 1978 export coarse English humour to the world. John F. Kennedy watched *Carry on Constable* in the White House.

When I told a friend that I was writing the *Mammoth Book of Sex Scandals*, he asked: "Do mammoths have sex scandals?" Do they, indeed, have sex? Not any more. That's how they died out.

As with the mammoths, sex scandals does not necessarily mean there was any actual sex going on. When two people disappear into a bedroom together, they usually come out with at least three different stories. What we are talking about here is sex that is reported in the press, or the history books, or wherever. The word "allegedly" will be used a lot. When push comes to shove, without a time machine and a predisposition for voyeurism one cannot check these things out.

This is an exercise in *Schadenfreude* or floccinaucinihilipilification. May contain nuts.

Nigel Cawthorne
Bloomsbury, November 2011

# 1

## Presidential Peccadilloes

### Barack Obama

When Barack Obama came to power in 2009, he was a breath of fresh air. With a beautiful wife and two young daughters, he was a young black man who was plainly virile. Within fifteen months of his arrival at the White House, the *National Enquirer* was printing scandalous rumours about the new president and attractive young campaign worker Vera Baker, who worked tirelessly to raise millions for Obama's US Senate race.

According to the US supermarket tabloid, a limo driver, who preferred to remain anonymous – discretion being the better part of valour – claimed he drove Ms Baker to a secret hotel rendezvous with the thrusting young senatorial hopeful. He said he chauffeured Vera "from a friend's home in the DC area to the Hotel George where I learned later that Obama would be spending the night".

The driver recalled that he "waited in the lobby while she went to change her outfit. But to the best of my knowledge she did not have a room at the hotel and she was not staying there so I thought that it was a bit odd." He said he also picked up Barack Obama at the airport and drove both him and Ms Baker to various locations where they were raising money.

"About 10.30 p.m., I drove them to the hotel and they went in together," he said. "My services for the evening were done."

So he left, but added: "There was absolutely no indication she was going to leave the hotel that night."

The *Enquirer* said the driver's account had been independently corroborated by investigators who believed the couple spent the night together there.

The story of the alleged affair had surfaced before. On 11 October 2008 – just three weeks before the presidential election – Britain's *Daily Mail* ran the rumour that Obama had a "close friendship with an attractive African-American female employee . . . who in 2004 was hired to work on his team for his bid to become a senator".

This caused problems in the Obama household, apparently.

"The woman was purportedly sidelined from her duties after Senator Obama's wife, Michelle, became convinced that he had developed a personal friendship with her."

The *Mail* also claimed that the rumours had first circulated in August, just two weeks before the Democratic Party convention where he finally wrested the nomination from Hillary Clinton. The newspaper went on to say that she had been "exiled" to a Caribbean island because Michelle Obama objected to her continuing to work with her husband on the 2004 campaign.

According to the *Mail*'s sources "she was removed from her position and the political scene because Michelle got wind of the fact that she had a close friendship with her husband. She disappeared, then she reappeared in the Caribbean."

The paper did not reveal the name of the mystery woman, but contacted her in the Caribbean.

"Nothing happened," she insisted. "I just left at the end of the campaign . . . I have no comment on anything. I switched careers. That's it. I'm a Democrat and I support Senator Obama . . . I don't have anything to say."

A lawyer representing the woman said: "Although her duties on the [2004] campaign changed over time, there was never any hint that Mrs Obama had any concerns about her relationship with the senator or played any role in recommending a change in her duties."

Plainly the *Daily Mail* was barking up the wrong tree as, on 12 October 2008, the *Enquirer* exclusively reported Barack Obama's long-time mentor and "father figure" was a "sex pervert". For seven years, he had a "father-son" relationship with Frank Marshall Davis, who the *Enquirer* said had confessed to having sex with children, sadomasochism, bondage and practising a wide array of deviant sexual activities. So this was supposed to have rubbed off?

In his 1995 memoir *Dreams from My Father*, Obama identifies his childhood mentor only as "Frank", but it has since been revealed that he was referring to Davis, a journalist and poet who was a pal of Obama's maternal grandfather, Stanley Dunham. Frank Marshall Davis admitted in his private papers that he had secretly authored a hard-core pornographic autobiography called *Sex Rebel: Black*, published in 1968. The author of the book is billed as "Bob Greene". But Davis later confessed to its authorship after a reader noticed similarities in style and phraseology between that book and Davis's poetry.

Neither allegation did anything to dent Obama at the polls the following month. But the *National Enquirer* was far from satisfied. In 2010, it claimed that "on-site hotel surveillance video camera footage could provide indisputable evidence . . . investigators are working to obtain the tape". And "top anti-Obama operatives are offering more than $1 million to witnesses to reveal what they know about the alleged hush-hush affair". Unfortunately, the tape never surfaced and the $1 million is, as yet, unspent.

## George Washington

Barack Obama would not have been the first president to have invited scandal. In 1775, during the War of Independence, George Washington found himself embroiled in the

"Washerwoman Kate Affair". In late July, Benjamin Harrison, a member of the Continental Congress in Philadelphia, had written to General Washington about "pretty little Kate, the washerwoman's daughter over the way, clean, trim and rosy as the morning" who he had "fitted for my general again his return". The arrangements were not quite complete as Mrs Harrison had intervened, but Harrison intended to meet Kate again to arrange an assignation because, as he told Washington, he was eager "to amuse you, and unbend your mind from the cares of the war".

The letter was published in the *Massachusetts Gazette and Boston Weekly News-Letter*. Then it was picked up by the *Gentleman's Magazine* in London. In the scandal that ensued, the story took the stage on Broadway in a play with the cumbersome title: *The Battle of Brooklyn: A Farce of Two Acts: As It Was Performed on Long Island, on Tuesday the 27th day of 1776, by the Representatives of Americans, Assembled at Philadelphia*. In the play, Lady Gates, wife of General Horatio Gates, a retired British general fighting for the revolutionaries, cross-questions her maid Betty about her relations with Benjamin Harrison who, it seems, had bought her services for fifty "hard" dollars, only to hand her over to Washington. But Betty was not unhappy with the arrangement. She tells Lady Gates that she could not stand Harrison even for half a night. George Washington, by contrast, was the "sweetest, meekest, melancholy sighing gentleman; and then he is such a warrior – oh, mam, I shall always love the General". Washington then gave her a thirty-dollar bill – "he assured me that it would have been more, but that he was obliged to repay Harrison the fifty hard dollars."

True, the British press was out to discredit Washington, even running stories that he was a woman dressed in man's clothing – which explained why he had no children by his wife, Martha. This is almost certainly untrue as he had a number of mistresses, both black and white. But then he was an eighteenth-century gentleman and that was expected.

From his youth Washington had had a colourful sex life. While still a schoolboy, he loved to romp with one of the largest girls and love blossomed. At the age of sixteen, in embarrassing adolescent love poetry, he bemoaned that his "poor restless heart" was "at last surrendered to cupid's feather'd dart". This was addressed to Frances Alexander of Fredericksburg, though he could not bring himself to express his feelings in person. He soon moved on.

After a surveying expedition down the Shenandoah Valley, he frothed about a "Low Land Beauty". This may have been Miss Betsy Fauntleroy, Miss Mary Bland or Miss Lucy Grimes. Well, he was on a surveying expedition. Lucy Grimes went on to marry Henry Lee II of "Leesylvania", Virginia. Their son was the Revolutionary War hero General Henry "Light Horse Harry" Lee III, a favourite of Washington's, and her grandson was the Confederate General Robert E. Lee.

On his return, he met the love of his life, Sally Fairfax, the wife of his best friend, George Fairfax. Washington's patron, Lord Fairfax, noted that Washington was "beginning to feel the sap rising". She was two years older than Washington, and he found her beautiful, intelligent and utterly enchanting. To discourage the affair, George Fairfax spread the scandalous rumour that Washington was a mulatto.

At the time, Washington was staying at Fairfax's estate, Belvoir. He wrote to a friend: "My place of Residence is at present at His Lordships where I might was my heart disengag'd pass my time very pleasantly, as there's a very agreeable young lady lives in the same house . . . but as that's only adding fuel to the fire, it makes me the more uneasy for, by often and unavoidably being in the company with her, revives my former passion for your Low Land Beauty, whereas was I to live more retired from young women, I might in some measure alleviate my sorrows by burying that chaste and troublesome passion in the grave of oblivion or eternal forgetfulness".

The sap was definitely rising.

Washington was involved in another local scandal in the summer of 1751. When he went swimming in the Rappahannock River, two women stole his clothes. They were arrested. One turned state's evidence. The other, Mary McDaniel, was convicted of "robbing the clothes of Mr George Washington when he was washing in the river" and was given fifteen lashes on her naked back. But Washington did not wait around to witness the punishment. He had escaped another scandal by sailing for Barbados in September 1751.

Washington had a friend named Captain John Posey, owner of the "Rover's Delight", who borrowed a great deal of money from him which he never repaid. In 1750, Posey's wife Elizabeth died in childbirth. There was enduring speculation that the child, Thomas Lloyd Posey, was in fact Washington's. When he grew up, he was extraordinarily tall, like Washington, who paid for his education and nurtured his career. He rose through the ranks of the Continental Army with inordinate speed. Although Washington had no children with Martha, he prided himself on his virility and only seems to have become sterile after catching smallpox in Barbados.

In the Caribbean, he met "an agreeable young lady" named Miss Roberts. They went to see the fireworks on Guy Fawkes Night. He found the women there "generally agreeable but by ill custom or what effect the Negro style".

Within weeks of his return from Barbados, Washington was pressing his suit with fifteen-year-old Miss Betsy Fauntleroy again, in the hope of a "revocation of her former cruel sentence". She had rejected him in favour of the son of a wealthy planter.

In 1753, Washington indulged his lifelong passion for uniforms and joined the Virginia Militia. Sally Fairfax was there to see him march off with General Edward Braddock to retake Fort Duquesne, in what is now downtown Pittsburgh, from the French. A coquette, Sally could not help flirting with the general. In anguish, Washington fired off a letter to her that night. She did not reply, so he fired off two more. When they provoked no response, Washington wrote to her brother and sister, imploring them to get Sally to write to him. Her sister-in-law got wind of this and she wrote to Washington, rebuking him. But Washington's ardour would not be thwarted. When Braddock sent him on an errand to Williamsburg, he stopped off at Belvoir to see Sally. She begged him to stop writing to her. But he continued, even though she did not respond.

However, his passions were not wholly engaged with Sally. In a letter, a fellow officer mentions a "Mrs Neil", saying: "I imagine you by this time plunged in the midst of every delight heaven can afford and enchanted by charms even stranger to the Ciprian dame." The "Ciprian dame" means Venus who was said to have risen from the water near Cyprus where her cult of temple prostitution later flourished.

There was only one thing on the minds of these young officers. George Mercer, then a captain in the Virginia Regiment, later Washington's aide-de-camp, wrote to him from Charleston lamenting the quality of the women there: "A great imperfection here too is the bad shape of the ladies, many of them are crooked and have a very bad air, and not the enticing heaving throbbing alluring ... exciting breasts come with our Northern belles." Another talks of his brother officer softening "his austerity in the arms of some fair nymph – could he reconcile the toying, trifling, billing sports of love to the solemnity and gravity of his deportment – amusements and joys unbecoming of his philosophic temper".

Washington had a particular affection for Native American squaws. He noted that to ingratiate himself with Queen Aliquippa he gave her "a match-coat and a bottle of rum". Encamped at Wills Creek, his detachment came across some Delaware Indians. Their young squaws were fond of hanging around Braddock's camp. It was reported that "they were not destitute of attractions; for the young squaws resemble the gypsies, having seductive forms, small hands and feet, and soft voices". What caught Washington's attention was "one who no doubt passed for an Indian Princess". Her name was Bright Lightning. She was the daughter of Chief White Thunder. And it is clear that the intercourse between the Indian women and the soldiers was not entirely chaste. The secretary of the expedition wrote to Gouverneur Morris, later one of the authors of the Constitution and no stranger to the "Ciprian mystery" with his French mistress: "The squaws bring in money aplenty; the officers are scandalously fond of them."

The braves got jealous and Bright Lightning and the other squaws had to be barred from camp. But this did not stop them from meeting elsewhere. Eventually, for the sake of peace, Bright Lightning and the other squaws were sent home to Aughquick.

While skirmishing along the Ohio River, Washington had already provoked the French and Indian War, which burgeoned into the Seven Years' War – essentially the first world war, fought between Britain and France in North America, the Caribbean, Europe and India, everywhere the two countries had territorial interests. In North America, it was known as the French and Indian War. It was the levying of taxes to pay for this war that sparked the American Revolutionary War.

At the Battle of Monongahela, or the Battle of the Wilderness, Braddock's column was ambushed and he died later of wounds. Washington discharged himself bravely. He had two horses shot from under him. Four musket balls tore through his clothes, but he remained miraculously unhurt. Just twenty-three, he took over command of Braddock's Virginia Regiment and returned home a hero. Sally immediately wrote, saying that if, even after a good night's sleep, he did not have the strength to come and visit her, she would come to him. But she would not be alone. A second note was also signed by Ann Spearing and Elizabeth Dent. And a letter from a leading Virginian named Archibald Cary said that "Mrs Cary and Miss Randolph join in wishing you that sort of glory which will most endear you to the fair sex". Plainly, hearts were aflutter.

To avoid the crush, Washington found the strength to ride to Belvoir to see Sally. Now, it seems, his feelings were reciprocated. They began a long and intense correspondence – though she repeatedly urged him to observe certain proprieties. She was a married woman and insisted that he communicate with her through a third party. He took no notice. Even so, she began to undertake wifely chores for him, such as having his shirts made.

But still he was playing the field. In 1756, Washington was sent to Boston on military business, but tarried in New York for ten days on his way there and a week on his way back. He had met Mary Eliza Philipse, who was known as "the agreeable Miss Polly". His accounts show that he spent sundry pounds "for treating ladies". His tailors' bills soared. But neither treats nor clothes won her heart. She later married Colonel Roger Morris, who had been with him on the Braddock expedition. He was a prominent Tory – that is a supporter of the king, rather than a Whig who upheld the rights of the revolutionaries (on both sides of the Atlantic). During the War of Independence, Morris had to flee. Washington took over their house in 1776 as his headquarters. He met Polly there again and there are indications that they had an affair. She was certainly a looker: "Although slim, Polly was also statuesque; her delicate features were somehow expressive of cool strength; her full mouth was both sensuous and firm."

Washington returned in 1790, after the war was over. But all trace of her had gone and the house had been confiscated by a local farmer.

As it was, his dalliance in New York in 1756 invited scandal. The *Virginia Gazette* accused Washington and his officers of "all manner of debauchery, vice and idleness". While Washington may have been a rake, he was also a stern disciplinarian. To his men, he meted out brutal floggings of up to five hundred strokes.

Towards the end of 1757, Washington fell ill. The doctor put him on a diet of "jellies and such kinds of food". But strangely, among the fourteen slaves he had inherited from his brother – including a woman and her child – and the six he had bought, no one could make such confections. So Sally rode to the rescue.

At the time, her husband was away in England. Sally visited Mount Vernon to nurse Washington. From then on, they corresponded frequently. Washington scrupulously destroyed all of Sally's letters during this period and urged her to do the same, saying that the "world has no business" knowing his thoughts in this matter. Sally, who remained childless, kept his letters though. Early in the twentieth century the financier J. P. Morgan bought Washington's letters and burnt the smutty ones. However, the surviving letters are loaded with innuendo. In one, he said he felt "the force of her amiable beauties in the recollection of a thousand tender passages". Tender passages – oo-er, missus.

He admits to being a "votary to love" and that he wishes to obliterate his feelings for her "'till I am bid to revive them – but experience alas! sadly reminds me how impossible this is". He went on to make an allusion to Juba, an African prince, who loves Cato's daughter Marcia, in the play *Cato*, by Joseph Addison, which spawned some of the American Revolution's most memorable quotes, such as "Give me liberty or give me death" and "I only regret that I have but one life to lose for my country."

He says that he would be "doubly happy in being Juba to such a Marcia as you must make". In the play, Marcia is asked why she hides her love for Juba. She replies: "While Cato lives, his daughter has no right to love or hate, but as his choice directs."

This letter caused a scandal when it was published by the *New York Herald* in 1877. It was dated 12 September 1758, four months after Washington had become engaged to Martha Dandridge Custis, the richest widow in Virginia.

Washington already knew their love was doomed. The situation was impossible – George Fairfax had returned from England. In 1758, there was no way that Sally could divorce her husband and marry Washington. It would have caused an immense scandal, leaving them both social outcasts. Continuing a clandestine affair could easily have had the same result. Either way, Washington would expose himself to a ruinous lawsuit from her aggrieved husband. Both he and Sally would have remembered when George Washington's half-brother Lawrence had prosecuted a neighbour for allegedly raping his wife, Sally's sister-in-law Anne Fairfax, before her marriage. The court proceedings were reported in salacious detail in newspapers in Virginia, Maryland and Pennsylvania. Before it was over, everyone wished that Lawrence had kept quiet.

However, Washington could still aspire to Sally's social class. In an effort to climb a few rungs in the social ladder, he had begun wooing Martha Custis. The daughter of a plantation owner, she had been a wild thing in her youth, once riding her horse, Fatima, up and down the stairs of her uncle's house. At eighteen, she married the wealthy planter Daniel Parke Custis and moved into the Custis family home, called, ironically, the White House. Twenty years her senior, he gave her four children, though two died in infancy. Her husband died in 1757, after seven years of marriage. Washington began wooing her the following year. At twenty-six, he was eighteen months her junior. On his first visit, they sat in the parlour and talked, then he stayed the night. He visited again the following week.

News of their impending nuptials spread quickly. Sally wrote to congratulate him. He replied tetchily: "If you allow that any honour can be derived from my opposition to our present system of management, you destroy the merit of it entirely in me by attributing it to my anxiety to the animated prospect of possessing Mrs Custis."

After professing his love for her, he tells Sally: "But adieu to this, till happier times, if I ever shall see them."

At 1 p.m. on 6 January 1759, after what would have been considered a whirlwind courtship, they married in front of forty guests. The ceremony was brief, the reception formal. Marriage brought money and Washington was having the house at Mount Vernon renovated, so the couple honeymooned in the White House. When they moved back into Mount Vernon, George and Sally Fairfax were frequent visitors. What had gone on before was politely ignored.

The couples went their separate ways in 1773, when the Fairfaxes returned to England on family business. They were Tories and could not return after the Revolution. George Fairfax died in 1787. The following year, Sally wrote to her sister-in-law, saying: "I know now that the worthy man is to be preferred to the high-born who has not merit to recommend him . . . when we enquire into the family of these mighty men we find them the very lowest of people." And Washington confessed again in a letter to Sally in later life that she was the passion of his youth. She died in 1811. Among her possessions was found Washington's letter ruing that he was going to marry Martha. Indeed Martha was no great beauty like Sally. She was plump, dowdy and rather shy, and once described herself as "an old-fashioned housekeeper". Later, he compared the "domestic felicity" he found in marriage unfavourable to "the giddy round of promiscuous pleasure" he had enjoyed in his youth.

Washington was plainly discontent. In a letter to his stepdaughter he said: "Love is a mighty pretty thing, but, like other delicious things, it is cloying; and when the first transports of the passion begin to subside, which it will assuredly do, and yield, oftentimes too late, to more sober reflections, it serves to evince that love is too dainty a food to live on alone."

But Washington's passion had not subsided. Should Martha die, he speculates that he would marry a "girl" and sire an heir. So plainly he felt capable.

He warns his step-granddaughter: "In the composition of the human frame there is a great deal of inflammable matter, however dormant it may lie. When the torch is put to it, that which is within you may burst into blaze." But in marriage, he says, "the madness ceases and all is quiet again. Why? Not because there is any diminution in the charms of the lady, but because there is an end of hope."

There were other ways he could sate his passions. He was as brutal with his slaves as with his troops. Runaways were hunted down and severely flogged. Female slaves were also whipped. In his diaries, Washington refers to this or that slave woman as "a wench of mine". When he was president and one ran away from his home in Philadelphia, he wanted her hunted down and punished for "ingratitude".

At Mount Vernon, stern punishments were handed out for "nightwalking". This, he complained, left his servants and field hands "unfit for the duties of the day". He knew what was going on as there is every indication that, like many Virginia planters of his day, Washington visited the women in the slave quarters at night. As he told his step-granddaughter: "Men and women feel the same inclinations to each other now that they always have done, and which they will continue to do until there is a new order of things, and you, as others have done, may find, perhaps, that the passions of your sex are easier raised than allayed . . . there is no truth more certain than that all our enjoyments fall short of our expectations; and to none does it apply with more force than the gratifications of the passions."

If Washington was leading the relatively restrained life of a colonial gentleman, his stepson was not. Endeavouring to be a good father to Martha's son Jack, Washington employed a live-in tutor. When that did not work out, he sent the boy to a school run by the Reverend Jonathan Boucher, who wrote that he had never met a lad "so exceedingly indolent, or so surprisingly voluptuous". The boy showed a "propensity to the female sex, which I am at loss how to judge, much more how to describe. One would suppose that nature had intended him for an Asiatic prince."

Quitting school without his parents' permission, he enrolled at King's College, later Columbia University, where he got engaged to Nelly Calvert, the daughter of an illegitimate son of the fifth Lord Baltimore, again without consulting his parents. To avert a scandal, Washington wrote to Mr Calvert, telling him that Jack must finish his education before he got married. But at nineteen, he wed anyway, but not to Nelly. In the American Revolution, he was aide-de-camp to Washington and died of "camp fever" – typhus – shortly after the Battle of Yorktown.

Meanwhile, Washington's surviving brother shared his overactive libido and married five times. But Washington was not left to rusticate. Fate intervened. Sent to represent Virginia at the Continental Congress in Philadelphia in 1774, he was chosen to command the Continental Army the following year and the War of Independence gave him plenty of opportunities to play away from home. He was away from Mount Vernon for eight years during the war. Martha paid a conjugal visit to the front on an average of one week a year. So he had fifty-one weeks a year to play around.

During the war, he billeted himself in various well-appointed mansions – including that of "the agreeable Miss Polly" – and enjoyed the attentions of the pretty women of the household. Even at Valley Forge, where Washington and the Continental Army spent the bleak winter of 1777–8, the Revolutionary forces did not go without sex. General Charles Lee, Washington's rival as commander-in-chief, was caught smuggling local girls into the camp. Others brought their mistresses. Then there was the ravishing nineteen-year-old Margaret "Peggy" Shippen, the wife of Benedict Arnold, who ran around Washington's headquarters half naked when crazed by her husband's defection to the British. She claimed that there was "a hot iron on her head, and no one but General Washington could take it off". When he went to comfort her, she appeared topless in a dressing gown. Could it be that she was demonstrating her loyalty by not turning her coat? According to another account, she was in bed when he went to comfort her and the distraught woman pulled back the bedclothes, "revealing her charms".

Washington did not hide his proclivities from his wife. A French officer at Morristown said that he "admires pretty women . . . notices their gowns and how their hair is dressed. He does it quite openly, and before his wife, who does not seem to mind at all." However, a neighbour, Mrs Martha Daingerfield Bland, the wife of a Virginia colonel, wrote to a friend, saying that he was in "perfect felicity when she is by the side of her 'Old Man'", but when Martha was not around he "throws off the hero and takes on the chatty, agreeable companion. He can be downright impudent sometimes – such impudence, Fanny, as you and I like".

She also noted that he was their "noble and agreeable commander, for he commands both sexes, one by his excellent skill in military matters, the other by his ability, politeness and attention . . . from dinner until night he is free for all company".

According to Marvin Kitman, author of *The Making of the President 1789*, Washington was an accomplished womanizer. His A-list of possible lovers included the aptly named Lucy Flucker Knox, who abandoned her Tory family to rally to the Revolutionaries; Mrs Clement Biddle, wife of the leader of the "Quaker Blues"; Mrs George Olny, who when Washington grabbed her in public told him to mind his hands; Theodosia Provost Burr, wife of Aaron Burr, who was knocking off their maid at the time, siring two illegitimate kids by her; Lady Kitty Alexander Duer, New York party girl; Lady Stirling, Lady Kitty's mother, who was often seen in Washington's arms on the dance floor; Elizabeth Gates, who often wore men's clothing and was called "a daemoness" by General

Charles Lee; Phoebe Fraunces, serving wench at the tavern owned by her father Black Sam Fraunces and Washington's only nod to egalitarianism, in his love life at least; Elizabeth Willing Powel, the young widow of the mayor of Philadelphia and notorious political groupie; society hostess Mrs William Bingham, another of the Willing clan; Mrs Perez Morton, poetess known in literary circles as "the American Sappho"; and the ubiquitous Kitty Greene, "a younger version of Sally Fairfax," an intimate remarked.

Colonel Freeman said of Kitty: "She enlivened many a black night in the revolutionary headquarters."

An orphan, she was bewitchingly pretty and grew up to be the belle of Providence, Rhode Island. In 1774, she married General Nathaniel Greene, but remained a notorious flirt. With the outbreak of war, she rushed to the front, while other generals' wives were being packed off home. At Valley Forge she became the mistress of General Lafayette, the French marquis who rallied to the revolutionaries' cause. She said so herself, remarking in a letter to Colonel Wadsworth that she was "sleeping with the Marquis".

She also slept with her husband's business partner, Colonel Kósciuszko and General "Mad" Anthony Wayne. It was soldiers she loved most of all. In a letter to a friend in March 1779, General Greene complained that Washington had danced with his wife non-stop for three hours, a gross breach of etiquette. Washington himself remarked in a letter home to Martha how fond he was of Kitty. Add the off-the-record statement of an anonymous coach-driver and that would have been enough for the *National Enquirer*.

On Kitman's B-list are the two daughters of a Mrs Watkins of Passaic, New Jersey, who "entertained" Washington before he visited the then widowed Theodosia Provost; Mrs Bache, Benjamin Franklin's goddaughter, who danced the night away with Washington at his twentieth wedding anniversary; Mary Gibbons, whom Washington met during the war and reportedly "maintained genteelly in Hoboken, New Jersey"; and unemployed seamstress – and "beautiful young widow" – Betsy Ross, who is credited with making the first American flag. Did she run it up his flagpole first?

Washington was also approached by the renowned poetess Annis Boundinot Stockton, then a handsome widow. She sent him a poem and begged his absolution for writing it. He wrote back saying that if she would dine with him "and go through the proper course of penitence, which shall be prescribed, I will strive hard to assist you in expiating these poetical trespasses on this side of purgatory". One imagines *la belle* Stockton on her knees.

If his intentions were not clear enough, he continued: "You see, Madam, when once the woman has tempted us and we have tasted the forbidden fruit, there is no such thing as checking our appetites, whatever the consequences may be."

When Washington became the first president of the United States, Martha reluctantly moved with him to New York, then Philadelphia. She hated being first lady, saying the role would suit "many younger and gayer women". No doubt Washington thought so too. At that time, he was receiving the adulation of women throughout the country. His diary makes frequent references to them.

Once of his closest confidantes while he was president was Henrietta Liston, the young wife of the British minister to the United States. Elizabeth Willing Powel, whom he had first met in Philadelphia in 1774 when he had attended the Continental Congress there, was still at hand. She persuaded him to stand for a second term, though he had been unwilling to do so. In her letters to him, she teases him about his "continence to the ladies". In response, he implies that he would be unconcerned about being caught in adultery. A greater sin would be to have "betrayed the confidence of a lady".

When an epidemic of yellow fever broke out in Philadelphia in 1793, he invited Elizabeth Powel and her husband to come with him to Mount Vernon. They refused. So Washington risked his life staying behind in Philadelphia too. But it was Samuel Powel that came down with the disease and died.

Washington quit office in 1797 and left Philadelphia amid a flurry of letters to the widow Powel. In the move back to Mount Vernon, the Washingtons found they now had too much furniture and put some of it up for sale. Mrs Powel bought a desk and found in a draw what she said was a bundle of "love letters to a lady" – though she claimed not to have read them. Washington denied that the letters professed "enamoured love". If they had, he said, he would have burnt them.

In 1798, he wrote again to Sally Fairfax in England, begging her to return to Virginia, now that she was a widow. Neither the revolution nor his period in high office seems to have quenched his ardour.

"None of these events, however, nor all of them together, have been able to eradicate from my mind those happy moments, the happiest in my life, which I have enjoyed in your company," he said.

His correspondence with Elizabeth Powel continued and, eighteen months after retiring from office, he returned to Philadelphia for a month-long visit. During his stay, she shunned other friends. He would visit her in the afternoons and they would take long walks together. And, in one letter, she let it slip that they had breakfast together at her house. One can only surmise.

Six months later, Washington died after catching a chill. American school children are told that he caught the chill while out horseback riding in the snow. However, Harvard historian Karal Ann Marling said that he came down with the fatal chill "after an assignation with an overseer's wife in the Mount Vernon gardens on a cold afternoon", while the distinguished British historian Arnold Toynbee said, more bluntly, that Washington caught the chill "visiting a black beauty in his slave quarters". History does not record whether her name was Vera Baker.

## John Adams (and Benjamin Franklin)

The second president of the United States, John Adams, was, of course, above reproach. He was married to Abigail, a minister's daughter, for fifty-four years. However, in 1778, he was posted to join that old reprobate Benjamin Franklin in Paris. Initially, he was shocked by the forwardness of French women. He wrote home to his wife, complaining of the plague of sexual promiscuity that was engulfing Europe. While tut-tutting about the "profligate women" of Paris, he was slowly seduced by the city.

Soon he was writing to Abigail: "To tell the truth, I admire the ladies here. Don't be jealous. They are handsome and very well educated. Their accomplishments are exceedingly brilliant. And their knowledge of letters and arts exceeds that of the English ladies, I believe."

Perhaps Abigail could read the signs for, in the summer of 1779, he quickly returned home – only to be ordered back to Paris by the Continental Congress. Abigail was unable to join him until 1784. All that time, Adams was under the sway of Ben Franklin. He was a bad influence. At the age of twenty-four, Franklin had an illegitimate son with a "low woman". He was raised by Franklin's common-law wife – they could not marry as she was already wed. This was, of course, scandalous at the time.

At the age of thirty-nine, Franklin wrote to a young male friend, recommending taking an older mistress rather than a younger one. The advantages include: "when women cease to be handsome, they study to be good"; "there is no hazard of children"; "they are more prudent and discreet"; they "prevent his ruining his health and fortune with mercenary prostitutes"; "the pleasure of corporal enjoyment ... is at least equal, and frequently superior, every knack being by practice capable of improvement"; "the sin is less [than] debauching a virgin"; "the compunction is less ... having made a young girl miserable may give you bitter reflections, none of which can attend the making an old woman happy"; "and lastly they are so grateful". After all, "in the dark all cats are grey".

In England, Franklin had been a friend of Sir Francis Dashwood, founder of the Hell Fire Club. He attended its meetings where prostitutes, local girls in search of excitement and even society ladies seeking titillation indulged in orgies. They began the evening, at least, dressed as nuns. Dashwood was also thought to have the largest collection of pornography in England and Franklin was a bibliophile. He was one of the first Americans to own a copy of John Cleland's *Fanny Hill; or the Memoirs of a Woman of Pleasure* and, as a bookseller, carried such lurid titles as *The Arraignment of Lewd Women* and *The Garden of Love*.

In eighteenth-century Paris, Franklin was in his element. According to Adams, he could never get to see Franklin before breakfast to read the diplomatic correspondence. Then the rest of Franklin's morning was taken up with visitors, some of whom were "philosophers, academics, economists, but by far the greater part were women". No work was done in the afternoon either as "Madam Helvétius, Madam Chaumont, Madam Le Roy, etc., and others I never knew ... were complaisant enough to depart from the custom of France as to ... make tea for him". Then Franklin would spend his evenings "hearing the ladies sing and play upon their piano fortes". Dr Franklin's life, Adams complained, was "a scene of continual dissipation".

In fact, Franklin would spend most evenings with the Brillons. Monsieur Brillon would be accompanied by his mistress, while Madame Brillon sometimes brought another lover. Adams was surprised that they did not cut each other's throat.

Adams was even more shocked by his behaviour at the Auteuil household, where Franklin tried to seduce Madame Auteuil and her two daughters. He called Madam Le Roy, the diminutive wife of a scientific collaborator, his "pocket wife" and Madame Filleul would send a carriage to collect him, along with a note saying how she "looked forward to kissing him". Then there was Mademoiselle de Passy, the exquisite young daughter of the *seigneur* of the village outside Paris where Franklin lived. She was "his favourite and his love and his mistress, which flattered the family and did not displease the young lady".

But Adams could not be too hard on Franklin because he was in his seventies and had "neither lost his love of beauty nor his taste for it". Indeed, Franklin was so popular with the women at court that they had their hair done *à la Franklin*. In an age of powdered wigs, embroidered coats and lace cuffs, Franklin stood out with straight unpowdered hair and the brown cloth coat of an American farmer.

He was lauded as a philosopher and entertainments were laid on in his honour. At one, three hundred women were present to smother him with kisses after the most beautiful placed a crown of laurels on his head. Adams wrote: "My venerable colleague enjoys a privilege here that is much to be envied. Being seventy years of age, the ladies not only allow him to embrace them as often as he pleases, but they are perpetually embracing him."

Abigail was afraid that the influence of the dissolute Franklin might rub off on the resolute John, likening herself to Penelope, left at home in Ithaca while her husband Odysseus was out having all the fun – perhaps being entertained by the nymph Calypso on the idyllic island of Ogygia for seven years. So, after a separation of five years, Abigail arrived in Paris.

She was immediately shocked by the behaviour of Madame Helvétius who, when she came to dine with Dr Franklin, complained that she had not been told other women would be present. But that did not stop her kissing the good doctor. Fortunately, Abigail did not have to put up with this for long. Thomas Jefferson arrived in Paris to replace Adams, while he moved on to England to be the United States' first minister to the Court of St James, before returning to America.

Untainted by his time in Paris, John Adams became vice president in 1789 and president in 1797. In 1800, he lost to Jefferson. Eventually Franklin was also recalled, to die "a stranger in my own country," he lamented.

John Adams was still around in 1820, when his daughter-in-law Louisa, wife of John Quincy Adams, wrote to him saying she had just learned that the orphan asylum would need more space because "the fathers of the nation had left forty cases to be provided for by the public".

Forty pregnant women left behind by the 16th Congress – and there were only 232 members! Furious, asylum trustee Louisa Adams huffed: "I recommended a petition to Congress next session for that great and moral body to establish a foundling institution" and use the $2-a-day pay increase they had voted themselves to fund it. Of course, that never happened.

## Thomas Jefferson

In 1998, the University of Leicester did DNA tests on the descendants of former slave Eston Hemings, which proved that Thomas Jefferson had had sex with one of his slave girls. America was scandalized. This was the smoking, er, gun. One of the founding fathers had been caught with his hand in the ... As George Washington demonstrated, sex across the colour line was going on in the eighteenth century.

But it was not just a scandal in 1998, pre-Obama times. It was a huge scandal at the time. The man who broke the story was James T. Callender, the editor of the *Richmond Recorder* in 1802, who had already exposed the affair the Secretary of the

Treasury Alexander Hamilton was having with Maria Reynolds, a married women. Twenty-three-year-old Maria approached the thirty-four-year-old Hamilton, who was also married, asking for the fare back to New York after her husband James had abandoned her. Hamilton consented and delivered the money in person to Maria later that night. As Hamilton himself later confessed: "I took the bill out of my pocket and gave it to her. Some conversation ensued from which it was quickly apparent that other than pecuniary consolation would be acceptable." They began an illicit affair that would last over three years. When James Reynolds discovered this, he charged Hamilton more than $1,000 to allow him to continue sleeping with his wife. A scandal ensued and Hamilton was forced from office in 1795.

Jefferson had financed Callender as a pamphleteer, but Callender's outspoken attacks on John Adams ended with his prosecution under the Sedition Act. When Jefferson became president in 1801, he pardoned Callender, who expected to be made the postmaster of Richmond as a reward. Instead he went to work for the Federalist *Richmond Recorder*. There he turned on his patron, revealing that Jefferson had paid for the anti-Adams pamphleteering. In response, Jefferson's supporters smeared Callender, saying that he had abandoned his wife while she was dying of venereal disease. It was then that Callender brought the big guns out, publishing a series of articles about Jefferson and his child by his slave girl Sally Hemings. It was a sensation.

Not only was Sally Hemings Jefferson's slave girl, she was the half-sister of his dead wife Martha. Callender also published details of Jefferson's sexual relations with Betsy Walker, a married woman he had stalked in his twenties. Her husband demanded an apology and Jefferson was forced to admit "when young and single I offered to love a handsome lady. I acknowledge its incorrectness".

As a youth, Jefferson had been very close to another young man named Dabney Carr, the son of a wealthy Virginia planter who went on to marry Jefferson's sister. They swore to be buried together. Carr died young, shortly after Jefferson was married, and was interred at Monticello, Jefferson's Virginia estate. When Jefferson himself died at the age of eighty-three, he was indeed buried alongside his young friend.

Jefferson married a young widow named Martha Wayles Skelton. They had six children, but only two survived infancy. When Martha's father John Wayles died, Jefferson inherited his slaves including the children of Elizabeth Hemings, a slave woman the widowed Wayles had taken as his mistress. One of them was a young beauty named Sally.

As Martha lay dying after giving birth in 1782, Jefferson promised that he would never marry again. Later that year, he was posted to Paris, where his behaviour with the local women caused a scandal. Alexander Hamilton, Jefferson's political rival, called him a "concealed voluptuary . . . in the plain garb of Quaker simplicity". But then Hamilton was not above a bit of how's-your-father. In Paris, Jefferson had taken up with the artist Maria Cosway, wife of the renowned English miniaturist Richard Cosway, who had a lucrative sideline in painting pornographic snuff boxes and was perpetually unfaithful to her with his models. When Maria left Paris he poured out his feelings in the famous romantic colloquy *A Dialogue between Head and Heart*. But he soon found consolation with Hamilton's sister-in-law Mrs Angelica Schuyler Church.

In 1787, Jefferson's nine-year-old daughter Polly arrived in Paris. Accompanying her as maid was fourteen-year-old Sally. While she was in Paris, Jefferson paid Sally a wage. He also paid for her brother James to train as a chef. When Jefferson returned to the United States in 1789, they could have stayed behind in Paris, where they would have been free. But Sally was already pregnant and agreed to return to Monticello as his mistress on the condition that their children would be freed. In Albemarle County, their relationship was hardly a secret. Many southern planters took their slave women as concubines. But in 1802, Jefferson was playing on a national stage. Callender called Sally Jefferson's "black Venus", though another slave described her as "mighty near white ... very handsome, long straight hair down her back" and Jefferson's grandson called her "light coloured and decidedly good looking". Nevertheless, Callender claimed that Jefferson could be seen frolicking at Monticello with his "black wench and her mulatto litter" while he was supposed to be attending to the affairs of the country.

The scandal seized the public imagination and Callendar upped the ante, claiming that Jefferson maintained a "Congo harem" in the Executive Mansion and that there was a slave named "Yellow Tom" at Monticello who was the spitting image of Jefferson, only somewhat darker, and who pretended to be president. It was even said that Jefferson had driven Sally's sister into prostitution in Baltimore.

The opposition Federalists had a field day. The Federalist poet William Cullen Bryant wrote:

> Go wretch, resign the presidential chair,
> Go scan, Philosophist, thy Sally's charms,
> And sink supinely in her sable arms,
> But quit to abler hands the helm of state.

The Tories in Britain were still smarting from the loss of their American colonies and the English poet Tom Moore wrote:

> The patriot, fresh from freedom's council come,
> Now pleas'd, retires to lash his slaves at home;
> Or woo some black Aspasia's charms
> And dreams of freedom in his bondsmaid's arms.

Aspasia was the mistress of the Athenian statesman Pericles. The revolutionary Tom Paine rose to Jefferson's defence, only to be accused of sleeping with "Dusky Sally" himself and cuckolding his friend.

Jefferson himself maintained a dignified silence. The scandal did him no harm and he was re-elected by a landslide in 1804 and the Democractic-Republican party he founded dominated the political scene for decades to come. Jefferson's relationship with Sally continued and she had two more children by him after that, making six in all, though one died in infancy.

Despite the crude invective hurled at her, Sally Hemings was not dark at all. Her mother Betty was mixed race, the daughter of an English sea captain and an African slave woman. So Sally herself was a quadroon. Jefferson gave certain privileges to his light-skinned slaves. He only sold one of the family, Sally's sister Thenia, who was purchased by James Monroe, who went on to become the fifth president of the United States.

Two of Jefferson's children with Sally were allowed to "run away" – he gave them the money to escape to the north, where they were light enough to pass as white. The other two offspring who had survived into adulthood were freed in Jefferson's will. Sally herself was freed by Jefferson's legitimate daughter, Polly's older sister Patsy.

The story never went away. In 1873, Madison Hemings – Sally's next to last child born in 1805 while Jefferson was president – gave an interview to the *Pike Country Republican*, a newspaper in Ohio, claiming that he and all Sally Heming's children were fathered by Jefferson. This was confirmed by Israel Jefferson, a former slave from Monticello and a long-time friend of Sally's. Madison was said to resemble Jefferson and also claimed that he had been named by Dolley Madison, wife of the fourth president of the United States, who had visited Monticello.

However, the year after Madison's interview, James Parton published *The Life of Thomas Jefferson*, where he claimed that Peter Carr, son of Jefferson's adolescent pal Dabney, was the real father of Sally Hemings's children. It was also alleged that Peter's brother Samuel was the father as he was "the most notorious good-natured Turk that ever was the master of a black seraglio kept at other men's expense," according to Jefferson's granddaughter Ellen Randolph Coolidge.

But then in 1968, in *White Over Black: American Attitudes Toward the Negro, 1550–1812*, the author Winthrop Jordan pointed out that Sally only became pregnant when Jefferson was at Monticello – he was away over two-thirds of the time. On the other hand, new scholarship revealed Jefferson as a virulent racist, insisting that it was impossible to sustain a biracial society in America. Strict segregation had to be maintained, he believed, so that African slaves and their descendants could eventually be returned to Africa.

With the development of DNA profiling it would be possible to put the matter to the test. However, white descendants of Jefferson and his wife Martha did not exist and his body was dug up. But it was possible to compare the Y-chromosome of descendants of Jefferson's paternal uncle and the descendants of Sally's oldest and youngest sons. The Y-chromosome is passed intact down the male line. They matched. The chance of the match happening randomly is around one in a thousand. There was no match with the Y-chromosome taken from the male descendants of the Carr family, so they are out of the picture.

However, what was seen as scandalous in 1802 – and even more so after the introduction of the Jim Crow laws following the Civil War – no longer seems so scandalous now. Even the word miscegenation had fallen out of every day usage. With Barack Obama in the White House, race mixing is not an issue. However, Sally was just fifteen and Jefferson forty-three when they first had sex – though that would have not been illegal in France or the US at the time, so we can't accuse him of being a paedophile. These days, though, there are strict prohibitions on employers using their position to coerce an employee into having sex. But in Virginia in the eighteenth century, that's what slave girls were for. The worst we can say against Jefferson in light of the DNA evidence was that he was a hypocrite – preaching racial segregation while banging the coloured maid. But then what else is new? He was a politician. On the other hand, in the Declaration of Independence, he did say that all men were born equal, so maybe he was practising what he preached.

## John Quincy Adams

Coming from a strict Unitarian family, the sixth president of the United States can be seen as an austere figure. But in his youth he was a wild child. He joined an outfit called the Crackbrain Club and spent his time drinking and going with prostitutes. His diaries reveal that he met with unknown people in strange places late at night. But his marriage at the age of thirty in 1797 put paid to that.

He did however retain one habit from his youth – skinny-dipping. Even when he was in the White House, he would regularly nip out at 5 a.m. for a quick dip in the Potomac *au naturel*. It is said that Anne Royall, thought to be America's first professional woman journalist, heard about this and secured an interview with the president by gathering up his clothes and sitting on them.

The president swimming in the Potomac nude would certainly be a scandal today. On the other hand it would enliven press conferences.

## John Tyler

Widowed in office, John Tyler caused a sensation when he married a woman thirty years his junior. What's more, his bride was a model. Julia Gardiner was nineteen when she scandalized polite society in New York, posing for an advertisement for a department store alongside an elderly dandy. A great beauty, she was dubbed the "Rose of Long Island". A poem singing her praises by one "Romeo Ringdove" appeared on the front page of the Brooklyn *Daily News*. It contained these immortal lines:

> When gallants buzz like bees around
> Who sweets from flowers suck,
> Where shall the man so vain be found
> As hopes this rose to pluck?

The answer was, of course, the White House. They met at a reception there in 1842. He was instantly smitten, paying her "a thousand compliments" such that those present "looked and listened in perfect amazement". Julia was plainly used to this treatment. She noted "the silvery sweetness of his voice . . . the incomparable grace of his bearing, and the elegant ease of his conversation". But her sister Margaret dismissed him as a jolly old man.

Tyler had rivals for her affections though – his two sons. John Jr bombarded her with erotic verse. He was attempting to divorce his wife at the time. Robert was rejected because he was not so handsome.

The next time Tyler met Julia, it was at a whist drive and he demanded to know how many beaux she had "in the name of the president of the United States".

Robert's father-in-law Thomas Cooper remarked: "Do you see the president playing old sledge with Miss Gardiner? It will be in the *Globe* tomorrow."

Miss Gardiner and her sister visited the presidential apartments and kisses were exchanged. Tyler then took the two of them and their father on a cruise down the Potomac on the steam frigate *Princeton*. Unfortunately their father died in a freak accident and Tyler comforted her.

At a ball to celebrate George Washington's birthday on 22 February 1843, Tyler saw Julia dancing with a young naval officer. As commander-in-chief, Tyler pulled rank. He asked her to marry him, though his first wife had only been dead five months. She refused him. At the time she was being pursued by Judge John McLean, but at fifty-seven, he was even older than the president. McLean stood aside and, the following month, they had come to a "definite understanding". Julia's mother was still against the match though, as she was nine years younger than her prospective son-in-law.

Friends advised against marrying her. But on 26 June 1844, the fifty-four-year-old John Tyler married the twenty-four-year-old Julia Gardiner in New York. The thirty-year age difference drew a great deal of public interest.

The wedding had been kept secret until after the event. The pro-Tyler *Madisonian* merely announced the day before that the president was taking a temporary absence from his "arduous duties' in Washington for a few days' "repose". The *Herald* remarked: "We rather think that the president's 'arduous duties' are only beginning. 'Repose' indeed!"

Tyler's daughters were upset because he had not told them of his intentions. Only weeks before, he had written to them saying he had nothing interesting to report. The eldest daughter, Mary, was five years older than the bride. The second daughter Letitia Tyler Semple, who had been acting as first lady since her mother had died, never accepted Julia as her stepmother. And it was three months before twenty-one-year-old Elizabeth could write: "My dear Mrs Tyler . . . even now it is with difficulty that I can convince myself that another fills the place which was once occupied by my beloved mother."

But his sons eagerly embraced their new stepmother.

The honeymoon was a triumphal procession back to the White House via Philadelphia and Baltimore. Back in Washington, Tyler began to complain that his wife had trouble getting out of bed in the morning and constantly demanded his attention rather than letting him get on with his work. Even sister Margaret urged Julia to leave her husband alone during business hours.

"Business should take precedence over caressing," she said, "reserve your caressing for private leisure and be sure you let no one see it unless you wish to be laughed at."

A difficult election was coming up. Nevertheless on 1 July, they took a boat to Old Point Comfort on the tip of the Virginia Peninsula where they stayed in what Julia called a "true love cottage". Colonel Gustavus A. De Russy, commanding officer of Fort Monroe, had been put in charge of bedroom matters and the couple were provided with "a richly covered high post bedstead hung with white lace curtains looped up with blue ribbon, and the cover at the top of the bedstead lined also with blue – new matting which emitted its sweet fragrance, two handsome mahogany dressing tables, writing table and sofa". These are details of a couple's bedroom arrangements one would hardly expect today.

Rather than preparing for the 1844 election, he spent his time writing poems to Julia. She even set one of them to music. After a visit to his plantation, Sherwood Forest in Virginia, Tyler realized that there was more to life than politics and decided not to stand again.

Soon after the inauguration of Tyler's successor James T. Polk, Julia gave birth to their first child. The newspapers began running stories about a separation and possible divorce. But they stayed together and had seven children.

# 2

## British Bonking

### John Profumo

One of the biggest sex scandals in British political life took place, ironically, in the swinging sixties, when everyone was supposed to be at it – except for government ministers of course. When it was discovered that Minister of War John Profumo had been sleeping with a prostitute who had also been bonking the naval attaché at the Russian embassy and had lied to the House of Commons about it – an unforgivable sin – he was forced to resign. The government was badly damaged by the scandal. Soon after the prime minister resigned and the following year the Conservatives were swept from office after thirteen years in power.

The scandal centred around Christine Keeler who, at the age of fifteen, quit her home in the Buckinghamshire village of Wraysbury for the bright lights of London. Within months, her self-confidence and good looks had taken her from being a waitress in a Greek restaurant to being a part-time model and a topless dancer in Murray's Cabaret Club in Soho where she earned £8.50 a week. There, fellow show-girl Mandy Rice-Davies, a perky seventeen-year-old from Birmingham, introduced her to her friend Stephen Ward.

Ward was a thin and elegant man in his late forties. He was a talented artist but he earned a living as an osteopath. He numbered among his clients several high-ranking members of the establishment. These included Lord Astor, who let him a cottage in the grounds of his Cliveden estate for the peppercorn rent of £1 a year, and the editor of the *Daily Telegraph* Sir Colin Coote, who was closely associated with Sir Roger Hollis, the head of the British counter-intelligence service, MI5, that spycatcher Peter Wright would name as the fifth man in the Cambridge spy ring.

Ward liked doing favours for people. He also liked drugs and the company of pretty women, including prostitutes. Christine Keeler and Mandy Rice-Davies moved into his London flat in Wimpole Mews and would go down with him to Cliveden at weekends for parties in his cottage.

In June 1961, over lunch at the Garrick, Coote introduced Ward to the Soviet naval attaché Yevgeny Ivanov. MI5 had singled Ivanov out as a man who might succumb to the temptations of the West. The counter-intelligence service thought that a weekend party with some of Ward's attractive young female friends might be just the thing to turn him. The defection of such a high-ranking Russian official would be quite a prize. Specifically, MI5 wanted Ward to "honeytrap" Ivanov with Christine Keeler.

Ward invited Ivanov down to Cliveden on Sunday 9 July 1951. He took Keeler down there the night before. The Astors were holding a dinner party in the house. Keeler wanted to go swimming and Ward dared her to go in the nude. When she did, he stole her swimming costume.

Lord Astor and John Profumo were out in the gardens for an after-dinner stroll when they spotted the beautiful naked nineteen-year-old in the swimming pool. Christine realized that they were coming and struck out for the edge of the pool. She emerged nude and grabbed a small towel to cover herself moments before the two men caught up with her.

The two middle-aged men were fooling around with the near-naked girl when suddenly the floodlights were turned on. The rest of the guests – including Profumo's wife – came out into the garden too and Christine was introduced. Later, Profumo managed to give her a guided tour of the bedrooms at Cliveden.

At forty-six, Profumo was a rising Tory politician. The son of a successful barrister, he was independently wealthy and lived the life of a Tory squire. Educated at Harrow and Oxford, he served on the staff of General Alexander during World War II, rising to the rank of lieutenant-colonel. He was elected to parliament as a Conservative for Stratford-upon-Avon in 1950, joined the government in 1952 and became Secretary for War in 1960. In 1954, he had married the actress Valerie Hobson.

The day after Christine Keeler met Profumo, Ivanov turned up at Cliveden. Ward laid on a swimming party as a way to introduce him to Christine. She fancied Ivanov immediately, later telling the *News of the World*: "He was MAN. He was rugged with a hairy chest, strong and agile."

However, when they decided to have a piggy-back fight in the pool, it was John Profumo's shoulders she clambered on to, not Ivanov's. That evening, Christine left with Ivanov, but not before Profumo had asked her for her phone number. Christine was flattered and told him to contact Ward.

Back at Ward's flat, Christine and Ivanov demolished a bottle of vodka. Then he kissed her.

"Before I knew what was happening, I was in his arms," she said. "We left serious discussion and I yielded to this wonderful huggy bear of a man . . . He was a wonderful lover."

Two days later, Profumo phoned and came around. On his third visit, he began to kiss her and soon "I was returning his kisses with everything that I suddenly felt for him," she said.

Profumo would always call first before he came round for what Keeler called a "screw of convenience". They had to be discreet. With Ivanov, she went out on the town, but Profumo could not risk being seen out with her in a pub or restaurant. Occasionally though they went out for a drive. As well as having sex at Ward's flat, they did it in Profumo's red Mini and a black car he borrowed from the Minister of Labour, John Hare. And once, when his wife was away in Ireland, he took Christine back to their house in Nash Terrace near Regent's Park. It was late and the butler and staff were asleep. And he took her directly to the master bedroom.

Profumo had no idea that he was sharing his mistress with Ivanov. He soon became deeply attached to her. Profumo showered her with expensive gifts and money – ostensibly to buy her mother a birthday present. But she did not share his feelings. For her, sex "had no more meaning than a hand-shake or a look across a crowded room," she said.

After a month, MI5 learnt about Profumo's affair with Keeler. Fearing that it compromised their entrapment of Ivanov, Hollis asked the Cabinet Secretary Sir Norman Brook to warn Profumo. On 9 August 1961, in panic, John Profumo wrote a note to Christine Keeler:

> Darling,
>
> In great haste & because I can get no reply from your phone –
>
> Alas something's blown up tomorrow night & I can't therefore make it. I'm terribly sorry especially as I leave the next day for various trips & then a holiday so won't be able to see you again until some time in September. Blast it.
>
> Please take care of yourself & don't run away.
>
> Love J
>
> I'm writing this 'cos I know you're off for the day tomorrow & I want you to know before you go if I still can't reach you by phone.

It was this note that sealed his fate.

Despite the warning, Profumo continued seeing Christine Keeler for another four months. During that time, he took amazing risks. One evening an army officer turned up at the flat looking for Ward.

"I had to introduce him to the War Minister," said Keeler. "The colonel couldn't believe it. John nearly died."

Profumo only broke off the affair that December because Keeler refused to move out of Ward's flat and into a discreet love nest that he was going to buy for her.

MI5 began to lose interest in the plan to honeytrap Ivanov. They were finding Ward increasingly unreliable. Keeler had moved on too. While scoring marijuana for Ward, she met West Indian jazz singer Lucky Gordon and, through him, another black man named Johnny Edgecombe. She began sleeping with both of them. This led to a fight at an all-night club in Soho in October 1962 where Gordon got his face slashed. Keeler moved in with Edgecombe briefly. When things did not work out, she moved back into Ward's flat. One night Edgecombe came round to try to win her back. It was late and she would not let him in. So he pulled a gun and blasted the front door. The police were called and Edgecombe was arrested and charged with attempted murder.

After this incident, Ward asked Keeler to leave the flat. Turning to his patient Michael Eddowes, a solicitor, for help, she told him that Ward had actually been spying for the Russians and that he had asked her to find out from Profumo about British plans to arm West Germany with nuclear weapons.

She told the same story to former Labour MP John Lewis. He passed the information on to George Wigg, a Labour MP who disliked Profumo after he had bested him in the House of Commons. In January 1963, Paul Mann, a journalist, took Keeler to the *Sunday Pictorial*. Keeler showed the editor the note that Profumo had written and he offered her £1,000 for her story.

However, the newspapers were exceedingly cautious at the time. The previous year, the exposure of the spy John Vassall, an admiralty clerk who had been passing secrets to the Soviets, had led to a Tribunal of Inquiry that investigated the press's role in the affair. In the course of it, two journalists had been sent to prison for refusing to name their sources.

The *Pictorial* contacted Ward, who managed to convince them that Keeler's story was a pack of lies. In retaliation, Keeler went to the police and told them that Ward procured call girls for his rich clients. A few days later, Profumo found himself being questioned by the Attorney General Sir John Hobson, the Solicitor General Peter Rawlinson and the Chief Whip Martin Redmayne. He denied any impropriety with Keeler. Although sceptical, they chose to accept what he was saying.

Prime Minister Harold Macmillan was briefed. A man of the world, he said that if Profumo had had an affair with Keeler he had been foolish, but sleeping with a pretty young woman, even if she was a prostitute, was hardly a sacking offence. Everyone hoped that that was the end of it. But on 8 March 1963, a small-circulation newsletter called *Westminster Confidential* ran a piece about the story the *Pictorial* had dropped and revealed that both the War Secretary and a Soviet military attaché, one Colonel Ivanov, were the clients of the same call girl.

On 10 March, George Wigg, who by this time had a bulging dossier on the relationship between Profumo and Keeler, took it to the Labour leader Harold Wilson. Wilson urged caution. But events now had a momentum of their own.

On 14 March, Johnny Edgecombe came up for trial at the Old Bailey. The key witness, Christine Keeler, was on holiday at the time and it was rumoured that she had been sent out of the country to keep a lid on the scandal.

Next day, the *Daily Express* ran the headline: WAR MINISTER SHOCK. It claimed that John Profumo had tended his resignation for "personal reasons". Down page was a picture of Christine Keeler under the headline: VANISHED.

The *Express* later claimed that the juxtaposition of the two stories was purely coincidental. But everyone put two and two together.

On 19 March, during a debate in the House of Commons on the Vassall case, George Wigg used the protection of parliamentary privilege to raise the rumours circulating about the War Minister. He was supported by the Labour firebrand Barbara Castle and opposition frontbencher Richard Crossman. The government were flustered. The Home Secretary Henry Brooke told the Labour critics that, if they wanted to substantiate their accusations, they should use a different forum, one that was not shielded from the laws of libel by the cloak of privilege.

Profumo had one supporter though, a Labour backbencher named Reginald Paget.

"What do these rumours amount to?" Paget asked rhetorically. "They amount to the fact that a minister is said to be acquainted with an extremely pretty girl. As far as I am concerned, I should have thought that was a matter for congratulation rather than an inquiry."

Profumo was grilled again by the Chief Whip, the Leader of the House Iain Macleod and Bill Deedes, Minister Without Portfolio and future editor of the *Daily Telegraph*. Profumo again insisted that he was innocent. He then made a parliamentary statement.

In it he admitted knowing Christine Keeler, but he said he had not seen her since December 1961. He said he had also met Stephen Ward and Yevgeny Ivanov. He denied that he was in any way responsible for Keeler's no-show at Edgecombe's trial and stated categorically: "There was no impropriety whatsoever in my acquaintanceship with Miss Keeler." And he threatened anyone who repeated the allegations outside parliament with a libel writ.

A few days later, reporters caught up with Christine Keeler in Madrid. She repeated what Profumo had said. But George Wigg would not leave it at that. He went on the *Panorama* programme and said that Ward and Ivanov were security risks. The next day Ward met Wigg and tried to convince him it was not true. He failed. More than ever, Wigg believed that Profumo had lied about his relationship with Keeler. He wrote a report of his meeting with Ward and gave it to Harold Wilson, who passed it on to Macmillan.

Although the Vassall case was keeping the British press subdued, there was no such reticence in the foreign papers. Profumo issued writs against *Paris Match* and *Il Tempo Illustrato* who both said that he had been bonking Christine Keeler.

In an attempt to salvage the situation, the Home Secretary told the Metropolitan Police to try to find something on Ward. This was highly irregular. The police are supposed to investigate crimes and find out who committed them, not investigate people on the off chance they had committed a crime.

It soon became clear to Ward's friends and clients that he was in serious trouble. They deserted him in droves. Mandy Rice-Davies was arrested on trumped-up charges and held in prison until she agreed to testify against Ward.

Ward desperately wrote to everyone he could think of, protesting his innocence. Harold Wilson received a letter. He showed it to the Prime Minister, who agreed to set up a committee of inquiry under Lord Dilhorne. Profumo was on holiday at the time. When he returned, he realized that the game was up. He could not face a committee of inquiry and lie again, so he went to see the Chief Whip and Macmillan's Parliamentary Private Secretary, told them the truth and resigned.

His letter of resignation and Macmillan's reply were published the next day.

"I misled you, and my colleagues, and the House," Profumo wrote, but, he explained, "I did this to protect my wife and family."

Macmillan's reply said tersely: "I am sure you will understand that in the circumstances I have no alternative but to advise the queen to accept your resignation."

The very day this exchange appeared in the paper, 5 June 1963, there was more drama. Christine Keeler's other West Indian boyfriend Lucky Gordon came to court on the charge of assaulting her outside a friend's flat. Keeler turned up in court in a Rolls-Royce. From the dock, Gordon accused her of giving him a sexually transmitted disease. She responded with an outburst from the public gallery. The newspapers lapped it up. Gordon was sent down for three years, which was overturned on appeal.

Ward appeared on television on 9 June and denied that he had encouraged Christine Keeler to have an affair with John Profumo because he had a friend in the Soviet Embassy. The following day he was arrested and charged with living on immoral earnings.

By that time, newspapers worldwide were running the scandal on the front page. Mandy Rice-Davies told the *Washington Star* about society orgies in London. She mentioned that, at one dinner party, a naked man wearing only a mask waited on table. The hunt for the masked man was on. Was it a senior judge, a Cabinet minister or a member of the royal family?

Under the headline PRINCE PHILIP AND THE PROFUMO SCANDAL, the *Daily Mirror* vehemently dismissed the "foul rumour" that Prince Philip was involved – though he was, of course. The queen's consort was a member of a gentlemen's association called the Thursday Club, which also boasted Stephen Ward among its membership.

Allegations flew thick and fast. Everyone in any position in society was now a target. The Bishop of Southwark, Mervyn Stockwood, appealed for calm.

Politically, the question came down to: How had John Profumo managed to lie about his affair for so long? Macmillan, who had taken a lenient attitude to the matter back in January, was now in the firing line. Colleagues began to sense that his tenure of office was drawing to a close. The portly Lord Hailsham quit his title to become a contender for the premiership as Quintin Hogg. He threw his hat into the ring by appearing on television and condemning Profumo for lying. Again Reginald Paget rallied to Profumo's defence.

"When self-indulgence has reduced a man to the shape of Lord Hailsham," he said, "sexual continence involves no more than a sense of the ridiculous."

Milking the situation for all it was worth, Mandy Rice-Davies told the *Sunday Mirror* that the Soviet military attaché and the War Minister had missed bumping into each other at Ward's flat by a matter of minutes on a number of occasions.

Michael Eddowes issued a press statement, saying that he had warned the Prime Minister of the security risk as early as 29 March. Meanwhile, Christine Keeler sold her "confessions" to the *News of the World* who began serializing them.

*The Times* attacked the Conservative government for its lack of moral leadership. To which, Lord Hailsham responded petulantly: "*The Times* is an anti-Conservative newspaper with an anti-Conservative editor."

Even the *Washington Post* got in on the act, saying that "a picture of widespread decadence beneath the glitter of a large segment of stiff-lipped society is emerging".

Labour went on the offensive. In a debate in the House of Commons on 19 June, Harold Wilson said that the Profumo scandal had "shocked the moral conscience of the nation". Pointing the finger at the Prime Minister, he said that for political reasons he was gambling with national security.

Macmillan could not even count on the support of his own backbenchers. Conservative MP Nigel Birch rehearsed the simple facts of the case.

"I must say that [Profumo] never struck me as a man at all like a cloistered monk," he told the House. "And Miss Keeler is a professional prostitute. There seems to me to be a basic improbability that their relationship was purely platonic. What are whores about?"

Addressing the Prime Minister directly, he said: "I myself feel that the time will come very soon when my Right Honourable friend ought to make way for a much younger colleague."

Macmillan survived the debate, but was badly wounded. Four days later, he announced an official inquiry under Master of the Rolls Lord Denning. It did not save him. Macmillan resigned in the early autumn, shortly before the party conference. He was replaced by Sir Alec Douglas-Home, but the Conservative government was tainted by the scandal and was swept from office the following year.

Although Lord Denning was supposed to look into possible breaches of security caused by the Profumo scandal, he concentrated on the salacious aspects – so much so that, when he cross-questioned witnesses, he often sent the official stenographer out of the room to save her, or perhaps his own, blushes.

When Ward went on trial at the Old Bailey, the world's media were there in force. Again the salacious details were played up. One newspaper in New Zealand was prosecuted for indecency for merely reporting the case.

The star of the show was undoubtedly Mandy Rice-Davies, whom the judge mistakenly addressed as Marilyn Monroe. When it was put to her that Lord Astor denied that he had met her at his house parties at Cliveden, she said: "Well, he would, wouldn't he?"

That remark is now in the *Oxford Dictionary of Quotations*.

In his summing up, the judge pointed out that none of Ward's high-born friends had come to testify on his behalf.

"One would have thought from the newspapers that this country has become a sink of iniquity," he told the jury. "But you and I know that the even tenor of family life over the overwhelming majority of the population goes quietly and decently on."

He might as well have been putting the noose around the defendant's neck. Ward was not just guilty of introducing rich and powerful people to a couple of attractive and available girls, the judge was implying that he was responsible for the general loosening of moral standards that many people felt was engulfing the country. Ward knew that he was being made a scapegoat.

"This is a political trial," he told a friend. "Someone had to be sacrificed and that someone is me."

On the night of 3 July 1963, Ward took an overdose of sleeping tablets. He left a suicide note saying that, after the judge's summing up, he had given up all hope. He asked that resuscitation be delayed as long as possible, adding, somewhat bizarrely, that "the car needs oil in the gearbox".

With Ward unconscious in St Stephen's Hospital, the jury found him guilty on two counts of living on immoral earnings. He died on 3 August, without regaining consciousness. Even after he was dead, the newspapers kept vilifying him.

There were only six mourners at Stephen Ward's funeral and only two wreaths. One came from his family. The other was from the critic Kenneth Tynan, playwrights John Osborne, Arnold Wesker and Joe Orton, singer Annie Ross, painter Dominick Elwes and writer Penelope Gilliatt. The card on it read: "To Stephen Ward, victim of hypocrisy."

When the Denning report was published in October 1963, it was an instant best-seller, selling over four thousand copies in the first hour. It too laid the blame squarely at the door of Stephen Ward who was in no position to answer back.

Profumo left political life and threw himself into charity work, for which he was awarded the CBE in 1975. He remained married to Valerie Hobson. Christine Keeler was jailed for six months for contempt of court for failing to appear at the trial of Johnny Edgecombe. Her autobiography *Scandal* was published in 1989 and was made into a successful movie.

Mandy Rice-Davies wrote a series of novels, became a film actress, opened two clubs in Israel and married a millionaire. George Wigg became chairman of the Horse Race Betting

Levy Board and later pleaded guilty to soliciting for prostitutes in Soho.

## Charles Parnell

For centuries, Ireland had provided Britain with its most intractable political problems. However, in 1889, Home Rule seemed to be in sight, only to be knocked off the political agenda for another thirty years by a scandalous divorce case involving the Home Rule Party's charismatic leader Charles Stewart Parnell.

Born in County Wicklow, the son of a Protestant landowner, Parnell had swallowed anti-British sentiment with his mother's milk. She was the daughter of Commodore Charles Stewart, a US Navy hero of the War of 1812. His parents had emigrated from Belfast before the War of Independence.

Parnell went to school in England, then on to Cambridge. But he was sent down after a drunken brawl with a local merchant. When he was arrested, Parnell tried to bribe the policeman, but mistakenly gave him a shilling instead of a sovereign. He was charged and sent down.

Returning home to Ireland, Parnell found it in the grip of the Fenians, who had taken up armed struggle against British rule. He allied himself with their cause and got himself elected to parliament in 1875. The following year, he told the House of Commons that three Fenians executed in Manchester for murdering a policeman were Irish martyrs, a sentiment that won him a huge following at home in Ireland.

In parliament he began to adopt the filibuster techniques that had been used effectively in the United States Congress to hamper government business. However, while in Congress it was permissible for a politician to read at length from a newspaper, in the British parliament a speaker was required to stick more or less to the point. Parnell managed to do this brilliantly and with interminable speeches managed to talk government bills out. He believed that he could hinder the British parliament to the point that setting up a devolved government in Dublin would seem like a blessing.

In 1878, Ireland faced another famine and Parnell allied himself with the Irish Land League, who resisted evictions and used violence against rent collectors. And in 1880, he was returned to parliament with eighty-five other Home Rulers. Parnell was then voted party leader with the support of Captain William O'Shea, member for County Clare.

A Dublin-born Catholic, O'Shea had served in the 18th Hussars before becoming interested in politics. He retired from the army at the age of twenty-six, then married Kitty Wood, the daughter of an English aristocrat. They had three children. Generous handouts from Kitty's aunt and the untiring entertaining of his wife allowed O'Shea to develop the connections needed to make a career in politics.

In 1880, the newly elected O'Shea sought to advance his career by holding a series of dinner parties at St Thomas's Hotel. Parnell was invited, but failed to show up and O'Shea sent his wife to Westminster to find out why.

"He came out, a tall, gaunt figure, thin and deathly pale," she recalled. "He looked straight at me smiling and his curiously burning eyes looked into mine with a wondering intenseness that threw into my brain the sudden thought: 'This man is wonderful – and different.'"

But first Kitty chided him.

"I asked him why he had not answered my last invitation, and if nothing would induce him to come. He answered that he had not opened his letters for days but, that if I would let him, he would come to dinner directly when he returned from Paris."

The tryst made, there then came a truly romantic moment.

"In leaning forward in the cab to say goodbye," Kitty wrote, "a rose I was wearing in my bodice fell out on to my skirt. He picked it up and, touching it lightly to his lips, placed it in his buttonhole."

Later he sealed it in an envelope with Kitty's name on it.

Kitty O'Shea pressed a number of buttons for Parnell. She was a short, stout woman with beautiful hair and her incessant chatter and quick wit reminded him of his mother. These maternal attributes helped him overcome the guilt he felt over the death of his first love, a beautiful farmer's daughter from County Wicklow. At the age of nineteen, when he had tried to break it off with her, she had committed suicide. He had been out in a boat on the river with his sister Fanny when he had seen a crowd pulling her body from the water. Ever since then, he had been dogged with dark depressions.

The O'Sheas' marriage had been only for show for some time. When O'Shea was not abroad, he spent most of his time in his pied-à-terre in Victoria, while Kitty lived in Wornersh Lodge in Eltham, Kent. Soon after they had met, when Parnell was worn out by campaigning, Kitty invited him to stay there. She nursed him and often slipped into his sickbed beside him. How much her husband knew about this is unclear.

A maid said that Parnell used the name Stewart when he visited. When she went to his mistress's room, she would have to knock and wait ten minutes before entering. And Parnell, she said, would escape down the fire escape if Captain O'Shea returned unexpectedly.

Certainly, their relationship was clandestine. When Parnell's support for the Land League led to charges of "conspiracy to impoverish landlords", she shielded him from arrest by hiding him in a dressing room next to her bedroom, taking his meals to him there herself to avoid involving the servants.

They also met in rented houses and communicated by coded letters and sign language. If he twisted his handkerchief during a speech in the Commons, it meant he would see her later.

One day in 1881, O'Shea returned home to find Parnell's portmanteau in the house and challenged him to a duel. But Parnell talked him out of it, explaining that he had to work closely with Kitty as she was a vital conduit to Prime Minister

William Gladstone, who had gradually become convinced of the case for Home Rule.

O'Shea threatened Kitty with divorce, but she pointed out that he had been unfaithful to her on no less than seventeen occasions. Although this was hardly an obstacle to divorce, O'Shea was dependent on Kitty's aunt's money and backed down.

Politically, Parnell was still on the ascendancy. In 1881, Gladstone had conceded the Land Act, promising all Irish tenants rights of tenancy and fair rents. However, by supporting the passage of such a sensible piece of legislation, Parnell was seen to be colluding with the British. So he returned to Ireland to stir up sedition and got himself arrested.

While he was in Kilmainham jail, Kitty gave birth to their first daughter, whom O'Shea nobly acknowledged as his own. The child only lived for two months, dying before Parnell was released. Later they had two more daughters, which took O'Shea's name.

Rural Ireland was in turmoil. The only person who could restore order was Parnell. Using O'Shea as an intermediary, Gladstone negotiated the Treaty of Kilmainham, which offered Parnell further concessions in return for an end to agitation.

Four days after Parnell was released, Lord Frederick Cavendish and his senior civil servant Thomas Burke, a Catholic, were gunned down in Phoenix Park, Dublin. The killings appalled even the nationalists. Parnell used the crisis to bring the growing nationalist movement under his control.

The killings also resulted in a tightening of security. Parnell was put under twenty-four-hour surveillance. Soon the Home Office became aware of his irregular domestic arrangements and the Home Secretary Lord Harcourt warned that the Treaty of Kilmainham would be seen as tainted if it was known that Parnell had negotiated it via the husband of his mistress.

Parnell never acknowledged O'Shea's part in his release. O'Shea grew resentful and it became harder for him to close his ears to the rumours about his wife's infidelity. On the stump during the elections of 1885, Parnell was asked about his relationship with Kitty O'Shea in front of a boisterous crowd. He refused to answer.

While Parnell was a troublesome supporter of Gladstone, O'Shea began to side with Joseph Chamberlain, who was hostile to Parnell's Home Rule plans. Even though, at Kitty's behest, Parnell had found him a safe seat as a Home Ruler, O'Shea was the only Irish nationalist to follow Chamberlain and the Tories into the lobby to vote against the limited 1886 Home Rule Bill, which was defeated.

Things began to go badly wrong for Parnell. In May 1886, while Captain O'Shea was away in Europe, Parnell's carriage collided with a market gardener's cart while he was travelling home to Eltham. The *Pall Mall Gazette* ran the story and pointed out: "During the sitting of parliament the hon. member for Cork usually takes up his residence at Eltham, a suburban village in the south-east of London. From here he can often be seen taking riding exercise round by Chislehurst and Sidcup."

Later that year, the Sussex *Daily News* reported that he was staying with Mrs O'Shea in Eastbourne. In an effort to keep a lid on things, Parnell adopted the alias Fox and they became a little more careful about their movements.

In 1889, the Home Rule Bill came up again. Negotiations went on throughout the summer and the prospects looked better than they had for many years. However, on Christmas Eve 1889, Captain O'Shea filed for divorce, naming Parnell as co-respondent.

"I fear a thundercloud is about to burst over Parnell's head," wrote Gladstone, "and I suppose it will end the career of a man in many respects valuable."

The divorce was a coup for O'Shea. The evidence against them was now so overwhelming that Parnell and Kitty did not show up in the court. Kitty's aunt had recently died, leaving Kitty her fortune. O'Shea won custody of the children, including Parnell's, and her money. Delivering his verdict, the judge condemned Parnell as "a man who takes advantage of the hospitality offered him by the husband to debauch the wife".

O'Shea's mentor Chamberlain was happy too. Parnell had been wiped off the map. In Ireland, the Catholic Church turned against him.

"I cannot but look forward with dismay to our interest, religious as well as civil, being placed under the guidance of a convicted adulterer," said the Archbishop of Armagh.

The nonconformist churches, which were the backbone of the Gladstone's Liberal Party, condemned him. Even the Irish newspapers turned against him. Parnell fought on, but only succeeded in splitting the nationalists. This ceded the field to the Conservatives and the increasingly militant Ulster Unions and took Home Rule off the agenda for another thirty years. In his disappointment, Parnell grew more outspoken, losing the support of the mainstream but feeding the aspirations of the fanatical nationalists.

In 1891, Parnell and Kitty married in a registry office. A few months later, when he was canvassing for a candidate in Cregas, he gave one last barnstorming speech in a rain storm. He stayed up all night chatting in his wet clothes. The following day he left Ireland. Seven days later he died in Brighton of "rheumatism of the heart".

As Parnell's coffin was being closed, ready to be shipped back to Ireland, Kitty slipped inside the rose that he had kept from their first meeting eleven years before. She was advised not to accompany the coffin to Dublin, where Parnell was given a magnificent funeral.

Ruined by the divorce and blamed for the downfall of Parnell, Kitty had a nervous breakdown and withdrew from public life. She published her memoirs in 1914 and died in 1921, at the age of seventy-six. She never remarried.

## David Lloyd George

The "Welsh Wizard" David Lloyd George was one of the greatest politicians of his age. In 1909, he introduced the old age pension and, in 1911, unemployment insurance. That same year he forced through the Parliament Act, which effectively stripped the House of Lords of its powers. He was prime minister during World War I and gave Ireland Home Rule in 1922. He was also a great political survivor, who was mired in sexual scandal throughout his career but, somehow, managed to emerge without a stain.

Elected to parliament for Caernarfon in 1892, Lloyd George was threatened with disgrace in 1897 when he was named in a divorce case. A friend and constituent of Lloyd George's, a Montgomeryshire doctor named Edwards, was suing his wife Catherine for divorce on the grounds of adultery, naming as co-respondent a man called Wilson. However, Catherine also confessed to sleeping with Lloyd George. She said that it had happened on the night of 4 February 1896. Lloyd George had been staying the night at the Edwards' house. When her husband had been called out, "criminal conversation", as the divorce laws at the time delicately put it, took place. Six months later, she gave birth to a child. Catherine Edwards claimed that Lloyd George was the father.

Although Catherine Edwards mentioned that they had slept together on other occasions, Lloyd George could prove that he did not have sex with her on 4 February. On that night, he had voted in the House of Commons. Lloyd George claimed that Catherine Edwards was a fantasist, a would-be political groupie. Her allegations against Lloyd George had to be withdrawn. As Dr Edwards had plenty of evidence of his wife's adultery with other men, it did not matter. He was granted his divorce anyway.

When Lloyd George became chancellor in 1908, the political journal *The Bystander* made a veiled reference to his womanizing. Then, fearing a libel suit, it donated £300 to Caernarfon Cottage Hospital. But the *People* followed up, citing the Edwards case and forthcoming divorce suit in which, the paper said, Lloyd George was going to be named as co-respondent.

This time Lloyd George sued. He hired as his attorney his most outspoken political opponent, the Tory MP F. E. Smith, who was also a close personal friend. Against them was Edward Carson KC, the man whose shrewd cross-examination had destroyed Oscar Wilde.

Lloyd George clearly perjured himself when he told the court that the *People*'s allegations were "an absolute invention, every line of them". Everybody knew that Lloyd George was a ladies' man. So to add weight to his denials he brought his long-suffering wife Margaret with him to court. According to their son Richard, this conversation took place between them before their court appearance:

"You must help me, Maggie. If get out of this I give my oath you shall never have to suffer this ordeal again."

"And you will give your oath that this story is untrue?" she asked.

"I have to."

Maggie then asked: "And you give me your oath that I shall not have to suffer this sort of thing again. How can I rely on your 'oath'?"

"One day," said Lloyd George, "I shall be prime minister. I shall be a force for the public good. If you help me you shall never forget your decision."

As it happened, Edward Carson did not embarrass the future prime minister's wife with any questions. On behalf of the *People*, he offered a sincere and heartfelt apology and £1,000 was donated to another Welsh charity.

Of course, Lloyd George's oath to his wife was no better than his oath in court. His continued philandering earned him the nickname "The Goat". In 1912, he took as his lover his daughter Megan's tutor Frances Stevenson, sleeping with her at Number Ten Downing Street. Thirty years later, after his wife died, they married.

Although in future Lloyd George did manage to stay out of court, he did not stay out of the way of scandal. In 1912, his involvement in the Marconi Scandal nearly brought the Liberal government down. Lloyd George and other members of the Cabinet did a little insider dealing after the government decided to set up six radio stations that would link the government in Whitehall directly to all quarters of the Empire. As it was, Lloyd George was not very skilled at playing the stock market and lost £213. Nevertheless he went on to become prime minister in 1916.

After winning the war, Lloyd George promptly embroiled himself in fresh scandal. In 1918, the Liberal Party split. Asquith, who commanded the bulk of the party's funds, returned to the opposition benches. The radical wing, under Lloyd George, stayed in government, continuing the wartime coalition with the Tories. But it found itself short of funds. He solved the problem by selling peerages and other honours.

However, the 1922 Honours List contained the names of a wartime tax dodger and a shipowner who had been convicted of trading with the enemy. In public Lloyd George defended himself, denying everything and setting up a Royal Commission to look into the matter. In private, he said the sale of honours was the cleanest way of raising money for a political party. As he had stripped the House of Lords of its powers, the titles he conferred were meaningless baubles. But his authority was weakened, his coalition government split and he resigned.

## Jeremy Thorpe

The charismatic Liberal leader Jeremy Thorpe revived the party's fortunes in the sixties and brought them within striking distance of power for the first time since the fall of Lloyd

George. But Thorpe was brought down by a scandal that involved rough sex and pillow-biting.

Both Thorpe's father and grandfather had been Tory MPs, but when the twenty-six-year-old barrister ran for election in the Tory stronghold of North Devon in 1955, he ran as a Liberal. He lost. But in 1959, he won the seat and held it for twenty years.

Educated at Eton and Oxford, where he was president of the Union, Thorpe was well connected and seemed set for a brilliant career. But early in his career as an MP he made one small slip that would result in disaster. Visiting a friend's riding stables in Oxfordshire in the autumn of 1961, he befriended a good-looking young groom named Norman Scott.

Scott was mentally unstable and latched on to Thorpe. Later he turned up to see Thorpe at the House of Commons, asking for his help as he was now penniless and unemployed after being sacked over the theft of a horse. According to Scott, Thorpe took him to stay at his mother's home in Oxted, Surrey. That night, Thorpe appeared in his bedroom. There, Scott said, Thorpe had anal sex with him while he bit the pillow to stifle his cries.

The following morning, Thorpe was the perfect gentleman, preparing his guest's breakfast, then drove him back to London. Scott said that Thorpe gave him money to rent a flat in Westminster and letters authorizing him to purchase clothes on his account. Thorpe denied this.

However, Thorpe did make an effort to find his young friend a job, putting ads in *Country Life*. Scott had also lost his national insurance card at the stables. Thorpe got him another, stamping it for a few months as his employer.

He arranged for Scott to spend Christmas in the Devon home of May and James Collier, who was a prospective Liberal candidate for Tiverton. Scott was highly unstable and neurotic and, after a few weeks, they asked him to leave.

Then in February 1962, Scott was accused of stealing a suede coat from Ann Gray, a woman he had met at a psychiatric clinic. Thorpe told the police that he was "more or less" Scott's guardian and insisted that the interview take place in his room in the House of Commons. Impressed, the police dropped the case.

Scott wanted to go to France to study dressage. To raise the money, Thorpe found him a job tending horses in Somerset. He wrote to him there enclosing more job offers from *Country Life* and saying: "Bunnies can and will go to France." Thorpe called him "Bunnies", Scott said, because that night when Thorpe had approached him in the bedroom of his mother's house he said he looked like a frightened rabbit.

Scott had told Thorpe that his mother had inexplicably disappeared and that his father had recently died in plane crash in South America. Thorpe thought that he might be due some compensation and had a solicitor look into the matter for him, only to discover that Scott's father was alive and well, and his mother was still living in the family home. She blamed Thorpe for the estrangement of her son.

Thorpe was livid that Scott had lied to him. Scott, in turn, went to Chelsea police station and made a statement, alleging that he had had homosexual relations with Jeremy Thorpe. Homosexuality was still against the law back then. It was only decriminalized in England and Wales in 1967. Scott submitted to a medical examination that he had indulged in anal sex and, to substantiate his story, he handed over two letters from Thorpe – one of which was the letter where Thorpe had addressed him as "Bunnies".

After the 1964 general election, Thorpe was returned to parliament with an enlarged majority. Scott contacted him again, saying that he had been offered a job in Switzerland. Thorpe paid for him to go. Scott hated the position and returned, losing his luggage along the way. Thorpe tried to retrieve it, but told Scott that he wanted nothing further to do with him.

In retaliation, Scott wrote to Thorpe's mother saying that he had had a homosexual relationship with her son and it had begun the night he had brought him to her house.

"With Jeremy that day, I gave birth to the vice that lies latent in every man," wrote Scott.

Thorpe's mother forwarded the letter to him. He showed it to his closest friend in parliament Peter Bessell, Liberal MP for the neighbouring constituency of Bodmin.

Bessell was a slick businessman and a Congregationalist lay preacher who amazed his Cornish constituents by campaigning in a Cadillac. Like all good MPs, Bessell was bedding his secretary. But to secure Thorpe's support, he pretended to swing both ways. Scott was in Dublin at the time and Bessell went to see him. He told Scott, disingenuously, that his letter to Thorpe's mother constituted blackmail and said that he had an extradition order in his briefcase. Scott promised to be a good boy and Bessell put him on a retainer. This kept him quiet for the next three years.

In 1967, Jeremy Thorpe was elected leader of the Liberal Party. The following year, he married his first wife Caroline Allpass, who gave birth to a son. However, by then, Bessell's companies were beginning to come apart at the seams. Scott's latest career venture – as a male model – had come to nothing and Scott ended up on Thorpe's plate again.

This time Thorpe tried to ship him off to the US, but the American embassy refused Scott a visa. It was then, Bessell claimed, that Thorpe snapped. Thorpe called him up at the Commons and said: "Peter, we have got to get rid of him . . . It's no worse than shooting a sick dog."

It was also alleged that Thorpe had asked his friend, the merchant banker David Holmes, to organize Scott's murder. However, they suddenly got news that Scott had married and his wife was pregnant. That, everyone hoped, would be the end of the matter.

The following year, the marriage broke up. Scott left his wife and child and moved to Wales, expecting Thorpe to pick up the tab. He contacted Thorpe and got no joy. So he called Bessell and threatened to take his allegations to the newspapers. Meanwhile, Scott poured out his heart to an elderly postmistress. She, in turn, wrote to her Liberal MP, Emlyn Hooson, warning of the dangers. Hooson passed the letter on to the Liberal chief whip David Steel.

A secret inquiry was set up under the Liberal peer Lord Byers. Before Scott flounced from the committee room "like a jilted girl", he had told Byers that he had been stopped by the police carrying a gun in the House of Commons in 1965. This was easily disproved. Thorpe presented himself as the victim of an obsessed and deluded young man.

That seemed to be the end of it. But, on his way out of the Palace of Westminster, Scott claimed that he was threatened with death by a mysterious stranger. Frightened for his life, Scott told his story to freelance journalist Gordon Winter. He touted it around Fleet Street but it was generally considered too hot to handle. However, the Mirror Group, which was run by Thorpe's friend Lord Jacobsen, bought the story and locked it in their safe. It would have gone no further, but Gordon Winters was also a spy for the apartheid regime in South Africa and he sent a copy to Pretoria.

Meanwhile, Scott moved into Thorpe's North Devon constituency and started telling his story to anyone who would listen. This brought Scott to the attention of MI5. The Devon and Cornwall police arrested Scott, ostensibly on the charge of stealing £28 from a hotel nine months before, but they questioned him about any documents he might have that could be used to blackmail Thorpe.

Thorpe was riding high at the time. Although his first wife, Caroline, had been killed in a car crash in 1973, he quickly remarried. His second wife was Marion, Countess of Harewood.

Peter Bessell was now out of parliament and had absconded to America to escape his creditors. In 1974, builders were working on Bessell's London office when they came across some photographs and papers – one of which was Scott's letter to Thorpe's mother. Again Thorpe was lucky. The builders took them to the *Sunday Mirror* and they joined Scott's confession in the safe.

The Conservatives, under Edward Heath, had narrowly lost the election in February 1974. Thorpe was summoned to Number Ten for preliminary talks. There were rumours that he might be offered the position of Foreign Secretary in a coalition government, but the party vetoed any such arrangement.

In 1975, it was alleged that the murder plot was revived. At the subsequent trial in the Old Bailey, it was said that David Holmes, then Deputy Treasurer of the Liberal Party, along with nightclub owner George Deakin and athletics coach John Le Mesurier, used a political donation to hire a hit man. The contract was worth £5,000, with another £5,000 on completion. The bungling assassin they chose to do the job was an airline pilot named Andrew Newton.

He was so incompetent that, when he was told that Norman Scott was in Barnstable in North Devon, he went to Dunstable in Bedfordshire instead. But in October 1975, he caught up with his quarry. Instead of fleeing, Scott greeted Newton as his saviour. He believed that a hit man was on his way from Canada to murder him and, perversely, assumed that Newton had been sent to protect him.

Scott got into Newton's car with his Great Dane, Rinka. Newton drove to a deserted part of Exmoor. When they got out, Newton pulled a 1910 Mauser and shot the Great Dane.

"It's your turn next," he said to Scott. But the gun either jammed or Newton pretended it had. He drove away, leaving Scott sobbing over the body of his dead dog.

Newton was arrested and a small item about the shooting of Scott's dog appeared in the *News of the World*. But then, on 14 November 1975, *Private Eye* ran this intriguing item:

"A Mr Norman Scott has sent me some very curious material concerning his close friend, the Liberal leader Jeremy Thorpe. If Mr Thorpe would send me my usual fee of £5, I will send him the dossier and say no more."

In January 1976, things began to unravel. Scott answered a summons in Barnstaple on charges of defrauding the Department of Health and Social Security. The magistrate was shocked to find the courtroom packed with journalists. Scott then announced that he was being hounded by the press because he had once had a sexual affair with Jeremy Thorpe. As the allegation was given as testimony in a courtroom, it could be reported without danger of a libel writ.

The Prime Minister Harold Wilson defended Thorpe in the House of Commons, saying that the regime in Pretoria was trying to discredit his government by attacking Thorpe, which was true. Thorpe himself stoutly denied that he was a homosexual, which was not.

In March 1976, Newton was found guilty and sentenced to two years for a firearms offence. Newton claimed that it was he, not Thorpe, who had been the victim of Scott's blackmail. But Scott stuck to his story.

When David Steel discovered that David Holmes had been given £20,000 that was intended for the Liberal Party as part of the alleged murder plot, he asked Thorpe to step down. Thorpe refused. But the tide was turning against him. The newspapers found out about the retainers Bessell had paid Scott. When they tracked Bessell down in America, Bessell denied that he had given Scott cash for Thorpe's benefit. But if his whereabouts had been discovered, his creditors also would know where to find him, so he needed money. He sold his story to the *Daily Mail*. It appeared on 6 May, under the headline I TOLD LIES TO PROTECT THORPE. In the story, Bessell said he had paid Scott to protect Thorpe. Worse, he said that Thorpe had wanted Scott dead and that the botched assassination attempt had resulted in the death of the dog Rinka.

At the same time, Scott's solicitor issued a summons for the return of the letters Scott had handed over to the police in 1962. Thorpe followed suit. The court ruled in favour of Scott, who was given the originals. Thorpe received copies. In a bold move, he published them in the *Sunday Times* on 9 May 1976 with a protracted explanation. The paper agreed to make no comment. On the Monday morning, T-shirts appeared in London's Oxford Street, bearing the slogan: "Bunnies can and will go to France." By the end of the day, Thorpe had resigned.

Thorpe blamed a press witch-hunt and the public backbiting – if not the pillow-biting – on ambitious colleagues. The speaker George Thomas agreed, condemned the Liberal members' "disloyalty just when their leader needed him the most". But the third act had not yet started.

First, though, there was an eighteen-month interval with Thorpe sitting quietly on the back benches. Then in April 1977, Newton was released from prison. He sold his story to the London *Evening News* for £3,000. It appeared under the headline: I WAS HIRED TO KILL SCOTT. In October, the *Sunday People* paid him a further £8,000 to photograph Holmes's business associate John Le Mesurier pay off the £5,000 owed on the murder attempt.

Thorpe held a press conference and denied everything once again. He denied that he had had a homosexual relationship with Scott, though their friendship had been "close, even affectionate". Then came the $64,000 question. A BBC correspondent asked if he had ever had a homosexual relationship.

It was then that Thorpe lost it.

"If you do not know why it is improper and indecent to put such a question to a public man you ought not to be here," he said.

But he did not say no. Although homosexual acts between consenting adults in private had by then been legalized by the 1967 Sexual Offences Act, homosexual frolics, especially among MPs, were still frowned on.

The police were busy putting a case together. Although Newton had admitted, at the very least, conspiracy and perjury in his last trial, he was offered immunity from prosecution if he turned Queen's evidence. Detectives also travelled to California to interview Bessell and offered him immunity too. Eager to profit from the situation, Bessell began touting a book. The *Sunday Telegraph* offered a massive £50,000 for the serial rights. A third of this would be paid upfront. The rest would be paid if Thorpe was convicted. If Thorpe walked, Bessell would receive only another £8,000.

When charges were drawn up, Thorpe, along with Holmes, Deakin and Le Mesurier, surrendered themselves to the police. Thorpe had already delivered a long written statement to the police denying everything. He said he had tried to help Scott who was "suicidal and unbalanced" but "my compassion and kindness towards him was in due course repaid with malevolence and resentment". He knew no more than that, he said.

On his formal arrest, Thorpe refused to answer any further questions on the grounds that the answers might be leaked and prejudice the case.

Even after being charged, Thorpe made a dramatic appearance at the Liberal Party Conference. It was beholden on the new leader David Steel to greet him. His appearance was a great embarrassment. It overshadowed coverage of the policy issues and, with an election only months away, it was the worst sort of publicity for the party.

Thorpe was still on bail when he fought the 1979 election. At campaign meetings, his once loyal followers stayed away in droves. The satirist Auberon Waugh stood against him as a candidate for the Dog Lovers' Party. Only one Liberal MP, John Pardoe, from a neighbouring seat, turned out to lend his support. Thorpe was resoundingly trounced by the Tories. Pardoe lost his seat too.

Five days later, Thorpe was in the dock of the Old Bailey,

charged with conspiring to murder Norman Scott and inciting David Holmes to commit murder. He pleaded not guilty.

Although the case against him looked strong, Thorpe's barrister George Carmen QC made mincemeat of the prosecution witnesses. Bessell's statement that in 1968 Thorpe had said "we have got to get rid of" Scott was the only evidence of the involvement of Thorpe in any plot. Carmen demonstrated that Bessell had given several different versions of how Thorpe had told him this on different occasions. He also pointed out to the jury that Bessell stood to profit considerably from the contract with the *Sunday Telegraph* if Thorpe was convicted. He similarly savaged Scott who was, admittedly, an easier target.

These points were not lost on the judge who, in his summing up, described Bessell as a "humbug" and Scott as "a crook, an accomplished liar, a fraud, a sponger, a whiner, a parasite and a spineless neurotic character addicted to hysteria and self-advertisement" – though the judge conceded "he could still be telling the truth".

The jury did not think so. They also thought that Bessell's evidence was tainted by the £25,000 he stood to gain if Thorpe went down. After two days' deliberation, they returned a verdict of not guilty.

There was some criticism of Thorpe for not appearing on the witness stand to tell his side of the story. But the people of North Devon were delighted. Even though he had been defeated in the election, 23,000 of them had still voted for him. A thanksgiving service was held for him and he was elected president of the North Devon Liberal Association, in due course becoming the president of the Liberal Democrat Association, following the Liberals' merger with the short-lived Social Democratic Party.

Thorpe stuck to his story of complete innocence. However, two years after his acquittal, David Holmes spilt the beans in the *News of the World* in exchange for the donation of a "substantial fee" to charity. He said that Thorpe was the inspiration behind various attempts to silence Scott because of the threat he posed to Thorpe's political career. The plan had been to frighten Scott, not kill him, and certain actions had taken place "after discussion with Jeremy and with his authorization".

But it was hard to see Thorpe as a sinister conspirator. Since the pillow-biting incident had been made public, he was a figure of fun.

## Lord Lambton and Lord Jellicoe

In 1973, two ministers in the British government, both lords, were forced to resign when it became known they enjoyed the company of prostitutes. Although they both did the right thing and tendered their resignations immediately, Lord Lambton, for one, was puzzled by the scandal his downfall provoked.

"Surely all men patronize whores," he said.

Lord Lambton was a career politician. First elected to parliament in 1951 as Conservative MP for Berwick-upon-Tweed, he served as parliamentary private secretary to Selwyn Lloyd from 1955 to 1957, when he resigned over the Suez Crisis. He was a critic of Macmillan during the Profumo affair, but returned to the government in 1970 as parliamentary Under Secretary for Defence, responsible for the RAF, on the recommendation of Lord Carrington, then Secretary of Defence.

The son of the Earl of Durham, Lambton was a wealthy landowner with an annual income of £100,000 from his 25,000 acres of farmland in Durham and Northumberland alone. He owned racehorses and was reputedly one of the best shots in the country.

In 1942, he married Belinda Blew-Jones. They had six children. However, by 1972, he and his wife were living practically separate lives. Commander Bert Wickstead of the Metropolitan Police Serious Crime Squad who investigated the allegations against Lambton remarked: "The most remarkable feature of his London home was that it had been divided precisely into two halves. Lord Lambton's half was almost Spartan in appearance, more befitting a bachelor than a married man. Lady Lambton's half, by contrast, was beautifully furnished and full of female fripperies."

Although Lambton was serious about politics and conscientious in his ministerial role, he lived the life of a man about town. He made frequent use of a high-class call-girl service. His favourite playmate was twenty-six-year-old Norma Russell, who would entertain Lambton alone – or with other prostitutes – in her Maida Vale flat. To put everyone in the mood, they smoked marijuana.

At first Lambton used the *nom d'amour* "Mr Lucas", but then became careless, even paying Norma for her services with a personal cheque. In November 1972, Norma married Colin Levy, an unemployed minicab driver with a drink problem and a criminal record. After five months of wedded bliss, they had a row and Levy went abroad. While he was away, Norma went to the police and told them that he was on a drug-smuggling trip. When he returned the police pounced. They found no drugs on him, but he told the police that his wife was a prostitute and that one of her clients was Lord Lambton. He had seen his name on a cheque.

The information was passed to the Serious Crime Squad, which was investigating a ring of high-class prostitutes at the time. MI5 were informed because of the security implications. The Home Secretary was also told. He informed the Prime Minister Edward Heath, who was ever alert to ministerial misbehaviour after the Profumo scandal.

Meanwhile, Levy tried to sell his story to the newspapers. He and an accomplice hid a ciné camera in his wife's bedroom. A microphone was hidden up her teddy bear's nose. They offered the resulting film to the *News of the World* for £30,000. Unfortunately, the pictures were not clear enough for publication, so the *News of the World* hid a photographer in Norma Levy's wardrobe, behind a two-way mirror. The resulting shots showed Lord Lambton with Norma Levy and a black nightclub hostess, cavorting on the bed. Nevertheless, the *News of the World* decided not to go ahead with the story and returned the material. Levy then tried to sell it to the German magazine *Stern*. The deal fell through so he went to the *Sunday People*, who promptly turned the pictures over to the police.

When Lambton was confronted with the pictures, he said: "She is a kind of prostitute. I liked her, but she played no important part in my life whatsoever."

He immediately resigned, issuing a statement about "this sordid story" of his "casual acquaintance" with a call girl and one or two of her friends. He added: "There has been no security risk and no blackmail and never at any time have I spoken of any aspect of my late job. All that has happened is that some sneak pimp has seen an opportunity of making money by the sale of the story and secret photographs at home and abroad. My own feelings may be imagined but I have no excuses whatever to make. I have behaved with incredible stupidity."

Although he could simply shrug off his use of prostitutes, from the tapes it was quite clear that he was also using drugs. Later that day he was arrested for the possession of amphetamines and cannabis, charged, convicted and fined £300.

But Lord Lambton was not the only casualty of the scandal. The same day he resigned, Lord Jellicoe tendered his resignation too. Son of the World War I naval commander Admiral Earl Jellicoe, Lord Jellicoe was a war hero in his own right, winning the DSO, MC, Légion d'Honneur, Croix de Guerre and the Greek Military Cross in World War II. He rose to become Lord Privy Seal and Leader of the House of Lords. He also had a weakness.

"He is not flamboyant but he was a hedonist," a colleague said.

His hedonism extended to hiring girls from two agencies advertised in the London *Evening Standard* in 1972 and 1973. He would take the women to dinner, then back to his London flat for sex.

Jellicoe was the soul of discretion. He dealt with the agencies under an assumed name and never revealed his true identity to his sexual partners. As a member of the Cabinet, he had access to secret material, but never discussed his work with the girls. However, while the police were investigating the allegations against Lord Lambton, they came across rumours about Lord Jellicoe's liaisons in passing. Naturally, Ted Heath called Jellicoe in to ask him what he knew about the Lambton scandal and passed on the gossip.

"When you told me yesterday that my name was being linked with allegations about a ring of call girls," Jellicoe wrote, "I thought it right to tell you that, unhappily, there was justification for this because I had had some casual affairs which, if publicized, would be the subject of grave criticism. I also said that, since this must be a grave embarrassment to you and to my colleagues I felt I must resign."

Heath quickly accepted, remarking: "Your decision accords with the best traditions of public life."

When he heard of Jellicoe's resignation, Lambton said: "The way things are going it will soon be clear that Heath is the only member of the government who doesn't do it."

A lifelong bachelor, Ted Heath's sexual proclivities remained a matter for speculation. Heath was even criticized for being so quick to accept Lambton and Jellicoe's resignations.

"In the modern so-called permissive age," the *Daily Express* commented, "a splendid member of parliament and a junior minister have been cast into the wilderness ... can we really afford to discard men of talent, wit and patriotism because their personal lives fall short of blameless perfection?"

There were also rumours that other government ministers were involved with prostitutes. So Edward Heath had to issue a statement saying that all his other ministers were as pure as the driven snow and the Security Commission, under Lord Diplock, was asked to investigate.

Its report concluded that Jellicoe's affairs had been "conducted with discretion. There was no abnormal sexual behaviour, no criminal offence nor any risk of compromising photographs."

"Ordinary sexual intercourse" with a prostitute, the Commission found, did not pose a threat to national security. However, Lambton had "deviated from the normal" by having two girls at a time. This left him open to blackmail, though it was conceded that Lambton was not the sort of man to betray his country in those circumstances.

Lord Lambton withdrew from public life and went to live in Sienna, Italy, where he wrote a number of novels. Lord Jellicoe moved from the corridors of power into the boardroom, taking directorships in a number of large public companies.

## William Ewart Gladstone

One of the greatest parliamentarians of the nineteenth century, William Ewart Gladstone was a loving husband and father of eight. But his addiction to prostitutes almost brought him down. In the nineteenth century, they were plentiful – there were an estimated 80,000 prostitutes in 1850 in London alone. And he took pity on them. When Gladstone was prime minister, he would even bring young prostitutes that he had picked up on the streets back to Number Ten Downing Street, even though other members of the Cabinet begged him not to.

Apologists point out that Gladstone was a fierce moralist and a lay preacher, and contended that all he did with his "erring sisters" was read them an uplifting passage from the Bible. Indeed, he did manage to guide some of the young women he brought home into honest employment. However, Gladstone admitted in his own diaries that his motives were partly, at least, "carnal".

He began visiting prostitutes when he was a young man at Oxford in the 1820s. Tormented by guilt, he would scourge himself afterwards. But this did not seem to stem his appetite as he writes of returning to sin "again and again".

He married in 1839. It did not help. In 1843, when he joined Robert Peel's government as President of the Board of Trade, he wrote in his diary that he was "fearful [of] the guilt of sin returning again and again in forms ever new but alike hideous". Conscious of his position, he avoided prostitutes. Instead, like many another Victorian gentleman, he indulged himself in pornography. But, by 1851, his diary shows that he was visiting a prostitute named Elizabeth Collins regularly – sometimes every other day. Afterwards, he notes, he always scourged himself. This continued when he became Chancellor of the Exchequer in 1852.

And there were others. A man named William Wilson saw Gladstone picking up a prostitute near Leicester Square and tried to blackmail him. Gladstone handed over the blackmail demand to the police and Wilson went down for twelve months' hard labour.

There had been another brush with scandal with a courtesan named Laura Thistlethwayte. They exchanged passionate letters and he visited her regularly, both in her London town house and in her cottage in Hampstead. But Gladstone grew wary when she began showering him with gifts to the point that he feared her extravagance would ruin her husband, Colonel Thistlethwayte.

As prime minister, Gladstone had a close friendship with the Prince of Wales's mistress, the actress Lillie Langtry. And in the 1870s there were rumours that he was having an affair with Madame Olga Novikov, who advised him on Russian affairs.

However, he could not give up prostitutes. In 1880, when he was seventy, he was still visiting brothels to do what he called "rescue work". The situation became more ticklish in 1882, when the threat of assassination over the Home Rule Bill meant that he had to have a twenty-four-hour police guard. Lord Rosebery, then a junior minister in the Home Office, warned him of the danger of some lowly paid policeman taking advantage of the situation and selling the story to the press. It did no good. Three months later the Tory MP Colonel Tottenham saw Gladstone talking to a lady of the night and decided to make some political hay with it in the House of Commons. Gladstone answered Colonel Tottenham's allegations with studied dignity.

"It may be true that the gentleman saw me in such conversation," he said. "But the object was not what he assumed or, as I am afraid, hoped."

He survived, and even this close call did not stop him. In July 1886, his private secretary Edward Hamilton warned him that another blackmailer was at work. Gladstone promised Hamilton that he would stop, but his diaries record that he was still seeing prostitutes in 1892, though they may have accosted him rather than the other way around.

In 1896, two years before his death, Gladstone sought to set the record straight. He wrote a statement and sent it to his son Stephen, who had become a clergyman. In it, Gladstone said that he had "not been guilty of the act which is known as that of infidelity to the marriage bed".

But as we shall learn from the case of Bill Clinton that leaves an awful lot of room for misbehaviour. When one young prostitute came home with him for a second time, he wrote that he had "certainly been wrong in some things and trod the path of danger".

Maybe he just liked to watch. Some of the girls called him "Glad-eyes". Others called him "Daddy-do-nothing" – but he was eighty-two when he gave up visiting whores. His reputation, though, was far more formidable.

"Gladstone founded the great tradition," ran one obituary, "in public to speak the language of the highest and strictest principle, and in private to pursue and possess every sort of woman."

Gladstone's great political rival Benjamin Disraeli could not help teasing him over his predilictions. He is reputed to have said to Gladstone: "When you are out saving fallen women, save one for me."

## Benjamin Disraeli

Disraeli also weathered his share of scandal. After a tour of the Middle East in the 1870s, he returned a changed man. Always a dandy, he was now positively effeminate, dressing in green velvet trousers and ruffles. He spoke openly at dinner parties of his passion for the East and, according to the painter Benjamin Haydon, "seemed tinged with a disposition to palliate its infamous vices . . . sodomy". Disraeli's biographer Jane Ridley concurred. "Bisexuality came as naturally to Disraeli as did Tory Radicalism," she said.

He then had a series of affairs with older women, some of whom were married. His affair with Henrietta Sykes became a public scandal. She was much older than him and had been married for eleven years to the ailing Sir Francis Sykes, who was the father of her four children. Her letters to Disraeli were signed "your mother".

Despite the gossip they were seen out together at parties and the opera. Her husband turned a blind eye because he was having an affair with Clara Bolton, another of Disraeli's former lovers, at the time. Clara was jealous and encouraged Sir Francis to break up the affair. He did so. But soon after, he found his wife in bed with Disraeli's successor. In a fit of pique, he kicked her out of the house and placed a notice in the newspapers advertising her adultery and causing a scandal that tainted Disraeli, along with everyone else involved.

How much the scandal harmed him is hard to say as he seemed completely unelectable anyway. Voters did not appreciate his dandified dress and his Jewishness counted against him. On the hustings he was greeted with cries of "Shylock" and he was pelted with rotten chunks of pork and ham.

He was elected for Maidstone on his fifth attempt by bribing the electorate. Which is not to say he paid up. When Maidstone lawyer Charles Austin protested, he responded with scandalous allegations. Austin sued. Disraeli went to court where he apologized effusively. His court costs were paid by the latest woman in his life, Mary Anne Wyndham Lewis, the widow of his late rival for the Maidstone seat. It was a masterstroke. This fresh scandal eclipsed the bribery allegations. Disraeli then married Mrs Wyndham Lewis. Though she was twelve years older than him, she was rich.

As Disraeli climbed the greasy pole in the Conservative Party, his electoral ambitions were thwarted by another sex scandal. In 1864, the seventy-nine-year-old Liberal leader Lord Palmerston was cited in the divorce case of the attractive thirty-year-old Mrs O'Kane. Disraeli said that it was a pity that this had got out because Palmerston would sweep the country. With the unofficial party slogan "she was Kane and he was able", the Liberals won by a landslide the following year.

Disraeli had difficulty competing with this. When he became leader of the Conservative Party, he only managed to hold on to the position of prime minister for a matter of months. But after his wife died in 1872, he began a romantic liaison with two sisters, Lady Bradford and Lady Chesterfield, which he maintained until his death in 1881. Under this new arrangement, the electorate warmed to him. He won the election in 1874 and stayed in office for the next six years.

## Sir Charles Wentworth Dilke

While the careers of Gladstone, Disraeli and Palmerston seemed to thrive on sex scandals, the new rising star of the Liberal Party Sir Charles Wentworth Dilke, whom many saw as a future prime minister, was destroyed by it – even though the allegations against him were never proved.

In July 1885, he was the youngest Cabinet minister and privy councillor, and tipped as Gladstone's heir apparent. Then he was named in the divorce case of twenty-two-year-old Virginia Crawford, sister of his brother's widow.

Virginia was quite a gal. The daughter of a Tyneside shipowner, she had been forced to marry Donald Crawford, a Liberal MP, who was twice her age. But that did not inhibit her. For years, she and her sister Helen entertained themselves with medical students from a nearby hospital. They also visited a brothel in Knightsbridge where they both entertained one Captain Henry Forster.

Dilke and Virginia may well have been lovers. He visited her while her husband was away. But he was certainly the lover of her mother, Mrs Eustace Smith. Things were seldom as strait-laced in the Victorian age as one imagines. But when Virginia's husband filed for divorce, Dilke feared that his political career was over.

"In the case of a public man, a charge is always believed by many, even though disproved, and I should be weighted by it throughout life," he wrote.

However, he was determined to fight. He was engaged to be married at the time to Mrs Emilia Patterson, the widow of the rector of Lincoln College, whom he had been wooing for ten years. This was scandalous enough as, for most of that time, her husband had been alive.

Virginia's husband Donald Crawford knew nothing of his wife's affair with Captain Forster or her other dalliances. But he had received a series of anonymous letters telling him to "beware of the member from Chelsea" – Dilke.

Dilke and his fiancée Emilia had also been receiving anonymous letters which sought to disrupt their marriage plans. A staunch republican, Dilke had spoken out against the royal family and suspected his harassment was an establishment plot, though there were other suspects.

"In my belief the conspiracy comes from a woman who wanted me to marry her," Dilke wrote to his fiancée. The suspected conspirator was a Mrs Rogerson, a friend of Virginia Crawford's who may well have been another of Dilke's lovers.

When Crawford received a fourth letter naming Forster as his wife's lover, he confronted her. She denied that Forster was her lover but, seemingly eager for divorce, admitted to adultery with Dilke. She also alleged that Dilke had also had a string of other lovers, including her mother – which was true – and one of his maids called Sarah Gray. Dilke was plainly a busy man, and not just in Whitehall.

Even though Dilke was being cited in a divorce case, Emilia went ahead and married him in Oxford in October 1885. The following month, after writing to his constituents denying the charges of adultery, Dilke was re-elected as MP for Chelsea. However, as he had not yet cleared his name, Gladstone, a stickler for impropriety – in others, at least – dropped him from his government.

When the case opened in February 1886, Virginia Crawford was not present. However, Crawford said that he had wrung a confession from her. He told the court that his wife admitted going to an "assignation house" off Tottenham Court Road with Dilke. She had also visited him at his house in Sloane Street and entertained him in her own home when her husband had been away. But she was sketchy on the detail. What turned the trial from an ordinary divorce case into a huge Victorian scandal was one new and sensational allegation. Crawford said that Dilke had forced his wife into a threesome with a serving girl called Fanny Stock and had taught her "every French vice". Asked who Fanny was, his wife had said that she was Dilke's mistress. Virginia had also said that Dilke had compared Fanny to her mother.

All this was hearsay evidence. It was simply Crawford repeating what he alleged his wife had said. He had no evidence, such as a love letter or a note arranging an assignation in Dilke's hand. The only witness he could produce was his wife's parlour maid, Ann Jameson. She said that when Mr Crawford was out of town, Mrs Crawford stayed out at night. Dilke had also visited Mrs Crawford at her house. Under cross-examination though, it transpired that these were normal social visits. Captain Forster also visited, and Ann had handled correspondence between Mrs Crawford and Captain Forster. There was none with Dilke.

As the redoubtable Fanny had disappeared, the only witness the defence could call was Dilke himself. But he did not want to take the stand and have to answer questions concerning his relationship with Mrs Eustace Smith.

Explaining his client's reluctance to take the stand, Dilke's barrister, the Attorney General Sir Charles Russell said: "In the life of any man there may be found to have been possible indiscretions."

He moved to have Dilke's name stricken from the petition. The judge agreed to do so. He granted a decree nisi, finding that, while Mrs Crawford had committed adultery, there was no admissible evidence to indicate that she had done it with Dilke. And he ordered that Dilke's costs be paid for by Mr Crawford as he had accused Dilke of adultery without reasonable grounds for suspicion.

Legally, Dilke was not guilty of adultery. But Russell's decision not to put his client on the stand was a fatal error of judgement. Although Dilke had repeatedly denied sleeping with Mrs Crawford, verbally and in writing, that was not the same as saying it in the witness box while under oath.

The press seized Russell's remark that "In the life of any man there may be found to have been possible indiscretions", but

omitted the word "possible". In Victorian England, this was
tantamount to admitting that Dilke had committed adultery
with someone if not the errant wife in the Crawford case. And
the case stayed in the news because Mrs Crawford had been
guilty of adultery with someone and the papers wanted to
know who.

The *Manchester Guardian* condemned Dilke's behaviour at
the trial and said: "To ask us on the strength of this evasion to
welcome him back as a leader of the Liberal Party is too strong
a draft on our credulity and good nature."

A Liberal Association in Scotland passed a resolution
condemning any move to have Dilke back in a Liberal Cabinet,
saying it would condone things that were "unrighteous and
wrong". But it was the campaigning editor of the *Pall Mall
Gazette* and fiery moralist W. T. Stead who pulled out all the
stops. He wrote: "Grave imputations were stated publicly in
open court, but there was no detailed reply. Far from having
been disproved, they have not even been denied in the witness
box."

He was backed in his moral outrage by General Booth,
founder of the Salvation Army, who condemned the Dilke
scandal as "a shameful combination of lust, fraud and
falsehood". With Booth's blessing, Stead called for the member
for Chelsea's resignation.

"We are willing to believe that the more terrible part of
the charge brought against him is exaggerated," Stead wrote,
charitably. "But if that charge in its entirety were true, we
should not exaggerate the universal sentiment that the man
against whom so frightful an accusation could lie is a worse
criminal than most of the murderers who swing in Newgate."

Dilke considered a libel suit, but was afraid that a courtroom
would simply give Stead another soapbox. Stead was a man
who enjoyed martyrdom. He had recently been to jail for three
months for buying a thirteen-year-old girl for £5 from her
parents to expose child prostitution.

In an effort to clear his name, Dilke went to the Queen's Proctor who had the power to annul a decree nisi before the decree absolute was granted. Dilke persuaded him to intervene on the basis that the divorce had granted on the grounds of adultery, over an act which the judge had admitted in court had not taken place.

The Proctor ordered a second hearing. Dilke was optimistic. Fanny Stock had been found and she was willing to deny the three-in-bed romp. He also had powerful new evidence about Mrs Crawford's affair with Captain Forster, which she still sought to deny.

But Dilke and his lawyers had made another mistake. As the judge in the original case had stricken Dilke's name from the petition, he was no longer party to the action. His lawyers could not cross-examine Mrs Crawford, nor could they call any witnesses.

In the general election of 9 July 1886, Dilke lost his seat. Seven days later, the trial started. Dilke then found himself at another unforeseen disadvantage. As Dilke was trying to overturn a decree nisi granted on the grounds of adultery, the prosecutor had to try to prove that there had been no adultery while Mrs Crawford, who now wanted a divorce, made the case that there had.

Dilke was the first witness to be called to the stand. In front of a packed courtroom, he denied sleeping with Mrs Crawford. He also denied sleeping with Fanny Stock and Sarah Gray. But when he was asked whether he had slept with Virginia Crawford's mother Mrs Eustace Smith, he refused to answer. The judge ordered him to. Eventually, he had to admit to the affair.

Then Mrs Crawford was called to the stand. This time she had her story together. The assignation house where she had gone with Dilke was in Warren Street, off Tottenham Court Road, she said. She even sketched a plan of the bedroom there. She also remembered the dates and places of other assignations. And she stuck to her story that she had had a threesome at Dilke's Sloane Street home with Fanny Stock.

This time, she also admitted adultery with Captain Forster, but denied that she had invented the story about having slept with Dilke to protect him. Forster was called and confirmed that they had had an affair, but denied that they hoped to marry. He was engaged to a Miss Smith Barry at the time. Mrs Crawford called three other witnesses who said that they had seen Dilke go into the assignation house at 65 Warren Street on other occasions with other women. Dilke had no opportunity to refute these fresh allegations and no lawyer to probe them during cross-examination. His reputation was now irreparably damaged.

The trial lasted a week. It reached its climax in a summing-up from Mrs Crawford's barrister, Henry Matthews QC. By Mrs Crawford's confession, he said, Dilke "was charged not merely with adultery, but with having committed adultery with the child of one friend and the wife of another . . . he was charged with having done with an English lady what any man of proper feeling would shrink from doing with a prostitute in a French brothel, and yet he was silent".

At this point Russell leapt to his feet to object, but the judge ordered him to sit down. Dilke was not a party to the case and had no right to legal representation.

"The burden of proof was on the Queen's Proctor who, in order to be successful, must show conclusively that Mrs Crawford had not committed adultery with Sir Charles Dilke," Matthews continued. "The jury could only give a verdict against my client if they believed that Mrs Crawford was a perjured witness and that a conspiracy existed to blast the life of a pure and innocent man."

By this time, Dilke's character had been so irredeemably blackened that no one believed him to be a "pure and innocent man".

The prosecution was left with an impossible task. How could it prove that Dilke had not committed adultery with Mrs

Crawford? Mrs Crawford had already admitted adultery with Captain Forster, who had admitted it too. So Mr Crawford could have his divorce. What did it matter if Mrs Crawford had committed adultery with two people, or only one?

For that matter, Dilke had admitted adultery with Mrs Eustace Smith, why not with Mrs Crawford? What did it matter, if he had had extramarital sex with two people, or only one?

The judge hammered the last nail into Dilke's political coffin. He drew the jury's attention to Dilke's reluctance to take the stand in the first trial and asked: "If you were to hear such a statement made involving your honour . . . would you accept the advice of your counsel to say nothing? Would you allow the court to be deceived and a tissue of falsehoods to be put forward as the truth?"

Upstanding Victorian gentlemen to a man, the jury took just fifteen minutes to answer no. They found that the decree nisi was not pronounced contrary to the justice of the case. Dilke had failed to get it overturned. Although no real evidence had ever been put that he had committed adultery, it was generally assumed that he had and was deemed to be lying.

Dilke did manage to get himself re-elected to parliament for the Forest of Dean in 1892. He remained in parliament until his death 1911, but never again held office. Virginia Crawford began a political career of her own. She became a writer and a Labour councillor, and was such a vociferous campaigner against Fascism she was blacklisted by Mussolini. She died in 1948.

## The Duke of Wellington

Britain's greatest general, the Duke of Wellington, spent most of his married life away from his wife, notably fighting Napoleon Bonaparte. After Boney was sent to Elba in 1814, Wellington went to Paris where he sought out two of Napoleon's mistresses, whom he bedded. One of them was Josephina Grassini, an opera singer Napoleon had first set eyes on in Milan in 1797, when he was doing his damnedest to be faithful to his first wife Joséphine. Three years later, he succumbed. She mocked him for his earlier indifference, saying:

> I was in the full glory of my beauty and talents. I was the only topic of conversation; I blinded all eyes and inflamed every heart. Only the young general remained cold, and all my thoughts were occupied by him alone. How strange it seems! When I was still worth something, when the whole of Italy was at my feet, when I heroically spurned all homage for a single glance from your eyes, I could not obtain it. And now, now you let your gaze rest upon me, today, when it is not worthwhile, when I am no more worthy of you.

He thought different and took her as his mistress. Later that day, he gave a lecture to two hundred Catholic priests on the need for morality. It was not a discreet affair and she became known as "*La Chanteuse de l'Empereur*". She followed him to Paris, where she sang an ode to the "liberation" of Italy at Les Invalides on Bastille Day 1800. This was the French equivalent of Marilyn Monroe singing "Happy Birthday" to President Kennedy. She also topped the bill at the celebration of Napoleon's famous victory at the Battle of Marengo. However, Napoleon refused to acknowledge her as his official mistress, so she took a lover, a twenty-two-year-old violinist from Bordeaux called Rode. Napoleon was magnanimous towards his love rival. But Joséphine grew jealous when he continued seeing his "Giuseppina" even when she herself was crowned Empress. Grassini is thought to have cost the French taxpayer seventy thousand francs a year between 1807 and 1814.

When Wellington caught up with Grassini later that year, she was forty-one. While she was no longer the tasty twenty-seven-year-old Napoleon had espied in Milan, she was still, by all accounts, tremendously sexy. She called him *cher Villianton* and he did not take three years to get her into bed. Nor was she a great burden to the British taxpayer. The Treasury was only presented with modest bills for millinery and dressmaking. Meanwhile, Wellington was free to flaunt the spoils of war around Paris, as the composer Felice Blangini recalled:

When Madame Grassini attended informal gatherings at Lord Wellington's she declaimed and sang scenes from *Cleopatra* and *Romeo and Juliet*. Alone in the centre of the salon, she gestured as if she was on stage and using a big shawl she dressed up in different ways. I cannot remember if, during these sessions, she sang arias which end with a *sguardo d'amor* [an amorous glance]; but what I am certain of is that Lord Wellington was enchanted, in ecstasy.

The affair banished any thought Grassini had of joining Napoleon on Elba. After Waterloo, Wellington was even more attentive, according to the Comtesse de Boigne. On one occasion, he:

. . . conceived the idea of making Grassini, who was then at the height of her beauty, the queen of the evening. He seated her upon a sofa mounted on a platform in the ballroom, and never left her side; caused her to be served before anyone else, made people stand away in order that she might see the dancing, and took her into supper himself in front of the whole company; there he sat by her side, and showed her attentions usually granted only to princesses. Fortunately, there were some high-born English ladies to share the burden of this insult, but they did not feel the weight of it as we did, and their resentment could not be compared with ours.

But *La Chanteuse* was left with one great regret. Until her death in 1823, she would look back on her time with Napoleon and say ruefully: "Why would he not listen to me and patch things up with *ce cher Villianton*?"

According to the historian Andrew Roberts: "To sleep with one of Napoleon's mistresses might be considered an accident, but to sleep with two might suggest a pattern of triumphalism ..." The second of Napoleon's mistresses Wellington seduced was the actress Marguerite Joséphine Weimer. She was just fifteen when the thirty-three-year-old Napoleon, then First Consul, bedded her. On stage, she used the name Mademoiselle George. He called her Georgina. His technique was direct. He once pushed forty thousand francs down her cleavage, hopefully in notes.

Again poor Joséphine had to lump it, but as Napoleon explained: "Exclusivity is not in my nature." She faced a particularly public humiliation when he took her to see Mademoiselle George in the play *Cinna* at the Théâtre Français. In the play, La Weimer delivered the line, "If I have seduced Cinna, I shall seduce many more," and the audience rose to applaud the First Consul, though he was sitting in a box alongside his wife.

The affair ended after two years in 1804. As Marguerite put it: "He left me to become Emperor."

From 1808 until 1812, La Weimer was in Russia, and it would be nice to think that Napoleon invaded just to see her. Her presence was not lost on Tolstoy. An anecdote about her appears in the opening scene of *War and Peace*. When Napoleon abdicated in 1814, she fell from grace. Vilified in the press as "the Corsican widow", she was hissed at onstage. But the Duke soon rehabilitated her. She was twenty-seven when they began their affair. This time the Duke was more discreet, perhaps because Grassini was still on the scene. However, she has done history the favour of comparing the performance of the two rivals.

"*Monsieur le Duc était beaucoup le plus fort,*" she said – "The Duke was much the more virile."

This will come as a welcome relief to British readers who have long lived with the bitchy comment from another of Wellington's mistresses who said that one of Britain's greatest national heroes was "a cold fish". While to the French, La Weimer's comments will mean little, as Bonaparte had many more mistresses to keep his bed warm. Besides her fortunes went rapidly into decline. In 1855, she applied for the position of manager of the Lost Umbrella Office at the Paris Exposition. She did not get the job.

Wellington also had a thing about Napoleon's sister, the famously sexy Pauline, who made a show of being carried naked every day to her bath of milk by her black servant Paul. Wellington bought her house and kept her picture on his bedroom wall, next to that of Grassini. Between them was a portrait of Pope Pius VII – like "our Lord between the two thieves," remarked the Comte d'Artois. Unfortunately, the promiscuous Pauline was not around at the time. She was in Italy posing nude for the Italian sculptor Antonio Canova. Asked how she could pose naked, she replied: "Why not? It was not cold, there was a fire in the studio."

Wellington did not manage to get his hands on the statue, which ended up in the Villa Borghese. But he did manage to buy Canova's nude statue of Napoleon, as a youthful First Consul, which was installed in his London home, Apsley House. It cost 66,000 francs.

When Wellington went on to become prime minister he again courted scandal. The courtesan Harriette Wilson, whose other lovers included the Prince Regent, two other prime ministers and most of the dandies of Mayfair, planned to publish her memoirs. She wrote to everyone mentioned, asking for £200 to have their names blanked out. Wellington replied famously: "Publish and be damned."

## Winston Churchill

He was not always the potbellied, round-shouldered old man we remember. When he was young Churchill was a noted ladies' man. He was in the Indian Army at a time when they still had regimental brothels and he proposed to the actress Ethel Barrymore while she was having a lesbian affair with Tallulah Bankhead. He complained of being short of money because he spent too much on silk underwear. His cousin, a noted sculptress, Clare Sheridan, was one of Mussolini's many lovers. Then there was Churchill's gay affair.

You will find this tale told in any biography of the writer William Somerset Maugham. After Churchill fell from power, he went to visit Maugham in the South of France. Over lunch, Maugham, who was gay, was teasing Winston.

"Your mother," Maugham said, "told me that, when you were young, you went with other boys."

"It's a damned lie," said Churchill. "I only went with a man once, just to see what it was like."

The man, it transpired, was the singer-songwriter and matinee idol Ivor Novello.

"So how was it?" asked Maugham.

Churchill pulled the cigar from his mouth and said: "Musical."

## Alan Clark

Military historian and Tory politician Alan Clark revelled in sex scandals. He first found fame in 1961 with his book *The Donkeys*, which inspired the musical and movie *Oh, What a Lovely War!* He became an MP and rose to serve as a junior minister in Mrs Thatcher's government. But then, towards the end of his life, he published three volumes of his diaries which detailed his sexual exploits.

He certainly had a colourful sex life. When he first spotted his future wife, Jane, then fourteen, he noted in his diaries: "She is the perfect victim."

He was twenty-eight at the time. They married when she was sixteen. By the time she was seventeen, he was already planning to be unfaithful.

"How delicious to have a succulent little mistress," he wrote. "I must get one somehow this year."

From then on he pursued every woman he set eyes on. There was "darling, plump, pert, red-haired little Inge". He was so infatuated with a ballet dancer, at one point he followed her to Morocco. Then there was the twenty-two-year-old Labour candidate standing against him in Plymouth.

"I'm madly in love with Frances Holland," he wrote. "I suspect she's not as thin and gawky as she seems. Her hair is always lovely and shiny. Perhaps I can distract her at the count on Thursday and kiss her in one of those big janitors' cupboards off the Lower Guildhall."

He even fancied Mrs Thatcher – "Very attractive, I never came across any other woman in politics as sexually attractive in terms of eyes, wrists and ankles," he noted.

The most famous of Clark's conquests was Valerie Harkess, the wife of a South African judge, and her two daughters, Josephine and Alison, who were both virgins at the time. Clark less than chivalrously dubbed them "the coven". This revelation caused a scandal.

"I knew when the diaries were to be published in Cape Town there was no way I could keep this from my husband," said Mrs Harkess. "I knew it was time to tell him. He was heartbroken. I think the public and the rest of the government should see this man [Clark] for what he is: a depraved animal. Not content with having lured me into his lair, he ensnared my daughters, too."

The affair began after she met Clark at a ball at Grosvenor House in London. He rang her and asked her out for lunch, beginning their fourteen-year relationship. But he did not tell her how he had also seduced one daughter at his London apartment and slept with the other after she came to see him about a problem she was having.

She only discovered that the affairs were to be made public after buying a copy of the first volume of Clark's diaries while on a trip to England, intending to give the book to her husband as a present when she returned home. Then when she read it on the plane, she realized that their private lives were about to become very public. So she went to the *News of the World* herself.

"I expect no sympathy for my actions, nor for those of my daughters, but had it not been for these foul diaries, I might have taken the secret of my affair with Alan to my grave," she said.

She feared that her husband James might kill himself or leave her after she confessed to him.

"But he's a wonderful, tolerant and forgiving Christian man," she said. "Our marriage is intact. I know it will take years to build up trust again, but we intend to do it."

"There was no anger, I suppose a feeling of humiliation," said James Harkess. "If I'd known about it at the time I think I'd have horsewhipped Clark. The man is sick. But I was just relieved that at last I knew."

Clark agreed.

"I deserve to be horsewhipped," he said. "It all happened a very long time ago, and I am trying to keep a low profile. I probably have a different sense of morality to most people."

The Harkesses flew to London to cash in on the revelation and were thought to have made £150,000 from the story with the help of celebrity publicist Max Clifford. In an interview with Sky News, Josephine claimed that Clark had exposed himself to her and her sister when they were thirteen and fifteen.

"He showed his willy to us constantly," she said. "I was thirteen when I first saw Alan's private parts and my sister was eighteen months older. This was a pattern which went on throughout our teens. Alan, in a very gentle way – I won't elaborate on it – he would never force himself on us, he just sort of got a kick out of showing it to us. That was the thrill, to show it to us, a couple of young virgins, very young teenagers . . . This went on throughout our teens and developed into cupping our breasts, rubbing himself up against us."

Clark was the first man to show a sexual interest in her, she said. Clark denied the allegations.

"Of course I deny them, I have to deny them," he said. "It's virtually criminal. They are strong allegations and I think it's contemptible that they should follow Max Clifford's advice on that. I don't want to comment on that, I hate it. I'm not planning at this stage to take any legal action over these comments, I don't want to stoke this thing up. But presumably even Clifford's imagination is going to run out of ideas – he hasn't moved into electric flexes and rubber yet, has he?"

Clark also denied claims that he had set up a £100,000 offshore account for Mrs Harkess to hush up the affair. Josephine also accused Clark of seducing her when she was twenty-three, at a time when she was suffering from a severe drink and drugs problem that made her particularly vulnerable.

"I hope the girls got a good price for their story," said Clark.

However, Josephine's sister Alison, who was married to Sergei Kausov, a former KGB agent and ex-husband of Christina Onassis, wanted to stay out of the media circus.

Mrs Harkess admitted that her affair with Clark survived her daughters' confessions that they were also sleeping with her lover, whom she described as "a trusted family friend".

"I was very culpable in that," she said. "And I make no excuses for myself, except that I was in a vortex, a whirlpool. I simply could not swim strong enough for the shore."

She was, she said, "addicted" to Clark.

Clark's diaries even describe taking the three of them out together. On 13 June 1983, he recorded: "In London I collected the coven and off we went to Brook's for dinner. At intervals Joei said 'Gosh, Al, are you really a minister, zowee.' Valerie was less forthcoming. Ali sulked and sneered. Driving away we went past the Ritz and Joei said, 'Gosh is that the Ritz? I wish we could go in there.' 'Why?' 'To go to bed of course.' I was thoughtful; I have always been culpably weak in such matters."

Mrs Clark described her husband's many extramarital interests as tarts with short shelf lives and dismissed the Harkess women as "below stairs". However, she did admit: "He's a bit of a S H one T."

The Harkesses campaigned against Clark when he was seeking to be adopted as the Conservative candidate for the safe seat of Kensington and Chelsea. He won the candidacy and was returned to parliament in 1997. After he died in 1999, the BBC then took to the air with the diaries and the affair, making a TV series out of them.

However, in the diaries, Clark's last great love was identified only as "X". In 2009, his biographer revealed that she was his former private secretary Alison Adams. He was in his sixties; she in her twenties. At one point, his wife found the draft of a letter asking Alison to marry him. Jane threw an axe at him, locked him in a cupboard and walked out of Saltwood Castle, his estate in Kent. But after two days, she returned. Why should she leave, she reasoned; Saltwood was her home.

"I used to say to him: go and look it up in your dictionary – you are not in love, you are infatuated," she said. "But you see he was forever Peter Pan really, he never wanted to get old, and I think that's the whole trouble, isn't it? But that's the way men are. Men are so stupid, aren't they? You can see them coming a mile off!"

## David Mellor

In 1992, Prime Minister John Major appointed his friend and fellow Chelsea fan David Mellor Secretary of State at the new Department of Heritage, which was quickly dubbed the Ministry of Fun. It soon became known that the forty-three-year-old minister, who was married with two children, did not leave his portfolio in the office.

Part of Mellor's ministerial brief was to handle Sir David Calcutt's report on press intrusion into individual privacy. A Privacy Bill had already been mooted and Mellor had warned Fleet Street that it was drinking in the last chance saloon. But it soon appeared that Mellor was imbibing there himself.

The Minister of Fun was having his own private spot of fun with thirty-one-year-old actress Antonia de Sancha. This was extraordinary hubris as Mellor had been introduced to de Sancha three years earlier by *Private Eye* journalist Paul Halloran.

De Sancha was the only child of a Spanish father and a Swedish-born mother, who had both died shortly after they split up when she was in her mid-twenties. She made her living as a topless model and bit-part actress, whose starring role was in a soft-porn film called *The Pieman*. She played a one-legged prostitute who pays the pizza-delivery man in kind.

It took some time for the affair to develop, but by June 1992 they were lovers. Antonia wrote to her Swedish grandmother saying: "I am having a marvellous time at the moment. I have met a wonderful politician. I am very happy."

But she was already concerned about the possibility of exposure. Nosy neighbours, she feared, might spread gossip. Confiding her fears to a friend, she borrowed his flat in Finborough Road, west London, as a temporary love nest. The flat was bugged. Soon tapes of Mellor complaining that his nights of passion with the young actress were exhausting were being touted to the *News of the World*.

Early in July 1992, Mellor got a call from Sir Tim Bell, PR consultant and former government spin doctor. He informed Mellor of the story and the evidence that the *News of the World* had. Mellor denied that he was having an affair and expressed surprise that a newspaper could handle tapes that had been recorded in such an underhand fashion. This was just the sort of thing that his Privacy Bill would stamp out.

The moment that Bell was off the phone, Mellor phoned de Sancha and told her to keep her mouth shut.

Though they were not entirely convinced by Mellor's denials, the *News of the World* put publication on hold. The *People* had no such reservations. On Saturday, 18 July 1992, Mellor was tipped off that the *People* were going to run the story the next day. He phoned the prime minister and tendered his resignation.

John Major refused to accept it. He said he would stand by his friend and saw no conflict between his current plight and his handling of the Calcutt Report. But the press did. The very man who was threatening to shackle them had been caught with his pants down. What's more, because of Antonio de Sancha's career, they had plenty of juicy pictures to illustrate the story with.

Soon Antonia was besieged by the press. Mellor had to distance himself. He issued the obligatory statement saying: "My wife Judith and I have been experiencing difficulties in our marriage. We want to sort the situation out for the sake of each other and especially for our two young children." And there was the photocall with Mellor and his wife and children smiling outside their in-laws' house, before going in for a cosy family lunch. From a man demanding privacy, this reeked of hypocrisy.

By an unfortunate coincidence, the *Desert Island Discs* programme that Mellor had recorded earlier went out that weekend, keeping the story in the public eye. And Mellor's father-in-law, Professor Edward Hall, decided to attack his wife's errant husband in the media.

"If he'll cheat on our girl, he'll cheat on the country," he said.

In an effort to defend herself, Antonia de Sancha employed the publicist Max Clifford to handle the press for her. Soon the press was full of stories that Mellor liked to make love in a Chelsea strip and that he indulged toe-sucking as foreplay.

Clifford sold the serialization of de Sancha's story to the *Sun*. The paper even mocked up the tawdry scene for their readers, complete with the mattress on the floor where the couple had first made love, lurid red silk bedclothes and a bottle of cheap white wine.

Although Mellor had become a laughing stock, he may have survived the sex scandal. However, more serious allegations came to light. Mellor and his family had holidayed in the Marbella home of Mona Bauwens, the daughter of one of the founders of the Palestine Liberation Organization. While they had been there, Iraq had invaded Kuwait and the PLO backed Saddam Hussein. Mona Bauwens sued the *People* who carried the story for casting her as a "social outcast and leper".

Although the court case failed, it kept Mellor in the limelight. Valiantly, he fought on. He made endless rounds of TV studios and even took the time to attend the National Press Fund's annual reception.

"I was going through a quiet patch so it was good of you to invite me tonight," he told them.

But his sense of irony did not save him. He admitted that he had behaved foolishly and insisted what he had done was not a resigning matter.

"Who decides who is to be a member of the British cabinet, the prime minister or the editor of the *Daily Mail*?" he asked defiantly.

The answer was, of course, the editor of the *Daily Mail*. With the newspapers against him, Tory backbench support began to go soft. John Major then had no choice but to accept David Mellor's resignation, despite a letter of support in *The Times* signed by many senior figures in the arts whose work he championed in his ministerial post.

It was a case of FROM TOE-JOB TO NO JOB, as the *Sun*'s headline so succinctly put it.

There was no chance of him returning to office either. Two years later, the *News of the World* discovered that he had abandoned the wife who had stood by him and was having another affair, this time with Lady Penelope Cobham, a former adviser at the Department of Heritage. Mellor divorced his first wife and married Lady Cobham. He went on to build up a successful career in the media.

# 3

## Hollywood Hoopla

### Charlie Sheen

Movie actor Charlie Sheen has had a tumultuous career, both on screen and off. His scandalous sex life began early. He lost his virginity at fifteen, stealing his father's credit card to have sex with a hooker. When he was eighteen, he fathered a child by his girlfriend from high school, Paula Profit, whom he had since dumped.

His movie career was meteoric. At twenty-one he starred in Oliver Stone's *Platoon*. Then it crashed to Earth. "I went from making multimillion-dollar deals on movies and fucking Playmates to being unemployable and fucking a five-months-pregnant Mexican whore with caesarean scars, in a bar in Nogales," he told *Playboy* in 2001.

At twenty-five he took to the straight and narrow. He went to rehab and got engaged to actress and model Kelly Preston. But then he accidentally shot her. These things happen.

Charlie made the tabloids again when he got a taste for porn-film actresses. He dated Ginger Lynn Allen, a star in the adult industry who won numerous awards for her performance. She had a small part in *Young Guns II*. She did not say how big a part he had. Having been a long-time fan of her movie, he auditioned her himself on Valentine's Day 1990. The romantic couple celebrated in a strip bar, where Ginger bought Charlie a lap dance. It seems to have been the clincher.

According to Allen: "Three months later, he took his ring off and said, 'I've broken off my engagement with Kelly.'"

Nursing her wound, Kelly went searching for some stability in her life. She bedded George Clooney and married John Travolta. Meanwhile Charlie and Ginger spent a happy time in rehab together. They did not expect to be faithful to one another, but they did agree some standards.

"We'd always promised we'd be honest with each other," said Ginger.

But, as always, Charlie went too far.

"On his twenty-sixth birthday I got a call that the girls were over there – Heidi Fleiss's girls," said Ginger. "I loved the honesty but not the news. I put some of the things he'd given me in a pile and lit it."

Sure, he had not been monogamous, but the fact that he had spent $53,000 on prostitutes over fourteen months was an insult to a woman of her obvious and observable abilities. Sheen famously insisted that he never paid for sex, only paid to have the girls leave afterwards. When he was told how much he had spent, he wiped his brow and said, "Sheesh, it's starting to add up."

But he did not give up the porn stars. Next came Heather Hunter, known for her interracial and lesbian-themed movies. She and Ginger later appeared together in *Hustler*'s aspirational video *Can You Be a Pornstar?*

In 1995, he married model Donna Peele after they had filmed a cigarette commercial together in Japan. Hearing the news, the New York lap-dancing club Scores held a candlelit vigil and observed a minute's silence. They thought his roistering days were over. The marriage lasted six months. But you have to give the boy credit for trying. The following year, he announced that he had become a born-again Christian. It didn't help.

After Heidi Fleiss went to jail, Sheen called up-and-coming Hollywood madam Michelle Braun.

"I show up with three girls," Braun said. "I walk in, and he's in this amazing condo in Wilshire, laid out on the floor in silk pyjamas, embroidered C. MA SHEEN on the pocket, with some girl sitting on his face. There was, like, a buffet of drugs across the bar overlooking this amazing view of the city – every kind of drug you can imagine. I said, 'You like the girls I brought?' He gave me a cheque for twenty grand and said he wanted me to work for him exclusively, recruiting girls. What did he want? Two tits, a hole and a heartbeat. Charlie has an addiction for everything, especially women. He's the T-rex of consumption. I would send over five women at a time – porn stars, Playmates – at $10,000 each."

But it did not always turn out nicely. In 1997, porn star Brittany Ashland, a.k.a. Tanya Rivers, filed suit for assault. Sheen was given a year's suspended sentence, two years' probation and a £1,800 fine.

In 1998, he was hospitalized after a drug overdose. Looking back on the decade, he said, "I'd be drinking away, doing blow, popping pills, and telling myself I wasn't an addict because there wasn't a needle stuck in my arm." And he was not stinting in the sex department. In an interview with *Maxim* magazine in October 2000, Sheen estimated that he had slept with five thousand women.

Nevertheless he gave monogamy another go. In 2002, he married actress Denise Richards, who gave him two daughters. Four years later, she filed for divorce, alleging that her estranged husband was unstable, violent, addicted to gambling and prostitutes, and was surfing "disturbing" pornographic websites "which promoted very young girls, who looked underage to me with pigtails, braces, and no pubic hair performing oral sex with each other".

She also alleged that Sheen watched "gay pornography also involving very young men who also did not look like adults". But Charlie was not the sort of guy who liked to wait on the sidelines when it came to sex. Richards also said he discovered that Sheen "belonged to several sex search type sites" where he "looked for women to have sex with". His online profile, she said, included a photo of "his erect penis". Well, there's no harm in advertising.

Richards also claimed he threatened her and, as part of her submission, she attached the transcripts of six abusive phone calls he made when she was pregnant with their second daughter. In one of them, Sheen refers to Richards and her attorney as "two pregnant cunts . . . plotting against the rest of us". After an attempt at reconciliation, they divorced.

So Charlie was out on the town again. But, oh no, in 2008 he married actress and real-estate agent Brooke Mueller, who gave him twin sons. Two years later, the whole thing collapsed in a maelstrom of allegations. This time he admitted misdemeanour assault to escape more serious charges and it was back to rehab for Charlie. They divorced in May 2011.

Through the ups and downs of his private life, Sheen managed to resurrect his career. He made the jump to the small screen and became the highest-paid actor on TV with the hit comedy *Two and a Half Men*. The network stuck by him, even when he trashed a room after a reported cocaine and drink binge at the Plaza Hotel in New York with porn star Capri Anderson, who was paid a $3,500 "appearance fee". Denise Richards and their two children were also in the hotel. Richards, Anderson, Sheen, his assistant and possibly some other women had dinner together in a four-star restaurant. After two $5,900 bottles of 1959 Château Latour, washed down with vodka shots, Sheen and Anderson went to the restroom, where he allegedly snorted coke and demanded sex. She allegedly quoted what he felt was an exorbitant rate, reportedly $12,000. After that, the couple went to the Eloise Suite, where, Sheen would later claim, Anderson stole his $165,000 Patek Philippe wristwatch. She denied this, claiming she was the victim of a coke-fuelled rampage in which Sheen wrecked the room, threatened her life and called her a whore.

She fled, half-naked, into the bathroom and stayed there until the police arrived. Charlie denied everything. Anderson was similarly unforthcoming.

"First of all," she said. "I would never have sex in a bathroom, especially at such a nice establishment as Daniel, for any amount of money. I am a porn starlet, if you will, but I do have class."

Anderson sued Sheen for pain and suffering; he sued her for extortion, calling her "an opportunistic pornographic film star and publicity-hungry scam artist", and alleging that she had demanded at least $1m in exchange for not speaking to the authorities in the Mueller case. But the continuing scandal only fuelled the skyrocketing ratings of *Two and a Half Men*.

On 8 January 2011 he was at the annual porn expo in Las Vegas, where he reportedly spent $26,000 on three women from the CityVibe escort service. "Ginger. U are fabulous!" he emailed one escort at 8.37 a.m. on 10 January. "I'm an A-list actor that you mite like to meet." This was another Ginger, apparently a "fetching twenty-one-year-old". That weekend he also hooked up with porn star Rachel Oberlin, a.k.a. Bree Olson, winner of Best Anal Sex Scene 2008 and Best All-Girl Three-Way Sex Scene 2010.

Two weeks later, nineteen-year-old porn actress Kacey Jordan from Oregon, got a call offering her $5,000 to go to a party. This was five times Jordan's daily rate for a porn film. She said she slung on her "sluttiest" outfit and called a taxi.

When she arrived at the entrance to Sheen's Mediterranean-style villa, the gates opened and she was led in to the presence of Charlie himself. He was slumped in a chair, seemingly passed out, with wine stains on his white shirt. When he came to, he exclaimed: "Oh, my God, Kacey. I can't believe it's you!" And the thirty-hour sex binge started up again.

Also on hand were four other porn stars. Jordan dismissed them as "nobodies", newcomers to the industry who could not match her veteran status. She said she not only had sex with Sheen but got a cheque for $30,000 out of him.

After Jordan left, Charlie suffered excruciating abdominal pain and was rushed to hospital. The diagnosis was benign, given the excesses of the past few days. He had suffered a hiatus hernia, the press were told. Nothing leaked out about the drugs or porn stars, and there might have been no sex scandal at all if it had not been for hyper-aggressive agent, K-Bizzle, best known for peddling a sex tape of Paris Hilton.

"They call me the Whore Whisperer, because I'm really good at talking to these girls," said Bizzle. "I really care about these chicks. Most people consider them throwaway sperm receptacles, but these girls have a place in the world." After all, he makes money out of them.

Bizzle said he got wind of Jordan from "underbelly sources". She had barely unlocked the door of the house she shared with a friend in the environs of Los Angeles, which she called "the sticks, Bumfuck, Egypt", when her cell phone rang. It was the Bizzle.

"I know you were at Charlie's house last night," he said. "It's only a matter of time before the press knows who you are."

This was her big chance for fame.

"You have a story to tell, and I really believe we can save Charlie's life." He laid it on with a trowel. She had two choices, he said. She could run away and hide. Or she could sell her story to the media and persuade Charlie to get help.

"Look, you're a whore," he said, diplomatically. "I'm a whore. Take the money."

That night, he took her to dinner in a Hollywood restaurant where they met up with a reporter from TMZ, the celebrity news website, and recorded an interview.

"When I first saw him, he was just fucking wasted out of his mind, which I was trying to get to that point, too," she said to camera. "Trust me! I said: 'I can beat you! I'll beat you in drinking.' And he was like, 'Bullshit!' And I just gave myself like an all-vodka drink." She pantomimed pouring a drink as Sheen was snatching it from her hand. "I love the guy, right? Grabs it and he chugs it in, like, three seconds."

Then she described how Sheen received a large delivery of cocaine and smoked one pipe of it after another. He invited her to his home movie theatre to watch porn.

"This is the whole plan," said Jordan. "He had apparently gotten another girl a Bentley, and he was like, 'Well, what do you want?' He said, 'I'm gonna retire. I just want to go fucking crazy in this house, like a $20-million house, like twenty-seven rooms, and you're like the missing puzzle piece. We don't have a blonde. You're my blonde. Are you in?'"

Charlie already had a plan to create "a porn family" in a nearby mansion and stock it with "goddesses" on constant standby.

"I said, 'Of course I'm gonna be in! I want a blue Bentley!' Because the others got one."

So then they had sex.

"It was OK," Jordan said. "It didn't last very long."

By her count, Mr *Two and a Half Men* clocked in at just over two-and-a-half minutes. Afterwards, he made some "excuses" for his abbreviated performance.

"After sex we just sat in bed and he held on to me," she said. "He was sloppy but still functioning . . . wouldn't stop kissing my feet. He promised me he'd get me a Bentley."

Jordan claimed Sheen was so much the worse for wear that she felt bad leaving, but then she had to deposit the $30,000 cheque.

"He's the nicest guy, kind, sweet," she said. "But for my safety, if I didn't leave, I'll be on a stretcher in the hospital. I sent him a text asking for the other $25,000."

But she was not without a conscience. "I feel really bad," she confessed to camera. "I hope he's well."

The video went up on TMZ on 27 January. Then she told her story on *Good Morning America*, *Inside Edition*, *The Howard Stern Show*, E! Online and other outlets. By the time it was over, she had earned anther $70,000. All in all, it was a lucrative night's . . . work?

The morning after the TMZ interview appeared, executives from CBS and Warner Bros. arrived at Sheen's home. They found him sitting beside the pool. He was a little shaken from the hospital visit, but seemingly contrite. He gave a sheepish smile, showing off his real teeth – some gold, some broken – without the caps he wears in public. They told him they were shutting down the show until he got some help.

Two weeks later, Charlie said he was ready to go to work again. Production was due to resume on 28 February. However, on 14 February, the last episode they had in the can aired. At the end, the veteran writer Chuck Lorre, who created the show, posted one of his vanity cards – short, pithy statements that run with the credits. It ended: "I don't drink. I don't smoke. I don't do drugs. I don't have crazy, reckless sex with strangers. If Charlie Sheen outlives me, I'm gonna be really pissed."

Charlie took offence at this and did a ranting tour of the radio stations. Then he took off to the Bahamas on a private jet with Brooke Mueller, porn star Rachel Oberlin and graphic designer Natalie Kenly. Mueller returned early, citing threatening behaviour, and sought a restraining order. Charlie returned to file a $100-million lawsuit against Warner Bros. and Chuck Lorre.

He racked up a following of 3.6 million on Twitter and went on a planned twenty-city concert tour, which he called, "My Violent Torpedo of Truth/Defeat is Not an Option". It opened in Detroit with Oberlin and Kenly on stage kissing passionately. It was all downhill from there.

By then, forty-five-year-old Sheen was sharing his Beverly Hills home with Oberlin and Kenly, both twenty-four. These were his "goddesses," he said, dismissing Hugh Hefner as "an amateur".

"You've read about the goddesses," Sheen told ABC's *20/20*.

"They're an international sensation. These are my girlfriends. These are the women that I love that have completed the three parts of my heart."

Speaking of their ménage à trois, Kenly said, "It seems crazy to everybody else, but for us it works."

Oberlin explained: "Natty and Charlie have their own special connection, I have my own connection with Charlie and then Natty and I also have our own relationship."

Kenly said she "fell in love with his brain" and can't see her life without him, while Oberlin said she would love to marry the star. But Sheen has no plans to marry again, thank God.

"I tried marriage," he said. "I'm 0 for 3 with the marriage thing. So, being a ballplayer – I believe in numbers. I'm not going 0 for 4. I'm not wearing a golden sombrero." Then he reconsidered. "Maybe the three of us will get married. I don't know. I'm gonna say this. It's a polygamy story. All my guy friends are gonna like throw tomatoes at me. It's like an organic union of the hearts."

When asked why he liked porn stars, an unapologetic Charlie Sheen said: "You already know what you're getting before you meet them. They're the best at what they do and I'm the best at what I do. Sorry, Middle America."

And prostitutes?

"Who wants to deal with all the small talk and nonsense? And you're paying for something that eliminates that. And I don't know. It makes sense to me."

Sheen, Oberlin and Kenly, who call themselves "the wedge", said that his partying days were over. Shame. But there was other trouble on the horizon. Sheen's lawsuit against Warner Bros. and Lorre was denied a court trial by a California judge who ruled that the suit had to be settled in arbitration.

By summer, Charlie's goddesses had fled. But every cloud has a silver lining. Oberlin posed for *Playboy*, appearing on the cover beside the line: "Goddess Bree Olson Reveals All the Secret Sex Life of Charlie Sheen".

Sheen's role in *Two and A Half Men* was taken over by Demi Moore's husband Ashton Kutcher who was immediately plunged into a sex scandal of his own when an administrative assistant from Texas named Sara Leal claimed that she had spent the night with Kutcher in a hotel suite in San Diego. Heartbreak all around.

## Fatty Arbuckle

Hollywood's first sex scandal involved Roscoe "Fatty" Arbuckle. He had been a plumber's mate until he was discovered by the legendary Mack Sennett in 1913 when he came round to unblock the comedy producer's drains. Sennett usually searched for new talent on his casting couch. Aside from the Keystone Kops, he was famous for the Mack Sennett Bathing Beauties. Many of the legendary actresses of the era – Gloria Swanson, Mabel Normand, Norma and Constance Talmadge, Ruth Rich, Alma Rubens, Juanita Hansen and Barbara Lamarr – started their movie careers in swimsuits as Sennett Bathing Beauties, or rather out of them in Sennett's office.

Weighing 266 pounds, Arbuckle was as round as a butterball, but he was surprisingly agile when it came to throwing and dodging custard pies. Oh, those innocent days. By 1917, he was so popular with movie-goers that his salary had soared to $5,000 a week. To celebrate his pay rise, the studio laid on a party at Brownie Kennedy's Roadhouse in Boston. They knew Arbuckle's tastes and laid on twelve "party girls". A waiter peeked through a crack in the door and saw the girls on the table stripping.

As he had not been invited to join the fun, the waiter called the cops. Public decency had, apparently, been outraged. The studio ended up paying $100,000 in bribes to hush the whole thing up.

Four years later, on Labour Day Weekend 1921, Arbuckle was celebrating his new $1-million contract with Paramount with a party in San Francisco. Among the carloads of movie people who made the 450-mile dash up the coastal highway was raven-haired twenty-six-year-old Virginia Rappe, an ambitious young starlet who was living with actor-director Henry Lehrman. She had already made ten movies, starting with *The Foolish Virgin*, moving through *Paradise Garden*, *Fantasy* and *Wet and Warm*, to *The Adventuress* and *A Game Lady*. Her other claim to fame was that she had also given half of Mack Sennett's studio the crabs, forcing Sennett to have the place shut down and fumigated. Arbuckle seems to have had his eye on her for some time.

Fatty had taken three adjoining suites on the twelfth floor of the Hotel St Francis. He had filled them with bootleg liquor. The party began on Saturday and on Monday afternoon it was still going strong.

Soon after three, Virginia Rappe was found in Arbuckle's room. She had been drinking and her clothes were torn to shreds. Arbuckle gave her some water and applied ice – to her thigh or vagina, some said – to calm her down. It was generally agreed that she was drunk and she began screaming.

"Shut her up!" said Arbuckle. "Get her out of here. She makes too much noise."

People joked about whether Arbuckle had been having fun with her.

Suddenly Virginia began screaming at Arbuckle: "Stay away from me! I don't want you near me!"

She turned to her friend Maude Delmont, a woman well known to the police, and said: "What did he do to me, Maudie? Roscoe did this to me."

While others dunked her in a bath of cold water to calm her down, Arbuckle phoned for a doctor. When he arrived, he concluded that Virginia was drunk. She was then put to bed and the party resumed.

The hotel doctor looked in later and gave her a shot of morphine to put her to sleep. He gave her another shot the next day and inserted a catheter after being told she had not urinated for many hours. Meanwhile Delmont told the doctor that the trouble had started when Arbuckle dragged Virginia into his bedroom and tried to rape her.

Arbuckle checked out of the hotel on the Tuesday. Virginia stayed on. A couple of days later, she was taken to the hospital, where she died that Friday. The cause of death was peritonitis, an acute infection brought on by a ruptured bladder.

Yellow journalism was at its height and the newspapers went to town. Arbuckle was painted as a debauched sexual predator. Was his weight simply too much for the dainty Virginia? Could a bladder be ruptured during the normal sex act? Or had he indecently assaulted her with a champagne bottle or a jagged piece of ice? William Randolph Hearst told Buster Keaton that the *San Francisco Examiner* sold more newspapers because of the Arbuckle case than the sinking of the *Lusitania*.

"I don't understand it," said Arbuckle. "One minute I'm the guy everybody loved, the next I'm the guy everybody loves to hate."

Even Paramount did not have enough money to hush this one up. Morality groups called for Arbuckle to be executed. His films were withdrawn; his contract cancelled. However, Virginia's career had a posthumous revival with movie theatres across the country running her films, billing her as the victim of a sensational Hollywood murder.

Arbuckle was charged with first-degree murder. This was reduced to manslaughter. There was no evidence of rape, or attempted rape. The case went to trial three times. The first two trials ended with a hung jury. In the third, he was acquitted. Not only did they find Arbuckle not guilty, but that there was not the slightest evidence to connect him to any crime. And they issued a statement, saying: "Acquittal is not enough for Roscoe Arbuckle. We feel that a great injustice has been done him."

But the damage had been done. In the hope of diverting attention from other scandals, the studio heads got the new movie censorship tsar Will Hays to ban him from the screen. But he worked as a director under his father's name and enjoyed some success on the vaudeville stage. Arbuckle had been a mentor to Charlie Chaplin, Buster Keaton and Bob Hope. Thanks to a letter-writing campaign organized by friends, Arbuckle returned to the screen in 1932 in a series of Vitaphone shorts. He was about to sign a lucrative contract with Warner Bros. when he died in his sleep at the age of forty-six.

## Rudolph Valentino

Star of the early classics *Camille*, *The Sheik* and *Passion's Playground*, Rudolph Valentino was the silent screen's "Great Lover". However, off-screen he was a bit of a flop. He was forced to admit in court that his two marriages had both been left unconsummated.

Born Rodolfo Guglielmi di Valentina D'Antonguolla in the small town of Castellaneta, Italy, Valentino was widely admired for his beauty. Many locals thought he should have been born a girl. In 1912, he moved to Paris, where he was approached by an old pederast named Claude Rambeau. However, his interests lay elsewhere – in the female nudes of the follies. But his love of women was purely aesthetic. A friend lent him his girlfriend, but in the event she could not get him aroused and vilified him as a "queer". So he got drunk and went with Rambeau, though he did not seem to have enjoyed that experience very much either. The next day he left Paris for good.

The following year he moved to New York. There he anglicized his name as Rudolph Valentino and became a taxi dancer, earning $6 a day. Women would ply him with expensive gifts and fight over who was going to take him home. Soon he had a smart, two-bedroom apartment on

East 61st Street and a wardrobe of hand-tailored suits. He practised his smouldering-eyed look in the mirror, trimmed his waist with a corset and bowed and kissed hands in a way that many found effeminate. And no one was sure what he got up to in the bedroom. There was so little gossip about him, it was assumed he was celibate.

Maxim's hired him as an exhibition dancer. After his set he was to tango with the clients or sit at table with wealthy society ladies. When the New York Vice Squad began to crack down on gigolos, arresting several for prostitution, Valentino went on tour with a professional dance partner, culminating in a performance before President Woodrow Wilson. Back in New York, he was arrested in a vice investigation. Then to escape another scandal when his former dance partner shot and killed her husband, he took a job as a chorus boy in a musical comedy that was going on tour. It closed in the Midwest but instead of returning to New York he headed on to California.

He got a few jobs as an extra in Hollywood, setting up as a dance instructor to survive. He was invited to a "boys' night" at the notorious Torch Club, where he gave homosexuality a second chance, but blew his chance – or, rather, didn't blow his chance – when he fled from a prominent movie producer. He worked as a life model, and as a gigolo.

Movie star Mae Murray saw him dance and was smitten. Afraid of her husband director Bob Leonard's fiery temper, she knew that she could not risk having an affair with Valentino. Instead she got Leonard to offer him the role of leading man in her new picture, *The Big Little Person*. Their intense love scenes made the film an instant hit. They followed up with *The Delicious Little Devil* and Valentino's stardom was assured.

However, when he was invited to accompany actress Dagmar Godowsky to a dinner party given by Alla Nazimova, the great Russian star of the silent era was outraged.

"How dare you bring this gigolo to my table?" Nazimova demanded. "How dare you introduce that pimp to Nazimova?"

One of Nazimova's lesbian friends, Metro starlet Jean Acker, took pity on him. But when she refused to come home with him, he fell in love with her – he had never come across a woman playing hard to get before.

"I knew that I wanted her for my wife," he said.

He took her on a moonlit horseback ride through Beverly Hills and proposed. The following day, they were married by special licence. After their reception at the Hollywood Hotel, Jean was reluctant to leave with him. As he dragged her back to their room, she cried: "Slow down, give a girl time to think."

"This is no time for thinking," said Valentino, sweeping her up in his arms in proper leading-man style. "This is a time for action."

Other guests then overheard a furious row. Jean was screaming that the marriage had been a terrible mistake. She could not bear to have him touch her. The thought of his body on hers nauseated her. He pleaded for her to give it a try. But in the face of her furious onslaught, he was forced to retreat. Valentino separated from his wife after just six hours. The marriage, everyone in Hollywood soon knew, had not been consummated. The Great Lover was a laughing stock.

While people were sniggering behind his back, Lewis Selznick sent Valentino to New York to play the lead in the movies that were still being shot there. He returned to Hollywood a star in *The Four Horsemen of the Apocalypse* and women flocked to him once again. Jean Acker was put out and sued him for maintenance, claiming that he had deserted her. He counter-sued for divorce.

Meanwhile *The Four Horsemen of the Apocalypse* was a triumph. Even Nazimova was forced to eat crow. She visited him on the set of *Uncharted Seas* with another of her "friends", set and costume designer Natacha Rambova. Her real name was Winifred Hudnut, though she was known as "The Icicle" for her cold and aloof manner.

Valentino was now the hottest property in Hollywood. Nazimova wanted him to play opposite her in *Camille* and introduced him to Rambova. Soon "The Icicle" began to thaw. During the filming of *Camille*, they left Nazimova waiting on the set, while they went at it hammer and tongs in his dressing room. From the nadir of this marriage, his reputation as a Latin lover soared to new heights.

Rudy had learnt nothing from his disastrous marriage to Jean Acker. He ignored the accounts of the casting sessions that Rambova organized for Nazimova with lines of young women stripped to the waist being selected for all-girl orgies. He was determined to marry Rambova and have children with her. Rambova seemed keen too and sent nude pictures of them together to Acker as grounds for divorce.

Though a star, Rudy was still not making much money. So, to save money, Rudy and his flatmate French-born cameraman Paul Ivano moved into Rambova's tiny bungalow on Sunset. They shared the place with a lion cub that she had bought. One night it escaped. Without stopping to dress, Rambova chased after it and Angelinos were treated to the sight of a lion cub being chased down Sunset by a naked Amazon.

Then came *The Sheik*. It broke all box-office records. Some 125 million people saw it worldwide and women on five continents swooned. But Valentino's reputation as a lover was about to take a dent. Jean Acker told the divorce court Valentino had burst into her bathroom and beaten her when she was naked. She was asked why she had not let Valentino visit her when she was filming on location. Because she had been sharing her room with a girlfriend, she explained. Titters ran through the courtroom.

Then came the matter of non-consummation. Acker admitted that, a month after their wedding, they had even spent the night together in his apartment, but they had not made love then either. The divorce was granted. Valentino was ordered to make a one-off payment to Acker. The producer of *The Sheik*, Jesse Lasky, loaned him $5,000 as a down payment.

With the Arbuckle scandal at its height, Will Hays arrived in Hollywood to clean up the movie industry. The first thing he did was call Lasky to point out that his star, Rudolph Valentino, was a bigamist. On 13 May 1922, Valentino and Rambova had slipped over the border to Mexicali and tied the knot. The problem was that his divorce from Jean Acker was only an interlocutory decree. The decree absolute would not be issued for another year.

The happy couple were honeymooning in Palm Springs at the time. When the news of their legal slip-up reached them, Rambova took flight and went into hiding in the Adirondacks, while Valentino returned to LA to face the music. He surrendered to a Justice of the Peace and was thrown in the slammer. It was a Sunday and he did not have the $10,000 he needed for bail about his person. By the time his friends had rustled up the money, every pressman in Los Angeles was waiting outside the jail. He had erred, he admitted, but only because of his great love for Rambova.

The irony then deluged from the sky. The studio's lawyers told him that his only possible defence to the charge of bigamy was non-consummation of marriage to Rambova. Otherwise he faced one to five years in jail and deportation. Valentino hung his head in court when he said that, on his wedding night, instead of sleeping with his bride, he had slept in another room with two men. Nor had they shared a room in Palm Springs. Witnesses then testified that Valentino and Rambova had not been alone together for a single moment since the wedding.

Valentino was cleared, but humiliated. But the scandal did his career no harm. The moralists that were besieging Hollywood were delighted. Here was Valentino, the great romantic lead, who would not even make love to his wife – either of them. Lasky was delighted with the publicity. It was more than any money could buy. And Valentino's female fans adored him all the more. He was, perhaps, saving himself for them.

Not daring to risk getting arrested again, Valentino and Rambova lived in separate apartments in New York City, each with their own roommates, until the year was up. On 14 March

1923, they legally remarried and he got Paramount to take her on as a technical adviser.

By this time, Rambova had given up sex for spiritualism and encouraged him to do the same.

"It was a good thing for them that they had spiritual intercourse," said Rambova's friend Nita Naldi, who was Rudy's co-star in *Blood and Sand*. "I doubt if they ever had any other kind. Neither one of them liked that sort of thing – at least in a normal way."

Nita found it strange that he could rub her breasts and show passion in close-up on the set, but it never went any further off camera. However, Valentino's spiritualism did have its compensations. He consulted a beautiful African-American medium called Kitab. She told him to strip himself of all material things – that is, his clothes. Then she put him into a trance. While he was under, his body went into a spasm. When he awoke, he found himself lying on the floor with the beautiful young black medium on top of him.

Valentino was constantly propositioned by other women. A young prostitute named Adele used her charms to get his phone number and invited him to her apartment for a freebie.

"Don't be gentle with me," she begged.

"Let's not rush it," he said. "I want to savour the magnificence of your body."

But her passion became too much for him. It was all over in a second.

"That was wonderful, Rudy," she said. He knew that she was lying.

News of his un-sheiky performance got round the studio and Rambova began firing any woman that might take Rudy's fancy.

Old scandals continued to dog him. Jean Acker began appearing on stage as "Mrs Rudolph Valentino". Rambova filed suit without much hope of redress. Meanwhile, she began to tighten her grip on Rudy, even buying him a slave bracelet, though it was made of platinum. Colleagues refused to work with her; friends refused to visit. But she had a terrible hold over him.

"Natacha has threatened to tell the world that I am not a great lover," he confided to Mae Murray. "She has said that she will tell people what I am really in the bedroom. She will tell them that I am a freak, not a sheik."

This made the gossip columns and the papers branded him a wimp. To prove his manhood, Valentino wanted to give Rambova a baby, but she refused unless he gave up acting. United Artists then offered him a contract for $1 million, provided Rambova did not darken the studio doors. She was outraged and told him to refuse it. But he defied her. Suddenly, he was the Sheik again and signed.

"Your job is to have babies," he said. "Mine is to make films."

Rambova went into movie production with Nazimova with $50,000 she got from Rudy. Then she headed east to find a distributor. Press photographs caught their last kiss at Union Station.

Rudy began to think that he was incapable of love.

"Both my marriages have failed," he told friends. "Dear little Jean was my bride for only a month. And Natacha, she was never a wife at all."

Nita Naldi managed to get beyond the on-camera groping, but then damaged his reputation further by putting it about that Rambova had had three abortions while she was with Valentino. Meanwhile, he was seen publicly with Vilma Banky, the Budapest bombshell who was co-starring in his latest film *The Eagle*. Rumours they were having a passionate affair were denied. He protested that he was a married man. Nevertheless, Banky's fiancé, a Hungarian baron, threatened to kill him. When the two met, Valentino floored the baron with a single punch – he had been taught by heavyweight champion Jack Dempsey for the film *Cobra*. A duel was suggested. But

Valentino had been taught fencing by experts for on-screen swordplay and the baron thought better of it.

In 1925, Rambova filed for divorce. He did not contest it and was comforted by the ravishing Polish actress Pola Negri, who was wearing Charlie Chaplin's engagement ring at the time. They were a sensation on the dance floor. Afterwards, the great silent star seduced her wordlessly on a bed strewn with rose petals – also crushing the rumours that his two marriages to prominent lesbians meant he was impotent.

Still he was chided in the press for being unmanly. When a powder puff dispenser had been installed in the men's room of a dance hall, some witty editorial writer on the *Chicago Tribune* wrote a leader condemning the effeminization of the American male, blaming it all on Rudolph Valentino.

Valentino was beside himself and challenged the anonymous leader writer to a boxing match. There were no takers. However, in New York, the *Evening Journal*'s burly boxing correspondent Frank O'Neill offered to defend the honour of the profession. In a makeshift ring on the roof of the Ambassador Hotel, Valentino knocked the big man to the ground. Afterwards, Valentino was seen celebrating in a Prohibition strip joint that served a hundred-proof ginger ale with his ex-wife Jean Acker. Asked if they were considering getting married again, they said they were just good friends.

Later he collapsed with stomach cramps. These were not caused by bootleg booze or by the patent baldness remedy he had been guzzling, but by peritonitis and gastric ulcers. As he lay dying, Jean Acker was not allowed into the room as she was no longer his spouse. Neither was Natacha Rambova, whom he had left just $1 in his will.

The scandals that had punctuated his career had done little harm. A crowd of more than 12,000 people, mainly women, besieged the funeral parlour in New York where Valentino lay in state and more than 100,000 people filed past the coffin. At the funeral, Pola Negri looked near to collapse. Jean Acker fainted. Over three thousand miles away in London, an actress named Peggy Scott killed herself in her bedroom, surrounded by pictures of Valentino, though she had never even met him. For many years, a woman dressed in black laid red roses on his grave on the anniversary of his death. It was only discovered in 1945 that she was Marion Benda, a former Ziegfeld beauty whom Valentino had met shortly before he died. Later, she claimed to have married him.

## Charlie Chaplin

Throughout his life, Charlie Chaplin had a weakness for underage girls. This caused problems both with the law and with his public. And the scandals surrounding his sex life almost scuppered his career on a couple of occasions.

In 1916, when he was already well established as "the little tramp", Chaplin met fourteen-year-old child actress Mildred Harris, who had appeared practically nude in the notorious Babylonian scene in D. W. Griffith's *Intolerance*. Chaplin was immediately captivated. Her mother, a wardrobe mistress at the studio, knew of Chaplin's proclivities.

When Mildred was sixteen, her mother told Chaplin that the girl was pregnant. Fearing prosecution for statutory rape – penalty thirty years in jail – Charlie had no choice but to marry Mildred. But once they married, he discovered that she was not pregnant at all. This caused some friction in the Chaplin household. Louis B. Mayer was quick to cash in. He signed Mildred for a film about domestic strife called *The Inferior Sex*, starring "Mrs Charlie Chaplin". When Charlie upbraided Mayer over this blatant exploitation of his name in the foyer of the Alexander Hotel, Mayer responded by calling Chaplin a "filthy pervert". Charlie asked him to step outside. Mayer, a former scrap-metal dealer from New Brunswick, took off his glasses and punched the little tramp in the face right there.

In 1920, Mildred really did get pregnant, but gave birth to a deformed child that died after three days. The marriage collapsed amid charges of cruelty and infidelity. Mildred had suddenly noticed the stream of young starlets passing through Charlie's dressing room. But then she had quit the conjugal bed for that of Alla Nazimova. They divorced.

Charlie was on safer ground with Peggy Hopkins Joyce. A graduate of the casting couch of Flo Ziegeld of Follies' fame, she had five marriages behind her and $3 million in the bank, which she had earned in the conjugal bed and the divorce courts. It seems the term "gold-digger" had originally been coined in her honour.

On meeting Chaplin, the first thing she said was: "Is it true what the girls say – you're hung like a horse?"

The little tramp was enormously proud of his oversized appendage, which he called the "Eighth Wonder of the World". When they took off to Catalina Island, where they swam naked in a secluded bay, word soon got around that the world's most famous movie star was in the vicinity and the locals turned out on a nearby hillside to watch the couple's nude frolics. The local billy goats were soon nicknamed "Charlies" after Chaplin. But Peggy was more interested in money than sex and soon moved on to producer Irving Thalberg.

Chaplin's name was then linked with a number of other women, including Winston Churchill's cousin Clare Sheridan, who sculpted his bust. The affair was denied by Chaplin's press agent Carlyle Robinson who said: "Mrs Sheridan is old enough to be Mr Chaplin's mother." So she was not Charlie's cup of tea at all then.

Discarding a couple of other fiancées, Charlie hooked up with Pola Negri and called a press conference to announce the engagement of the King of Comedy to the Queen of Tragedy. Five weeks later, he announced he was "too poor to marry". Six hours after that, they announced that the marriage was on again.

Then when Chaplin and Negri were downstairs dining, his valet found a young Mexican girl in his bed. She said she had run away from her husband and crossed the border in the hope of sleeping with her idol. The following day, she was found lying in a flower bed in Chaplin's garden, claiming to have swallowed poison. When Pola turned up, the ensuing altercation became so heated that Chaplin had to douse the two women with a bucket of cold water. Soon the engagement was off again. At thirty, Negri was much too old for Chaplin.

Charlie met the second Mrs Chaplin, Lillita McMurray, when she was just six and, with the connivance of her mother, he groomed her for nine long years for a starring role in his life. Under the name Lita Grey, she was the "Angel of Temptation" in his movie *The Kid* at the age of thirteen. By 1923, she had filled out enough to be his leading lady in *The Gold Rush*. The studio said she was nineteen; she was in fact just fifteen.

She was expected to play his leading lady off screen too. In his hotel room, "he kissed my mouth and neck and his fingers darted all over my alarmed body," she wrote in her autobiography. "His body writhed furiously against mine, and suddenly some of my fright gave way to revulsion."

But she was not that revolted. As, after a naked romp around his house, Chaplin took her virginity on the tiled floor of the steam bath. Now Lillita was both surprised and flattered. He could have had any one of a hundred girls, she said.

"No, a thousand," he said, correcting her. "But I wanted to be naughty with you, not them."

He was twenty-one years her senior.

It was clear that her mother knew what was going on. Mrs McMurray had worked at Chaplin's studio when he had married Mildred Harris and promptly announced to the cast of *The Gold Rush* that her daughter was pregnant. He had been through this before and promptly dropped her from the film and urged her to get an abortion.

When she refused, her grandfather turned up with a shotgun. Charlie offered her $20,000 to marry someone else, but she wanted him. Her Uncle Ed, a lawyer, stepped in. When he mentioned a paternity suit, which would have brought a charge of statutory rape if Chaplin proved to be the father, Charlie realized that he loved Lita after all.

Chaplin was in enough trouble at the time as it was. He had been having an affair with the actress Marion Davis, mistress of the newspaper tycoon William Randolph Hearst. At a party on-board Hearst's yacht, the media mogul caught Chaplin and Davis making love and went to get a gun. Davis screamed and Chaplin fled. Hearing her scream, another guest, the producer Thomas Ince, came running. He put his arms around Davis to calm her. Mistaking him for Chaplin, Hearst shot him dead.

But Hearst was powerful enough to hush things up. The story was concocted that Ince had never turned up to the party due to an acute bout of indigestion. A compliant coroner signed a death certificate giving the cause of death as "natural causes". The body was quickly cremated. Ince's widow set sail for Europe $5 million the richer and a little-known journalist who had been at the party named Louella Parsons became a syndicated showbiz columnist on Hearst's newspapers, beginning her forty-year career as one of the most influential voices in Hollywood.

Taking a child bride was bad enough when Chaplin was twenty-six, but at thirty-six it was nothing less than scandalous, so they decided to have a quiet wedding across the border. On the way to the dusty town of Empalme, Chaplin suggested that Lita throw herself from the train. She didn't.

Hearst bore a grudge and, when they arrived at Empalme, the couple were besieged by reporters. Chaplin tried his best to smile. On the way back to Los Angeles, he remarked: "Well, boys, it's better than the penitentiary, but it won't last."

Oh, but it did. Lita gave birth to Charlie Chaplin Jr seven months later. Judging that her daughter was too young and inexperienced to run a household, Mrs McMurray moved in. But plainly having the mother-in-law in residence was not too much of a distraction. Nine months after the birth of Charlie Jr, a second son, Sydney, came along.

Meanwhile the entire McMurray clan had moved in. They had loud drunken parties after Chaplin returned from a long day at the studio. Eventually, he threw them out. Lita filed for divorce, asking for a $1 million settlement. While Chaplin was away in New York, he discovered that Uncle Ed had sequestered all Chaplin's assets in California. He countered by issuing a statement saying that he still loved his wife and wished to stay married.

But Uncle Ed figured he was on to a good thing. He responded by publishing the transcript of Lita's Bill of Divorcement as a fifty-page pamphlet. Tens of thousands were sold at twenty-five cents a copy. In it, Lita claimed that throughout their twenty-five-month marriage Chaplin had maintained at least five mistresses. He had suggested that they liven up the marriage bed by inviting another young conquest to join them. He wanted to film them having sex and suggested doing it in front of an invited audience. Worse, he suggested that she indulge in an "abnormal, against nature, perverted, degenerate and indecent act". This turned out to be fellatio.

"Relax, my dear, all married people do it," he said. However, oral sex was against the law in California.

That didn't matter, he said, and suggested that he employ a prostitute to show her how. He made light of the institution of marriage, read passages from the then banned *Lady Chatterley's Lover* and made persistent efforts to "undermine and corrupt her moral impulses and demoralize her rule of decency" – all in the name of "having some fun together". Bastard.

This proved an inspiration to enterprising film-makers. Stag film circulated, showing Chaplin lookalikes doing many of the things mentioned.

But Chaplin was in no position to fight. One of the five mistresses in the Bill of Divorcement was Marion Davis. The affair was still going on and he used to seek refuge in her beach house when there was trouble at home. The scandal could only get worse if Hearst took umbrage again. So he settled for $825,000, plus costs, which were estimated to have run to $1 million, largely going to Uncle Ed.

Chaplin consoled himself with another ex-Ziegfeld, later star of *Pandora's Box*, Louise Brooks. They spent their weekends in an exotic foursome with Louise's lesbian lover Peggy Fears and the impresario Alfred Blumenthal.

Louise recalled: "His passion for young girls, his Lolita obsession, left him deeply convinced that he could seduce a girl only with his position as a director and star-maker."

He had a brief fling with his secretary May Reeves, only to find that his brother Syd was bedding her too. Then he had a long relationship with Paulette Goddard, who co-starred with him in *Modern Times* and *The Great Dictator*. She had graduated from Flo Ziegfeld's casting couch at fourteen, married a millionaire at sixteen and walked away with a half-million-dollar divorce settlement at nineteen. She was definitely Chaplin's type of girl.

There is a dispute over whether they were ever married. If they were, Chaplin was less than faithful. In 1936, he planned an orgy to welcome Spanish surrealist director Luis Buñuel to Hollywood. Buñel recalled: "When the three ravishing young women arrived from Pasadena, they immediately got into a tremendous argument over which one was going with Chaplin, and in the end all three left in a huff."

After Chaplin and Goddard split, she signed with Cecil B. de Mille, but the story circulated that she had given her new lover a blow job at Ciro's in full view of the other diners. American audiences would not swallow this and her career faded.

He was seen out with Greta Garbo and Heddy Lamarr, who first came to fame through her full frontal nude scenes running through the forest in early Austrian films and her simulated orgasm on camera, though some say this was an early example of method acting. Now in his fifties, Chaplin's craving for young flesh was not quite so scandalous. He had an affair with twenty-two-year-old Carole Landis and Joan Barry, well known "party girls". Joan was, he said, "a big handsome woman of twenty-two, well built, with upper regional domes immensely expansive and made alluring by an extremely low décolleté summer dress, which ... evoked my libidinous curiosity". He groomed her for stardom, but she kept getting pregnant. Abortions were expensive, so he cut her wages from $100 a week to $25.

Joan took industrial action, drawing attention to her plight by dancing naked on his lawn. The police turned up and advised him to pay her fare back to New York. He was happy to pay her off, but this was not enough for her and she returned to his house with a gun. Curiously, this turned him on and he bonked her three times on the bear-skin rug without pausing for breath.

However, the fifty-three-year-old Chaplin had already met the love of his later life, seventeen-year-old Oona O'Neill, daughter of the Noble and Pulitzer prize-winning playwright Eugene O'Neill. He wanted to marry her. But Joan would not let go. She broke into his house and appeared naked in his bed. The cops were called and she got thirty days in jail.

While Joan was safely inside, Charlie and Oona married. But when Joan was released, she gave him an unwanted wedding present – a paternity suit. A worse scandal was to follow. FBI director J. Edgar Hoover hated Chaplin. He disliked the British and objected to the Communist sentiments that permeated his films. Chaplin was indicted under the Mann Act, a federal law which prohibited the interstate transport of women for "immoral purposes", designed to combat prostitution and the "white slave trade". Charlie had taken the LAPD's advice and given Joan the money to go back to New York. The charge sheet said that Chaplin "did willingly, unlawfully, and feloniously transport and cause to be transported Joan Barry from Los

Angeles to the city of New York with the intent and purpose of having her engage in illicit sexual relations with him".

Chaplin was very publicly arrested, fingerprinted and photographed. In court, Chaplin's lawyer argued that it was ridiculous to suggest that Chaplin would transport a woman three thousand miles just to have sex with her, when she was perfectly willing to have sex with him where he was. He was acquitted, but Hoover had succeeded in denting his image.

While he gallantly agreed to pay Barry's medical expenses, he denied that the child was his. The blood tests proved him right. Nevertheless, Barry's lawyer told the jury: "There has been no one to stop Chaplin in his lecherous conduct all these years – except you. Wives and mothers all over the country are watching to see you stop him dead in his tracks."

He convinced the court that the blood tests were inadmissible. Chaplin was ordered to pay $100 a week child support and Barry's child took the name Chaplin.

Throughout the court case, Hearst's newspapers whipped up a hate campaign against Chaplin, calling him "a pestiferous, lecherous hound", "a little runt of Svengli", "a cheap Cockney cad" and a "reptile who looked upon Joan Barry as so much carrion". In a case of extraordinary bad timing, Chaplin was working on a black comedy about the "modern-day Bluebeard", French sex killer Henri Landru, at the time. The film *Monsieur Verdoux* fell foul of the Hays Office. While killing the women was OK, the film implies that Bluebeard slept with them as well. When the film came out, it was butchered by the press and, in some places, boycotted.

Chaplin made one more film in Hollywood, *Limelight*. Many American cinemas refused to show it and when he went to London for the opening his re-entry visa to the US was revoked. Charlie and Oona went to live in Switzerland where they had eight children, the last being born when he was seventy-three.

## Errol Flynn

While Charlie Chaplin escaped charges of statutory rape, the great swashbuckling star Errol Flynn, star of *Captain Blood*, *The Adventures of Robin Hood* and *The Sea Hawk*, had his day in court.

Flynn was a drinker and a womanizer whose whole life was a scandal. But that was the way movie stars were expected to behave and as long as they kept it among themselves it didn't matter too much. However, in 1942, when Flynn was at the height of his career, *Life* magazine wanted a photo spread showing him in Catalina, surrounded by adoring females. Seventeen-year-old Peggy LaRue Satterlee seized the opportunity. The photographer delivered her to Flynn's yacht *Sirocco* and they spent the day sunbathing and swimming. That evening he took her out for dinner. Then, back on the yacht, he entered Peggy's cabin.

"At first, she said 'no'," he told a friend. "Then she said 'yes'. We happily went to bed."

When Peggy returned home, her mother took her to a doctor who said there was evidence of "forcible entry". Next stop, the DA. Flynn made a payment to the DA's staff. But Warner Bros.' lawyer Jerry Geisler warned him to be careful.

"You'd better check their birth certificates next time," he said.

However, at a party in the home of his friend Freddie McEvoy in Bel Air, seventeen-year-old Betty Hansen plopped herself unceremoniously in his lap. She was drunk. Later he found her on the sofa. She had been sick and he took her to the bathroom. Afterwards, she threw herself on the bed. To make her more comfortable, he loosened her clothing, then loosened his own. After they had made love, he invited the two friends she had come with – dancer Agnes "Chi-Chi" Toupes and nightclub singer Lynn Boyer – to join him in the shower. It was all entirely amicable. However, when Betty got home, she told her sister and ended up in Juvenile Hall, and the DA dusted off the Satterlee file.

Flynn was arrested for "having intercourse with a minor". It was a felony. He was dragged down to Juvenile Hall where Betty identified him. He was also arraigned for forcibly raping Peggy Satterlee on the *Sirocco* – twice.

The scandal drove the war off the front pages. Those close to Flynn knew that he had had sex with both girls, while among the public at large he had a reputation as a legendary seducer. But Geisler was a wily trial lawyer and managed to get nine women on the jury, figuring that women were more susceptible to Flynn's charm.

Taking the stand, Peggy Satterlee told the court that Flynn had come to her cabin, pulled her skirt up, her panties down and had sex with her. Afterwards, he brought her a glass of milk and called her JB – jailbait – and SQQ – San Quentin quail. Plainly he knew she was underage. The next occasion, she said, followed a day's swimming and photography. She was sitting on the deck looking at the moon. Flynn said it looked much prettier through a porthole. So she went to his cabin and got on the bed to look at the moon. Again, he had pulled down her panties and had sex with her.

The Assistant DA wanted to get this absolutely clear. "Did Mr Flynn insert his privates in you?" he asked.

"Yes," said Peggy emphatically. And on both occasions, she said she had stoutly resisted.

During cross-examination, Geisler established that Peggy often claimed to be twenty-one to get work as a showgirl in nightclubs. He then got her to admit that she had had sex with a married man and had an abortion. Then he capped this off by calling a renowned astronomer, who said that Peggy could not possibly have seen the moon through the porthole in Flynn's cabin. The moon was on the other side of the boat. Wherever she had been looking, it was not out of the porthole.

Betty Hansen took the stand wearing a tight sweater with

a poodle on the front. Despite this juvenile attire, it was clear that she was a well-developed young lady. She told the court that she thought Flynn was undressing her to put her to bed because she was not well. And the Assistant DA needed full details.

"Did he remove all your clothing?" he asked.

"All, except my shoes and stockings."

"And then what happened?"

"He undressed himself."

"Did he remove all his clothing?"

"Everything except his shoes."

"What happened next?"

"We, well . . ."

"What happened next, Miss Hansen?"

"We had an act of intercourse."

"You state that you had an act of intercourse with Mr Flynn right there in that upstairs bedroom?"

"Yes."

"And this act was forced on you. I mean to say, it was against your will."

"It was against my will."

"When you said before that you had an act of sexual intercourse with Mr Flynn – you meant, didn't you, that Mr Flynn inserted his private parts into your private parts?"

"Yes."

"Please speak up so everybody can hear you, Miss Hansen."

"Yes, it was like that."

"How long would you say the act of sexual intercourse took?"

"A half-hour. Maybe fifty minutes."

Afterwards she said she went into the bathroom to use a douche bag, so she had clearly come prepared.

Geisler used the standard means of attack and got her to admit she was provocatively dressed. Then he pointed out contradictions in her testimony. One minute Flynn was a nice man helping her to undress because she was ill; the next she said that he had stripped her forcibly. She also admitted that she hoped Flynn would get her a part in the movies.

Under Geisler's cross-questioning, she denied having sexual intercourse with her boyfriend, Armand Knapp, a studio messenger. Then he asked her if she had ever been to Juvenile Hall before. She had.

"Did you not admit, Miss Hansen, under oath before the grand jury that you have performed two acts of sexual perversion with a man?" he asked.

The courtroom erupted.

Sobbing helplessly, Betty Hansen admitted she had been charged with having oral sex with Knapp – and that she was suspected to have performed oral sex on several of his fellow messengers.

Fortified with five jiggers of vodka, Flynn took the stand and denied everything. In his summing-up, Geisler alleged that Flynn's two accusers were lying to deflect their own felony charges. The jury stayed out overnight. The women found him not guilty, figuring that rape on the narrow bunk on the *Sirocco* would be impossible. Two of the men thought he was guilty, but eventually gave way. Flynn left the court with a wave. In his autobiography, he wrote: "I yielded with a smile to the now complete legend of myself as a modern Don Juan."

Of course, no one really believed that Flynn was innocent and the expression "in like Flynn" entered the language. Critics said that his latest film *Gentleman Jim* should be renamed *Jim* – he was no gentleman because he had not taken his shoes off when servicing Betty Hansen. Then there was his classic *They Died With Their Boots On*.

After the trial, Flynn put a notice on his front door that read: LADIES: KINDLY BE PREPARED TO PRODUCE YOUR BIRTH CERTIFICATE AND DRIVER'S LICENSE AND ANY OTHER IDENTIFICATION MARKS.

But the scandal had hurt his career. Problems with his health meant that he could not join up and fight. He was criticized for playing war heroes in the movies when he had not served, but the studio could hardly admit that their great swashbuckler was unfit.

He certainly had not learnt his lesson. In 1957, when he was forty-eight, he met fifteen-year-old Beverley Aadland in Hollywood. It was plain that they were an item. They even met Stanley Kubrick to discuss the casting of *Lolita*, but it was decided that James Mason and Sue Lyon were to be used instead, because of the statutory rape charges against Flynn fifteen years earlier. According to Aadland, he planned to marry her and move to their new house in Jamaica, but during a trip together to Vancouver, British Columbia, he died of a heart attack at the age of fifty. Later she admitted that the incorrigible Flynn had committed statutory rape again. After she had met him in his dressing room, he had invited her back to his estate. There he gave her hot saki and invited her to lie down on a bearskin rug in front of a blazing fire with him.

"I knew next to nothing about sex," she told *People* in 1988. "With Errol I didn't know what was happening at first – I thought he was just trying to kiss me. He knew so many women who would say yes that when I was saying no, no, no, he thought I meant yes. I know that because I asked him about it later. I was scared. He was just too strong for me. I cried. At one point he tore my dress. Then he carried me off to another room, and I was still carrying on. What was going through my head was, what was I going to tell my mother? When it was all over, and he realized I was a virgin, there was a complete change. He started to cry."

He convinced Beverley that he was sorry about what had happened and she agreed to go out with him a few days later. They could not keep their hands off each other.

"We made love again," she said. "I started out being a plaything, but in twenty-four hours I no longer was."

He began to take her with him everywhere. When he had to go to Africa to make a movie, Beverley decided to tell her mother.

"How long has this been going on?" she demanded.

Beverley phoned Flynn and put her mother on.

"Mrs Aadland," he said. "I have to tell you, I'm in love with your daughter and she's in love with me."

According to Beverley: "Mom finally heaved a sigh of relief. She realized I was happy and that we were serious about each other."

She had a party for her sixteenth birthday at his ranch in Jamaica. They then co-starred together in *Cuban Rebel Girls* before he died. Beverley Aadland did not regret being Flynn's lover at such a young age.

"I'm still glad I had the experience," she said. "I was fifteen chronologically, but I was so much older. I believe Errol was trying to do the best for me. I don't blame him for anything."

## Heidi Fleiss

Hollywood madam Heidi Fleiss claimed that she was too lazy in bed to be a prostitute. So the twenty-seven-year-old turned to procuring instead. She charged a minimum of $1,500 an hour for sex with one of her girls. When she was arrested in 1993 on charges of pimping and the possession of cocaine, Tinseltown was engulfed in scandal. Everyone wanted to know who was in her little black book.

Heidi's problem was that she was too successful and competitors wanted to put her out of business. They began informing the police of her activities. Pressure was brought to bear and, eventually, the authorities set up a sting operation. A Beverly Hills police officer, posing as a wealthy Japanese businessman, contacted Heidi and arranged for four prostitutes to meet him and several colleagues at a room in the Beverly Hills Hilton. He would pay $6,000 for the girls' services. He also wanted cocaine.

On 8 June 1993, Heidi sent four of her best girls with thirteen grams of charlie. The room had been bugged. Hidden cameras were running and there were twenty more cops in the next room. When the girls arrived, the seemingly eager clients chatted to them about sex and showed them pornographic videos. Then each girl was asked explicitly for sex. When they had all agreed, a signal was given. The cops burst in from the adjoining room and the girls were arrested.

The following day, Heidi was taking the garbage out from her $1.6-million home in Benedict Canyon when she was arrested for pandering and the possession of narcotics. If convicted, she faced a minimum of three years in prison.

From the moment she was arrested, the news spread. Celebrity marriages were under threat. Careers could tumble. Everyone was on edge.

Daughter of a Los Angeles paediatrician, at nineteen, Heidi had gone to work for the flamboyant businessman Bernie Cornfield, then sixty-one. One of the wealthiest men in the world, he was a friend of Hugh Hefner and a frequent guest at the Playboy mansion. He famously lived with ten or twelve girls at one time. Heidi soon became one of them. But she tired of his womanizing and left. Bernie eventually mended his ways. In 1976, he married a model named Lorraine, but found it hard to settle to married life. Polygamy was "considerably simpler than monogamy," he said, "and a lot more fun."

At twenty-two, Heidi was dating the film-maker Ivan Naggy. He introduced her to Elizabeth Adams, a.k.a. Madam Alex, who ran the most prosperous prostitution service in Los Angeles. It catered to the rich and famous. Heidi worked as a prostitute for Madam Alex for a time. But the sixty-year-old madam was to retire. She had had trouble with the police and feared that if she were arrested again, she would go to jail. So Heidi stepped into her shoes and took over the running of the business.

Heidi revamped the operation. While clients included wealthy businessmen, oil sheiks, Hollywood producers and, of course, Charlie Sheen, many of Madam Alex's employees were ageing and average looking. Heidi recruited good-looking girls in their mid-twenties. Many seized on it as a way to meet rich men. Profits soared. Heidi was only on a small percentage of takings, but she could afford a house in Benedict Canyon where her neighbours included Elizabeth Taylor and Michael Caine. Her best friend Victoria Sellers, daughter of the late Peter Sellers and Britt Ekland, moved in and they hosted a birthday party for Mick Jagger where the house got trashed.

Heidi took a six-month sabbatical after a friend was killed. When she returned to work, she fell out with Madam Alex over her share of the profits, so she set up on her own. She was now so well known that ambitious young women – university students, would-be actresses, even a former Miss USA contestant – flocked to her at Victoria Sellers's nightclub, On the Rocks, where she hung out most evenings.

The deal was simple. Her girls got to keep forty per cent of the inflated fees that Heidi charged – anything from $1,500 to $1 million a customer – while Heidi took sixty. Her clientele was international and she jetted girls to London and Paris, making millions. The problem was, she was taking business away from other madams, including Madam Alex. They wanted her stopped.

The court case soon came to media attention and Heidi Fleiss was billed as "madam to the stars". It had all the makings of a juicy sex scandal. Her lawyers argued entrapment, but she was convicted on three of the five pandering charges. She was fined $1,500 and sentenced to three years, but remained at liberty on bail while the case was appealed. Meanwhile, she was indicted by a federal grand jury on fourteen counts of conspiracy, income tax evasion and money laundering. Her father was also indicted for having signed a bank loan for $1 million for Heidi to buy her Benedict Canyon home under false pretences. They pleaded not guilty.

Eventually, her father got three years' probation. Heidi was sentenced to thirty-seven months, serving twenty, plus a reduced sentence of eight months for pandering. She served twenty-one months in all.

Despite intense press speculation, Heidi did not reveal the names of her clients. However, two came forward – Charlie Sheen and Texas billionaire Robert T. Crow. Another name that came up was Australian media and cricket tycoon Kerry Packer. At Fleiss's trial, prostitute Judy Geller testified that Packer paid for her and at least eight other women to fly to Las Vegas with him in 1992.

After being released from jail, Heidi Fleiss moved to Nevada, where prostitution is legal. She planned to set up a male brothel called Studfarm, catering for women.

## Jody Gibson

Meanwhile back in Tinseltown, Heidi's place had been taken over by Jody "Babydol" Gibson. Taking a leaf out of Fleiss's book, her escort agency California Dreamin' employed porn stars and *Playboy* models, charging up to $3,000. Her area of operation was said to have covered sixteen states and Europe.

When she was arrested in a sting operation in 1999, her black book was seized. And when the case came to court, the names were blacked out. However, when her appeals were exhausted and she was sent to jail for twenty-two months, the court records were opened and the black book appeared unredacted. Among the names were actors Ben Affleck who had a "steamy night with a hot blonde", Mark Wahlberg, Bruce Willis and Gary Busey, Sex Pistols guitarist Steve Jones, film producers Steve Roth, Jon Peters and Don Simpson, as well as baseball legend Tom Lasorda, former Texas Lieutenant Governor Ben Barnes, one of the biggest donors to the Democratic Party, and Maurice Marciano, founder of Guess? Inc.

Marciano told the *Los Angeles Times* he "couldn't imagine how [his] name got mixed up in this". The *Times* reached Roth, who produced *Last Action Hero*, by dialling the number next to his name in Gibson's book. He hung up. Willis and Lasorda denied having anything to do with Gibson, while Jones, who was then working as a DJ at a Los Angeles radio station, admitted that he may have known her.

Barnes, the Texas politician and now lobbyist who controversially claimed he had helped a young George W. Bush avoid the Vietnam draft, denied knowing Gibson and could not explain how his mobile phone number found its way into her book.

When Gibson got out of jail, she pumped up the sex scandal even further with her autobiography *Secrets of a Super Madam*. "This book is about my life servicing the rich and famous . . . and their sex, sex, sex!" she wrote in the introduction.

## Hugh Grant

On 27 June 1995, foppish English leading man Hugh Grant hit the headlines after being arrested and charged with lewd conduct in a public place with beautiful black hooker Divine Brown.

Divine had flown in from her one-bedroom apartment in the San Francisco Bay area that night, following an argument with her pimp Gangsta Brown, in the hope of earning $1,500 needed to pay her bills. She was on Sunset Boulevard when she saw a white BMW circling. The driver had an LA Dodgers baseball cap pulled down over his face. She took off, fearing he may be a cop or a stalker.

"He kept circling the block and pulling up in front of me," she said.

Then he pulled into a side street and flashed his lights.

"Eventually, I built up enough courage to confront him," said Brown. "I said: 'I'm going to call the cops if you keep stalking me.'"

He said: "I want you. You're so beautiful. What's a beautiful girl like you doing on the street?"

She said he sounded a bit like Prince Charles but tried to cover up his accent. He kept calling her "Cherry Red" because her shoes were red, her clothes were red, even her underwear was red – and, more importantly, the lipstick on her large soft lips was red. Her nickname on the Strip was "Little Red Riding Hood" and it did not take her long to overcome her fear of the Big Bad Wolf. Perhaps she wanted to show him what she had in her basket. Besides, he looked nothing like Grandma.

"When I saw him up close," she said. "I could see he was a gorgeous guy. He kept talking about how pretty I was and how he was struck by my lips and my feet. I guess he has a foot fetish, too."

There were a lot of other women out on the street that night. "Why choose me?" she asked.

He said he was looking for a beautiful black woman. When she looked around she noticed all the other girls that night were white.

"You're so gorgeous," he said.

She was on top form that night. When she arrived in Los Angeles earlier in the day, she said: "I went out and pampered myself. I got my hair done, I had a facial and a pedicure and bought a pair of hot shoes."

He gave his name as "Lewis" and Hugh, the perfect gentleman, said, "Please come with me."

And she did.

For $100, he could have enjoyed the privacy of Ms Brown's hotel room. But he said he only had $60, so they had to make out in the car. Still, Hugh wanted a little romance. He asked if she could kiss him. Most prostitutes regard kissing as intimate. It is for lovers, not clients, and she refused.

So he said, "Well, can I kiss you?"

She told him he could, so he leaned across and nuzzled her. Then he said fatefully, "You really smell beautiful."

They drove somewhere quieter. But unfortunately, he left the ignition switched on when Ms Brown got down to business, so to speak.

It seems she put her heart and soul into it. They were about twenty minutes into it when they were interrupted by a tap on the window. At that rate she would be sucking for over eleven hours to make the $2,000 she normally expected to make on a Friday night, or over eight to cover her bills.

Two police officers had been on routine patrol of the red-light district when their attention was drawn to the brake lights of a BMW flashing on and off.

Hugh's foot was on the brake pedal and he kept pushing on it as he sighed, "Oh Cherry Red, Cherry Red, oh Cherry . . ."

"I guess he was having a really good time," she said.

The patrolman shone his flashlight on the back of her head. It was plain what they were doing. At first the happy couple thought it was just a mischief-maker knocking on the window. Then Divine looked up and Hugh said, "Oh shit."

The police were laughing.

Then one of them said, "Please step out of the car."

Ms Brown took her hand off the gear stick and Hugh reversed it back into the garage, as it were. The moment of bliss had passed and they were led away separately in handcuffs. At the precinct, they were both photographed, charged and released. Ms Brown still had no idea who her famous client was and was back working the streets trying to make up for lost time when her pimp saw her face on the TV. Hugh Grant's nocturnal misdemeanour had made the morning news. The police had also released her mugshot to the media. And she looked good. She had already had a facial. Then there were those big red lips. For the press, this was a real-life *Pretty Woman*. By the time she got back to San Francisco, reporters were camped outside her house.

In fact, the ensuing scandal helped both Grant and Brown professionally. Grant was in the US to promote his first major studio movie, *Nine Months*, and was already booked to appear on a number of chat shows. He did not cancel the interviews. Instead, he brazened it out, making no excuses. On *The Tonight Show with Jay Leno*, he said, "I think you know in life what's a good thing to do and what's a bad thing, and I did a bad thing. And there you have it."

Then on *Larry King Live*, he said: "I could accept some of the things that people have explained, 'stress', 'pressure', 'loneliness' – that that was the reason. But that would be false. In the end you have to come clean and say 'I did something dishonourable, shabby and goatish.'"

King recommended that he seek professional help to probe his psyche. Grant declined, saying that psychoanalysis was "more of an American syndrome", while he himself was "a bit old-fashioned". The American people found his honesty appealing and his movie was a huge hit. Rather than ruining his career, getting caught with a hooker put Grant's face in front of the public. He was now a big box office hit. The press agent could not have planned it better.

Unfortunately, Hugh's long-term girlfriend Liz Hurley could not see the funny side and dumped him. His very public infidelity was all the more embarrassing because Grant had told Brown that he liked her perfume. It was not Estée Lauder, which Hurley was being paid £1.5 million to promote. Brown said she found Estée Lauder "too sweet and sickly". Just to rub Hurley's nose in it, Divine Brown posed in the Versace "safety-pin" dress that Hurley had made famous.

In court, Grant pleaded "no contest" and was fined $1,180, given two years' summary probation and sent on an Aids-awareness course. Brown also entered a no-contest plea and was sentenced to five days' community service as well as attending an Aids-awareness course. Additionally, she was fined $1,350 and eventually went to prison for parole violations.

However, the $60 trick turned out to be worth over $1 million to Divine Brown. It took her off the streets and put her two daughters through college. She was an instant celebrity, appearing on a number of TV shows, including *The Howard Stern Show* and Danny Bonaduce's short-lived *Danny!* The British tabloids paid her a fortune for her story. She appeared in a television commercial promoting a Los Angeles radio station, a commercial for a Brazilian lingerie company, in semi-nude pictures for soft-porn magazines such as *Penthouse*, and as a presenter on UK porn channel Television X. In 1996 she played herself in an X-rated docu-drama based on the incident, *Sunset and Divine: The British Experience*. By then, she had a house in Beverly Hills, a Rolls-Royce and several wardrobes full of designer clothes.

"I was able to buy amazing things, beautiful gowns and dresses," she said. "I was always attracted to the glamorous life and that half an hour with Hugh Grant made me able to buy all the things I'd dreamt of having. That film *Pretty Woman* seemed to be what my life was about. Hugh Grant was my Richard Gere."

Gangsta Brown continued to "manage" her, but eventually they split. Divine Brown went to live in Atlanta, Georgia, under her maiden – maiden? – name, Stella Thompson. In 2011, she was running a music production company with her fiancé and was a member of the local PTA. Her scandalous past has been forgotten by everyone except the British newspapers who regularly run stories on how she is getting on. While she can hardly believe her good fortune, she feels sorry for Hugh, now over fifty and still unmarried. So maybe there is hope for him yet.

## Pee-wee Herman

Emmy-award-winning children's show host Pee-wee Herman retired in the spring of 1991 when he declined to sign a new television contract. He quit giving interviews, reverted to his real name – Paul Reubens – and went travelling. Explaining why he wanted to give up the creation that had made him rich and famous, he said, "I don't want to be a fifty-year-old man with a really bad toupee and a facelift doing this." He grew his hair and beard and turned into the old hippy he had been before he created the character of Pee-wee.

It was all going so well until he went to visit family in his hometown of Sarasota, Florida. Then on the evening of 26 July he went to the XXX South Trail Cinema to see the triple feature of *Tiger Shark*, *Turn Up the Heat* and *Nurse Nancy*. He could have rented the videos and watched them in the privacy of his own home, if he had not been staying with his parents.

The local police had been out that night on a drugs bust. But the lead they had been given did not pan out. So they went to the South Trail Cinema to see if they could catch someone violating Florida State Statute 800.03, which deals with the "Exposure of Sexual Organs". The police report says that at 8.25 p.m. and again five minutes later, the suspect was observed "with his exposed penis in his left hand". Detective William Walters allegedly saw a man "masterbate" – that's how it's spelt on the rap sheet. Reubens was arrested in the lobby as he was leaving the theatre.

Even then, all might have been well. The police were hardly likely to recognize the bearded, long-haired individual they had in custody as the clean-cut, childlike, bow-tie-wearing kids' TV star. But, true to form, Pee-wee was determined to put his foot in it. When the police were examining his driver's licence, Reubens said: "I'm Pee-wee Herman. Maybe I could do a charity benefit for the Sheriff's Office or something to take care of this."

Reubens later explained that he did not think he had done anything wrong.

In the movie theatre, he said, "I knew people fooled around with each other, but I thought it was OK to be by myself."

In court, Reubens pleaded no-contest, sparing himself a trial and the resulting publicity. He was fined and given community service. His lawyer said that the no-contest plea means that Reubens "can get on with his life and his career". Fat chance.

The moment a local reporter recognized his name on the arrest sheet, the scandal machinery went into overdrive. Even though he had not yet gone to trial and was protesting that he had in no way exposed himself or "engaged in any other improper activities", CBS had pulled the five scheduled reruns of his show *Pee-wee's Playhouse*. Disney-MGM Studios in Florida suspended a tape that Pee-wee had made from their studio tour and Toys-R-Us removed Pee-wee toys from their shelves. His then attorney announced "his career is over" and quit. Now the butt of jokes – including that one – Reubens went into seclusion.

Cyndi Lauper, voice of *Pee-wee's Playhouse* signature tune, rushed to his defence and Bill Cosby said: "This has been blown out of all proportion." Poor choice of words there, Bill.

There were protests against CBS pulling the show in New York, Los Angeles and San Francisco, where they had T-shirts printed bearing the words: "Hands off our Pee-wee". Again, that could have been better thought through. "We (love) U Pee-wee" was sprayed on the South Trail Cinema. And Corporal Joan Verizzo of the Sarasota sheriff's department, who had known Reubens for twenty-two years, found herself in trouble for lending Pee-wee $40 towards his $219 bail on the night of the arrest. She got a day's suspension for breaking departmental policy against posting bail for anybody except family.

In a telephone survey, callers supported Reubens nine to one. According to a Gallup poll taken after Reubens's arrest, only one-third of parents thought Pee-wee's TV shows and movies should be off-limits to children and forty per cent of people thought Reubens got a raw deal from the media. He made a subsequent public appearance as Pee-wee at the 1991 MTV Video Music Awards. He asked the audience, "Heard any good jokes lately?" and received a standing ovation. Throughout the nineties, Reubens took a number of small parts. The cable network Fox Family even ran *Pee-wee's Playhouse* again.

Then in November 2002, while filming the video for Elton John's "This Train Don't Stop There Anymore", Reubens's home was raided and the police took away his collection of vintage erotica, most of it gay. The district attorney maintained that some of the models were underage, but eventually dropped child pornography charges, and Reubens pleaded guilty to the possession of obscene material.

But Reubens bounced back again. In 2010 and 2011, he began appearing as Pee-wee again and even talked of making an adult Pee-wee with "a lot of *Valley of the Dolls* moments in it". The problem is that Reubens is now sixty, though it is not known whether he wears a toupee or has had a facelift.


## Angelina Jolie

When Brad Pitt and Jennifer Aniston split after Brad and Angelina Jolie filmed *Mr and Mrs Smith* together in 2004, Angelina denied that they had had an affair.

"To be intimate with a married man, when my own father cheated on my mother, is not something I could forgive," she said, taking the moral high ground. "I could not look at myself in the morning if I did that. I wouldn't be attracted to a man who would cheat on his wife."

For seven years Jolie and her father Jon Voight were not even on speaking terms. On Spanish TV she even denied being his daughter. Voight split from her mother, his second wife, actress Marcheline Bertrand, a year after Angelina was born and went to live with actress Stacey Peckrin who had a walk-on part as a hooker in *Coming Home*. So one can understand the delicacy of her feelings.

But before Brad, Angelina did not shy away from scandal. In 2001, she told the *Daily Mirror* that her mother had allowed her to move her first boyfriend in when she was fourteen, even giving up the master bedroom for the pubescent couple. The age of consent in California is eighteen.

"He was my first boyfriend at a time when I wanted to be promiscuous and was starting to be sexual," she said. "We were in my bedroom, in my environment, where I was most comfortable and I wasn't in danger."

They were at it for two years.

"That relationship felt like a marriage," she told the *Calgary Sun*. "It was a tough break-up, so I immersed myself in acting to get over it."

However, the *New York Daily News* printed allegations that, at sixteen, Angelina bedded Marcheline's live-in boyfriend, damaging her relationship with her mother.

At the age of twenty, while filming *Hackers*, she fell for English actor Jonny Lee Miller.

"I've always been at my most impulsive when English men are around," she said. "They get to me. When I was fourteen, I visited London for the first time and that's when I discovered my problem. English men appear to be so reserved, but underneath they're expressive, perverse and wild. All the insane moments of my life have happened with English men."

When Angelina and Jonny married the following year, she drew attention to herself with a bridal outfit of a pair of skintight black rubber pants and a white T-shirt with Jonny's name written across the back in blood. That's pretty perverse and wild, Angelina.

John Hiscock, the Los Angeles correspondent for a number of British newspapers, said: "Unlike many of her Hollywood contemporaries, she does not spare me the details of her love life – even though her revelations include tales of self-mutilation and a penchant for violence during sex."

Self-mutilation?

"You're young, you're drunk, you're in bed, you have knives, shit happens," she explained.

She also attended S&M parties. Andrew Morton's book *Angelina: An Unauthorized Biography* carries a picture of her practically naked with black tape over her nipples and a dog leash around her neck.

The marriage to Miller lasted less than a year with him going on to date and dump catwalk model Kate Moss and Natalie Appleton of All Saints.

"Divorcing Jonny was probably the dumbest thing I've ever done, but I don't dwell on it," she said. "Fortunately he lives over here while I'm in New York. But we're still very close. I was so lucky to have met the most amazing man, who I wanted to marry. It comes down to timing. I think he's the greatest husband a girl could ask for. I'll always love him, we were simply too young."

In between times she threw herself straight into a lesbian relationship with model-actress Jenny Shimizu, whom she met on the set of *Foxfire*.

"I would probably have married Jenny if I hadn't married my husband," she said. "I fell in love with her the first second I saw her . . . She's great. We had a lot of fun."

In 2005, Shimizu, who had already been "friendly" with Madonna and a host of other Hollywood stars she refused to name, said that her relationship with Angelina "lasted many years. I was dating her while she was seeing other people – she was that type of person; wonderful and open."

Guess what? In 2011, Shimizu turned up on the cover of *Diva* magazine with Rebecca Loos, fresh from her alleged affair with the English footballer David "Golden Balls" Beckham. Of course, Shimizu denied using her sexuality to get publicity.

"I never intended for my sexuality to be known. It was something others leaked to the papers," she said in a long lead article in Britain's leading lesbian magazine. Obviously, she was a very private person.

Meanwhile, Barbara Walters asked Jolie if she was bisexual.

"Of course," she said. "If I fell in love with a woman tomorrow, would I feel that it's OK to want to kiss and touch her? If I fell in love with her? Absolutely! Yes!"

"Honestly, I like everything," she told *Elle*. "Boyish girls, girlish boys, the heavy and the skinny. Which is a problem when I'm walking down the street."

Just to prove that she did like *everything*, she kissed her brother James Haven on the lips at the 2000 Oscars, causing an outcry that still made headlines ten years later.

"For some reason people thought it was more interesting to focus on something that was sick and disturbing rather than the fact that two siblings support and love each other," she said. "Unfortunately, it has put a distance between us, because Jamie now feels he has to keep a space between us."

Maybe you should give up with the knives.

In 1999, she co-starred with Billy Bob Thornton, playing husband and wife in *Pushing Tin*. At the time Thornton was living with his fiancée Laura Dern. But they weren't actually married at the time, so that's OK then, Angelina. Dern was a veteran of high-profile romances with Kyle MacLachlan, Nicolas Cage, Renny Harlin and Jeff Goldblum, while Thornton split from his fourth wife, *Playboy* model Pietra Dawn Cherniak and mother of his two sons, to move in with her. Oh, what a tangled web.

Billy Bob and Angelina opted for a quickie wedding in Las Vegas. There was hardly time to tell Laura. The bride wore a sleeveless sweater and jeans; the groom had matching jeans and his trademark baseball cap. She had already announced their coupledom to the world by having "Billy Bob" tattooed on her arm, and they carried each other's blood in vials around their necks.

Put the knife down, Angelina.

"I'm madly in love with this man," she told *Talk* magazine, "and will be till the day I die."

And just to make sure, she called his mother to find out where his family were buried, then reserved two lots so that, one day, they could be buried side by side. They also had matching tattoos. But, coyly, Angelina would not show them to anyone.

"He's an amazing lover and he knows my body," she told the *Mirror*. "He knows things that I don't know. We didn't belong any place until we met each other."

In *Lara Croft: Tomb Raider*, Jolie was reconciled with her father Jon Voight. Then she starred in *Original Sin*, which featured nudity and bedroom scenes with Antonio Banderas.

"We got to know each other quite well," she said. "He's like a strange brother." Not Jamie. So that's all right then.

In March 2002, Jolie and Thornton announced that they were adopting a son from Cambodia, then separated three months later. They had been together nearly two years – a lifetime in Hollywood.

"It took me by surprise, too," she told *Vogue* in 2004, "because overnight, we totally changed . . . one day we had just *nothing* in common. And it's scary but I think it can happen when you get involved and you don't know yourself yet. It's taken me a while to grow up, and I still think I'm not even close to it yet. So I've kind of had to check myself: Don't even consider a relationship for another seven, eight years."

Oh, Angelina. It was that very same year that you told the *New York Times* that you had fallen in love with Brad Pitt on the set of *Mr and Mrs Smith*. It has to be said, Brad had the habit of laying his leading ladies: Robin Givens (*Head of the Class*), Jill Schoelen (*Cutting Class*), and Juliette Lewis (*Too Young to Die?* and *Kalifornia*), who, at the age of sixteen, was ten years his junior when they started dating. Then there was his three-year romance and engagement to his *Seven* co-star Gwyneth Paltrow, which ended shortly before he hitched up with Jennifer Aniston. She also had something of a track record: her co-star in *Ferris Bueller* Charlie Schlatter, musician Adam Duritz, actor Tate Donovan. After the split from Brad, she began a relationship with actor Vince Vaughn, with whom she co-starred in *The Break-Up*, British model Paul Sculfor, singer John Mayer, actor-director Justin Theroux. Round and round goes the Hollywood carousel.

## Eddie Murphy

At 4.45 a.m. on 2 May 1997, Murphy was driving his wife's SUV down Santa Monica Boulevard in West Hollywood, an area known for homosexual prostitutes. He pulled over, and a transvestite hooker named Atisone Kenneth Seiuli got in. They drove off together, but didn't get far before he was pulled over by a Los Angeles Sheriff's Department squad car.

The officers spent half an hour talking amiably with Murphy, warning him about the neighbourhood – they were less than a mile from where Hugh Grant had been caught with Divine Brown. Murphy said he had been feeling "restless" and was out for a drive when he saw a person he thought was a woman needing help.

"I did nothing wrong," he insisted. "I simply stopped to give a lift to someone who appeared to be in distress."

The cops found nothing illegal had taken place and let Murphy go. But they arrested Seiuli because there was an outstanding warrant for violating probation on an earlier prostitution charge. He later appeared in court, where his lawyer referred to him as "she". He/she was jailed for ninety days and ordered to take an Aids test.

As soon as Seiuli could post bail, the story was in the tabloids. According to Seiuli, during their brief conversation in the vehicle, Murphy had put two hundred-dollar bills on her leg.

Seiuli said: "He asked me if I did this for a living, being a transsexual prostitute. I said yes. Eddie said, 'Do you like to wear lingerie?' I said yes. He said, 'Can I see you in lingerie?' I told him, 'Whenever you have the time.' He said, 'I'll make the time.' Then he asked me, 'What type of sex do you like?' I said I was into everything."

Murphy's version of the story is completely different, of course.

"I'm married with three children," he said. "I'm not going to be out there screwing hookers off the street or anything like that. I'm just being a nice guy. I was being a Good Samaritan. It's not the first hooker I've helped out. I've seen hookers on corners and I'll pull over and they'll go, 'Oh you're Eddie Murphy, oh my God,' and I'll empty my wallet out to help."

This seemed to satisfy Eddie's wife Paulette McNeeley, who said: "He told me there was this person on the corner crying, so he stopped to help. But I'm thinking, 'Well, why the hell did you let them get into the car?'"

The marriage lasted another eight years and they had two more children before they split, citing "irreconcilable differences".

The weekend after the incident, *Saturday Night Live* – the show where Murphy had initially come to national prominence – aired a sketch titled, "Good Samaritan Eddie Murphy", with Tim Meadows playing Murphy, ferrying transsexuals throughout metropolitan Los Angeles, out of the goodness of his heart.

A parade of local transvestite escorts told the *Globe*, the *National Enquirer* and *Gay & Lesbian Times* about assorted encounters, allegedly with Eddie. Several subsequently recanted their stories. Murphy sued the tabloids, but later quietly settled. Candace Watkins, a purported mother figure to several of the transsexuals involved, later wrote *In the Closet with Eddie Murphy* under the pen name Carnal Candy. The book was filled with tales from Watkins's girlfriends about their alleged liaisons with Murphy.

None of this helped his career and his next movie *Holy Man* bombed – which was a surprise, given what real-life televangelists get up to.

On 22 April 1998, Seiuli, wearing only a black bra, padded, and a leather bikini thong (both from Frederick's of Hollywood), was found dead under the window of her fifth-floor apartment. She had apparently locked herself out and, while trying to get in through an open window, had fallen to her death. Her demise was not linked to Murphy, who went on to date Spice Girl Melanie Brown, but dumped her when she fell pregnant.

## Paris Hilton

Publicity-hungry heiress Paris Hilton was largely famous for flashing her panties to the paparazzi, when she remembered to wear any. But then she showed off a whole lot more. In 2003, footage of her having sex with her ex-boyfriend Rick Salomon appeared on the internet, just weeks before her reality TV show *The Simple Life* aired.

Ms Hilton claimed that she was so embarrassed by its release that she did not want to go back to America. It went on sale under the delightful title *One Night in Paris*, and became the top-selling video of 2005. However, she claimed that she made no money from it and thought that Salomon should give any money he made to a charity for the sexually abused.

The incident shocked her mother and Paris was worried about what any children she had in the future might think. However, the one thing she did not complain about was overexposure.

# 4

## Foreign Parts

### Silvio Berlusconi

Scandal-ridden Italian politician Silvio Berlusconi first came to prominence as a media mogul whose TV channel featured "stripping housewives" game shows. Other programmes regularly feature scantily clad young women. His wife would later complain about these *veline*, but they made him a very rich man.

His second wife, the actress Veronica Lario, first caught his attention when she stripped off in a play in Milan in 1980. She was twenty years his junior. He divorced his first wife, Carla, who was the mother of his first two children, in 1985. By then, he already had one child with Veronica and, by the time they got married in 1990, she had given him two more.

In December 1993, he founded the political party Forza Italia – "Go Italy". It won the election the following year and Berlusconi became prime minister in May 1994. But the ruling coalition fell apart and he resigned in December. In May 2001, he became prime minister again.

Forza Italia lost the election in April 2006 and he was replaced as prime minister by Romano Prodi. In opposition, Berlusconi was first connected to a sexual misdemeanour. In 2007, Berlusconi was forced to issue a written statement apologizing to his wife for flirting with other women after she demanded a public apology. Later that year, transcripts of Berlusconi's bugged phone calls to Agostino Saccà, the director-general of the state public service broadcaster RAI, were published in the magazine *L'espresso*. While soliciting several political favours, Berlusconi asked Saccà to give a young woman a job, saying explicitly that she would serve as a conduit to a senator in the majority party, and this would help bring down the Prodi government. Journalists and politicians then accused Berlusconi of exploiting prostitutes to promote political corruption.

In his own defence, Berlusconi said: "In the entertainment world everybody knows that, in certain situations in RAI TV, you work only if you prostitute yourself or if you are leftist. I have intervened on behalf of some personalities who are not leftists and have been completely set apart by RAI TV."

In April 2008, Berlusconi was returned to power, but the following year his wife wrote an open letter condemning his selection of young attractive female candidates with no political experience to run in the European elections, claiming that they were there for "the emperor's amusement". She went on to say: "What emerges today, through the screen of female beauty and curves, is power's impudence and lack of restraint which offends the credibility of all women."

Berlusconi demanded an apology, saying, "It is the third time she has done this to me in the middle of an election. It's too much."

Nevertheless, the press was full of pictures of the women he had selected, calling them *verline* and saying: "Silvio brings a troupe of showgirls to Strasbourg." One, it was said, was considered as a candidate after appearing on *Big Brother*, and a pair of twins had been considered after appearing on another TV show, *Island of the Famous*.

Then Berlusconi attended the eighteenth birthday party of the daughter of a business associate, an aspiring starlet named Noemi Letzia, in Casoria, near Naples. Signora Berlusconi was outraged because her husband had failed to attend his own daughter's eighteenth birthday party. Signor Berlusconi was reported to have given the rising starlet a gold necklace studded with diamonds.

Noemi gave several interviews to the Italian press, saying that she had often spent time with Berlusconi in the past, that he said he could take care of her career whether she decided to be a showgirl or a politician, and that she called him *Papi*, or "Daddy".

"It's a joke," said Berlusconi. "They wanted to refer to me as 'Grandpa', *Papi* is much better. Don't you think? ... According to what the lady [Ms Lario] said, I would not date seventeen-year-old girls. It's something I can't stand. I am a friend of her father, that's it. I swear!"

But his wife was adamant. "I cannot remain with a man who consorts with minors," said Veronica. "I read in the papers about how he has been hanging around a minor, because he must have known her before she was eighteen, and how she called him 'Grandpa' and about their meetings in Rome and Milan. This is no longer acceptable. How can I stay with such a man?" She added: "He is not well."

And she filed for divorce.

Berlusconi then gave his own explanation of the incident to the media. He swore that he knew the girl only through her father and that he never met her alone without her parents, claiming that it was all a plot hatched by "the left party and its press that can't quite accept my popularity reaching seventy-five per cent ... It's all false, it's a trap in which unfortunately my wife also fell into. There are no girls. It's an absolute lie."

However, on 14 May, newspaper *La Repubblica* published an article pointing out the many inconsistencies and contradictions arisen so far and formally asking Berlusconi to answer ten questions in order to clarify the situation. When he did not answer them, they published the ten questions.

They included how had he met Noemi and how often did he see her? Did he take an interest in her career and did he promise to help her if she entered show business or politics? When had he met her father and what was his relationship with him? Did he discuss the European candidates with Signor Letizia, even though he was not a member of the party? "Veronica Lario said that you 'frequent underage girls'. Do you meet others or 'bring them up'?" "Your wife says that you are not well and that you 'need help'. What is the state of your health?"

Two months later, *La Repubblica* asked ten new questions. These included: "Have you frequented other minors and do you still do so?" "You stayed with a prostitute on the night of 4 November 2008 and, according to judicial investigations, dozens of 'call girls' have been taken to your residences. Were you aware that they were prostitutes?" "Has it ever happened that 'official government flights" without you aboard were used to take female party guests to your residences?" and "Would you still be able to attend a 'Family Day' demonstration or sign a law punishing the customer of a prostitute?"

Finally, Berlusconi became so irritated that he sued for defamation.

While Silvio kept his own council, Noemi's ex-boyfriend Luigi Flaminio spoke up in her defence, but mentioned in passing that she had spent a week without her parents at Berlusconi's villa on Sardinia around New Year's Eve 2009. This was later confirmed by her mother. Photographs of the event had been taken by a paparazzo, but were confiscated by the Prosecutor's Office of Rome for violation of privacy. However, a selection of those photos was published in the Spanish newspaper *El País* on 4 June.

Berlusconi countered that he had never had a "spicy" relationship with Noemi. He swore on his children's heads that nothing like that had happened and said he would resign straight away if it had.

The following month, forty-two-year-old escort and former actress Patrizia D'Addario surfaced, saying that she had been recruited twice to spend the evening with Berlusconi. On one occasion, she stayed the night and was paid €2,000. She claimed she was invited to two candlelit dinners at Mr Berlusconi's imposing mansion in central Rome, Palazzo Grazioli, where the prime minister assumed the role of a "sultan" to a "harem" of gorgeous young women.

On the first occasion in October 2008, she said he asked her to stay the night but she declined. The second time was a month later, when she agreed to go to bed with him. She said she was taken aback by the prime minister's stamina, given that he has had prostate cancer. "He didn't appear a bit tired, he kissed me again and again and again," she said.

She decided to reveal all about her alleged night of passion with the media mogul because she said he failed to live up to promises he had made to help her with the building of a hotel in her hometown of Bari, on Italy's Adriatic coast.

"I gave him my body," she said, "but he gave me nothing."

The police in Bari were looking into the matter but, she said, the prosecutors would only believe her account if she produced tape recordings of conversations she claimed she had with Mr Berlusconi in his bedroom.

On national television, she ridiculed Berlusconi's claim that the dinners he had in the Palazzo Grazioli, where dozens of glamorous starlets and showgirls drank champagne and went home with jewel-encrusted butterfly brooches, were party political gatherings.

"First of all, such a political club would have to consist only of young, beautiful women dressed only in skintight black dresses, because they were the only sort of person I saw," said Ms D'Addario. "Secondly, the party members let themselves be caressed, kissed and touched in an unequivocal manner by their boss? If this is how politics is now conducted, I'm well qualified."

She later wrote a 240-page book called *Prime Minister, Take Your Pleasure*. It is subtitled *The Whole Truth, by the Most Famous Escort in the World*.

Berlusconi said he could not recall Miss D'Addario and that he did not pay for sex.

"I have never paid a woman," he said. "I have never understood what satisfaction there is if the pleasure of conquest is absent".

However, he acknowledged that he loved beautiful women and was "no saint".

Other young women began talking to the press about the parties held in the Palazzo Grazioli. Photographs and transcripts of audio-cassettes circulated widely. This raised concerns about the lack of security at the prime minister's residence. The doors seem to have been wide open if you were young, female and attractive.

And presents were not restricted to money and jewellery. Berlusconi was accused of spending over $1.8 million of public money to promote the career of unknown Bulgarian actress Michelle Bonev at a time when the government's arts budget was being cut back.

More details were revealed of what went on at the parties in Berlusconi's private villas by teenage Moroccan belly dancer and alleged prostitute Karima El Mahroug, who worked under the stage name Ruby Rubacuori. She claimed to have been given €7,000 and jewellery and attended orgies at his villas, where an African-style ritual known as the "bunga bunga" was performed by twenty naked women. Berlusconi was thought to have got the idea from Muammar Gaddafi.

The relationship came to light when Ruby was arrested for theft by the Milan police. As she was under eighteen, she was sent to a shelter for juvenile offenders. Berlusconi got her out after making two phone calls to the authorities where he claimed that she was a relative of President Hosni Mubarak of Egypt and he was seeking to avoid any diplomatic incident. He sent

Nicole Minetti, a former *verline* on the show *Colorado Café*, to collect her. She went on to become Berlusconi's personal dental hygienist, before having a burgeoning career in politics.

A criminal investigation was opened, resulting in Berlusconi being indicted for abuse of office for using his influence to have Ruby released and for paying for sex with an underage prostitute. Berlusconi's lawyers called the allegations "absurd and without foundation", while Ruby denied having sex with the prime minister. TV anchorman Emilio Fede and celebrity agent Dario "Lele" Mora have also been indicted for running a vast pimping network for procuring underage girls to attend Berlusconi's "bunga bunga" parties. According to the prosecutors' dossier, Fede discovered Ruby when acting as a judge at a beauty pageant in Sicily in September 2009, and passed her on to Mora's offices in central Milan, which served as a "form of 'clearing centre' for women eager to enter the prime minister's circle in pursuit of money, gifts and help with their show business careers".

Berlusconi is an acknowledged master of getting himself out of tight legal situations, but the prosecutors had some stiff evidence. They reportedly had thirty bugged telephone calls where he describes his nights with prostitutes and other female guests supplied by an alleged pimp. Prosecutors taped the conversations during an investigation into Giampaolo Tarantini, an entrepreneur from Bari, who was alleged to have paid women to attend Berlusconi's "bunga bunga" parties.

"So how did it go last night?" Tarantini asked Berlusconi. The prime minister then described the sex he had with his guests. He also discussed who to invite to Palazzo Grazioli and quizzed Tarantini about each woman's "specialities" and "qualities". Tarantini then described the women meticulously – whether they were blonde or brunette, their age and their vital statistics, according to the newspaper *Il Fatto Quotidiano* that published some of the transcripts. It also said that Tarantini used a mobile phone exclusively for his calls to Berlusconi, calling it the "red-light hotline".

Among the women Tarantini supplied were Barbara Montereale, a model, and the former prostitute Patrizia D'Addario who, it transpires, spent the night of Barack Obama's election with Berlusconi in Rome. Some celebration that must have been. The conversations often focused on the money Tarantini gave to the women and spent on gifts, including clothes and jewels, on Berlusconi's behalf. Other tapes were said to include conversations between Tarantini and the prostitutes who attended the parties.

In another intercept, Tarantini told Valter Lavitola, a former newspaper editor, that when news about the parties became public "there'll be an earthquake". While Berlusconi has said he had no idea that some of his guests were prostitutes, in one call Lavitola told Tarantini: "What could be dangerous and could come out is that you tell him: 'Listen, you've got to give me €10,000 because we've got to pay those whores.'"

Prosecutors believe that more than €500,000 has changed hands.

Tarantini, who had already been convicted of drug offences, was the subject of two investigations. In Bari, he was suspected of criminal conspiracy, pimping and corruption. In Naples, Lavitola, Tarantini and his wife Angela Devenuto were suspected of obtaining €850,000 from Berlusconi in exchange for Tarantini testifying that Berlusconi had no idea the guests were prostitutes. However, the prosecutors in Naples were also investigating the possibility that Berlusconi was being blackmailed.

Eventually, extracts from 3,500 pages of transcripts were published in the Italian press, though the *Corriere della Sera* said it had decided not to publish "the roughest or most vulgar passages, including detailed sexual descriptions, out of respect for readers". The leaks show that, between September 2008 and May 2009, there was almost daily contact between Berlusconi and Tarantini focusing on parties that the prime minister has previously described as "elegant dinners". In

January 2009, Berlusconi told Tarantini how he had seen in the New Year.

"Yesterday evening there was a queue outside my room . . . there were eleven of them," he said. "I had only eight of them because I couldn't manage more."

Well, he was getting old.

"But this morning I feel good," said Silvio. "I'm pleased with the way I manage to resist the challenges of life."

But there was a problem.

"Listen, all the beds are full here . . . this lot won't go home, even at gunpoint," said the old warhorse.

"But how many girls are there?" Tarantini asked.

"Forty," Berlusconi replied. "Anyway, I've bought a house near here to have more room . . . there's room for twelve more."

One of Tarantini's associates was overheard complaining he would need a caravan to pick up all the girls, while in another conversation Tarantini said to a colleague: "Find a whore, please."

Not that one would do.

"Listen, Gianpaolo, now we need at most two each," said Berlusconi in one call. "Because now I want that you have yours, otherwise I will always feel I am in your debt. Then we can trade. After all, the pussy needs to go around."

It is easy to understand why Berlusconi told one TV showgirl that he was only "prime minister in my spare time". On more than one occasion, Berlusconi complained that his commitments interfered with his social life. In October 2008 he asked Tarantini to bring only one woman, not three, because "I'm pretty busy right now". He went on to explain: "This week is terrible because on Saturday morning I'm receiving the Pope at the Quirinale [presidential palace] with the president. On Saturday afternoon, I'm in Paris with [Nicolas] Sarkozy and [Angela] Merkel and Gordon Brown, and on Sunday evening I'm speaking in Milan."

Later that month, he told Tarantini that "perhaps there were too many" women at a party the previous night. "Let's have two each at the most." He also praised the "golden little bottom" of Maria Esther Garcia Polanco, a lingerie model.

His women were, he said, "well provided for". This was of concern to one woman named Vanessa Di Meglio who sent a text from Berlusconi's residence to Tarantini at 5.52 one morning, asking "Who pays? Do we ask him or you?"

Earlier, in September 2008, Berlusconi planned to invite two senior TV executives from RAI to a party, telling Tarantini: "These are people who can get jobs for whoever they want, so the girls will get the idea they are with men who can decide their destiny."

Berlusconi hit back against the release of the wiretaps in a letter published in the newspaper *Il Foglio*.

"My private life is not a crime," he said. "My lifestyle may or may not please, it is personal, reserved and irreproachable."

Irreproachable? Hmm.

He told President Giorgio Napolitano last week that "if certain things come out, it won't be just me and the government which will be brought down, but the country too".

Court papers included a claim that the man who provided women for the parties had offered a well-known Italian actor the chance to present the annual San Remo song contest if she agreed to sleep with the seventy-five-year-old prime minister. Manuela Arcuri, the star of a string of TV dramas, said she refused.

Testimony was also leaked from Fadile Imane, a twenty-seven-year-old Moroccan model, who went to a party at Berlusconi's villa near Milan in February 2010. She said Nicole Minetti, the showgirl turned politician, and Barbara Faggioli, a former model, dressed up as nuns and then stripped for the prime minister while pole dancing.

Minetti, now a regional representative, denied the claim, but was then photographed in the Milan fashion district, wearing a top emblazoned with the words: "I'm even better without the T-shirt."

Imane also said that Berlusconi told her he was "madly in love" with Catarina, a young woman from Montenegro. During a dinner in September 2010, Catarina, whom Imane described as "psychologically fragile", was taken ill and escorted away by Berlusconi. He returned later, followed shortly afterwards by Catarina. When she saw him with other female guests, "she threw herself down the stairs," said Imane.

*L'espresso* identified her as twenty-year-old Katarina Knezevic, a former Miss Montenegro. It said she had a twin sister, and that in 2009 the pair, both models, had been photographed in Sardinia in the company of Madonna's ex-husband Guy Ritchie.

Berlusconi mentioned that he had a regular lover to rebut claims that he had wild parties at his home outside Milan. But the witness, another Moroccan belly dancer who said she was a reluctant participant in "bunga bunga" sessions, confirmed the claims.

When George Clooney, actor turned UN peace ambassador, visited Berlusconi to talk about the famine in Darfur, he was astonished to hear the prime minister joke about the "bunga bunga" parties. And Berlusconi proudly showed him the four-poster bed Russian premier Vladimir Putin had given him.

When Clooney said that he was leaving, Berlusconi begged him to stay. "There's going to be a party," said Berlusconi.

But Clooney said, "No, I gotta go."

According to Vanessa Di Meglio, after Clooney left, Berlusconi withdrew with two women while Di Meglio waited alone.

"Later the two girls came to call me and I joined them in a bedroom where the prime minister was too," she said. "There were advances."

Silvio allegedly made unspecified "gifts" to the three women the next day. He has consistently denied ever paying women for sex or any other impropriety.

Berlusconi got himself into more hot water when he said that he was thinking of renaming his political party Forza

Gnocca, which translates as "Go Pussy". Swamped in scandal and mired in a financial crisis, his coalition was sliding in the opinion polls.

"Some of the polls say the best choice would be Forza Gnocca," he joked, according to the Italian daily *La Stampa*.

Berlusconi has used the word *gnocca* publicly before, describing Margaret Thatcher in 2007 as a "*bella gnocca*". There is no accounting for taste.

As I write, while Berlusconi has resigned from office, he has yet to be convicted of anything. But if only a tenth of the allegations are true, at seventy-five he must be on industrial-strength Viagra. Or perhaps he is just the living embodiment of the Latin lover.

## Dominique Strauss-Kahn

When it comes to Latin lovers, it seems that the French have been attempting to rival the Italians. But Dominique Strauss-Kahn could not even wait to get into office before he got himself embroiled in a sex scandal.

A potential presidential candidate for the French Socialist Party, DSK, as he was known, was thought to be the only leftist able to beat Nicolas Sarkozy in the 2012 election. He was a well-known ladies' man, but that is something the French can forgive – even applaud – in a man.

While out of office, DSK became the managing director of the International Monetary Fund in September 2007, with Sarkozy's blessing. Perhaps he thought that DSK might disgrace himself on the international stage, while Sarkozy himself was getting over a little local difficulty in the romantic department.

In 2005, Sarkozy's wife Cecilia had left him for his friend, French-Moroccan national Richard Attias, who heads the Publicis Events Worldwide agency in New York, complaining Sarkozy was "a womanizer" who "loved no one". Meanwhile,

Sarkozy himself was said to be having an affair with Anne Fulda, a journalist on *Le Figaro*. Cecilia returned to stand beside him during the election in May 2007, but they divorced in October, five months after he had come to power.

In February 2008, Sarkozy married Italian singer, model and all-round rock chick Carla Bruni. There were reports of difficulties in the marriage with both parties having affairs. But then in October 2011 they had their first child, while he was away seeing Angela Merkel at the time – though it would be hard to make out anything was going on there.

DSK married his second wife Anne Sinclair in 1991, after warning her not to accept his proposal. He was a womanizer, he admitted, and he was not going to change. But she saw potential, in the political sphere at least. Of his sexual frolics, she said, "It is important for a politician to be able to seduce." Then in 2008 she stood by him when he faced a scandal over a sexual liaison with a junior colleague.

"That one-night-stand matter is behind us now, we have moved on," she said.

But he was building up for bigger things in the future.

On 14 May 2011, Strauss-Kahn was arrested and charged with the sexual assault and attempted rape of thirty-two-year-old Nafissatou Diallo, a Guinean housekeeper at the Sofitel New York Hotel in Manhattan earlier that day. He had already left for the airport, but had called the hotel asking them to send the cell phone he had left behind. Instead the police turned up at John F. Kennedy Airport and took him from his Paris-bound flight minutes before take-off. He was charged with four felony charges – two of criminal sexual acts, allegedly forcing the housekeeper to perform oral sex on him; one of attempted rape and one of sexual abuse – plus three misdemeanour offences, including unlawful imprisonment. He faced up to twenty-five years in prison. The US State Department determined that Strauss-Kahn's diplomatic immunity did not apply in this case.

The housekeeper, an asylum seeker from West Africa, picked him out of a line-up and provided a detailed account of the alleged assault. She said he emerged naked from the bathroom, grabbed her breasts and tried pulling down her pantyhose, before forcing her to perform oral sex. Strauss-Kahn, who had agreed to a forensic examination, pleaded not guilty. The judge detained him without bail pending the grand jury investigation. However, after a week, he was released from jail on one million US dollars bail on the condition he be confined to a New York apartment under armed guard while he awaited trial. He also had to wear an electronic tag on his ankle, turn over his passport and post an additional $5-million bail bond.

On 24 May, it was reported that the DNA tests of the semen found on Diallo's shirt had shown a match with the DNA sample from DSK. But Strauss-Kahn did not deny that they had had sex. He merely insisted that it was consensual. He pleaded not guilty. His lawyer Benjamin Brafman, said: "In our judgment, once the evidence has been reviewed, it will be clear that there was no element of forcible compulsion in this case whatsoever. Any suggestion to the contrary is simply not credible."

Meanwhile, the attorney for Nafissatou Diallo, Kenneth P. Thompson, said, "She is going to come into this courthouse, get on that witness stand and tell the world what Dominique Strauss-Kahn did to her."

The scandal was quickly portrayed as a clash of cultures. Here was an amorous Frenchman doing what came naturally – indeed, what would be expected of him in France where no one would have turned a hair. The worst that could be said of him was that he was a libertine. On the other hand, here was a poor black woman, a maid in a hotel, who had been forcibly taken advantage of by this oversexed foreigner. He had to be taught that this sort of thing was positively un-American.

While both God-fearing right-wing Americans and liberals who sought to protect ethnic minorities frothed at the mouth, left-wing journalist Jean-François Kahn spoke for much of France when he said of Strauss-Kahn: "He just lifted the skirt of a servant."

Others spoke of him admiringly as "the great seducer", though it was generally conceded that he was "NSIT" – Not Safe In Taxi. Indeed, it was said that he was NS in a lift, NS in an office, NS in a garden and especially NS in a hotel bedroom. But there was outrage that he was not given bail. After all, no one had been murdered.

Not only was Strauss-Kahn's DNA found on Diallo's clothes, but also on the carpet where she spat it out. Haven't women in America been taught to swallow? But the Gallic lobby remained sceptical. If he had tried raping her orally, couldn't she have bitten him?

A French newspaper which supported Sarkozy then claimed to have a leaked police report that suggested Strauss-Kahn had once been caught kerb-crawling in a red-light district of Paris. Diallo's attorney Kenneth Thompson hired a Parisian lawyer to look for women in France who might also have been victims of Strauss-Kahn's sexual predations. They did not have to look far. Step forward journalist and novelist Tristane Banon.

She said that, in 2002, when she was twenty-two, she had gone to interview fifty-three-year-old Strauss-Kahn. He met her in an apartment, empty except for a bed and a video camera. She told her mother, Anne Mansouret, that he had attacked her violently, ripped her bra off and acted like "a rutting chimpanzee", but as a Socialist Party stalwart and close friend of DSK, Mansouret persuaded her not to go to the police.

However, during a television chatshow in 2007, she referred to the interview, saying: "It ended really badly. We ended up fighting. It finished really violently. We fought on the floor. It wasn't a case of a couple of slaps. I kicked him. He unhooked my bra and tried to open my jeans. I said the word 'rape' to scare him but it didn't seem to scare him much. He was like a chimpanzee in rut."

Other women journalists reported "disturbing advances" from Strauss-Kahn during interviews. Sarkozy had even been warned about this before he put Strauss-Kahn's name forward to be head of the IMF. The Brussels correspondent of the newspaper *Libération*, Jean Quatremer, wrote a blog begging President Nicolas Sarkozy to reconsider.

"The only real problem with Strauss-Kahn is his attitude to women," Quatremer wrote. "He is too insistent . . . he often borders on harassment. The IMF is an international institution with Anglo-Saxon morals. One inappropriate gesture, one unfortunate comment, and there will be a huge media outcry."

Quatremer's blog was immediately attacked in the French press for "crossing a yellow line". He was criticized for his comments by the media correspondent of his own newspaper, Daniel Schneidermann, who asked why French journalists felt able to make such allegations on the internet but not in print. But Schneidermann went on to admit that DSK's reputation as an aggressive womanizer was well known.

DSK almost admitted as much himself. He said he saw three obstacles to his ambition to become president: "Money—" thanks to his wealthy wife he is seen as a champagne Socialist "—women and my Jewishness."

However, big holes began to appear in the Manhattan rape case. The housekeeper admitted to prosecutors that she had lied about what happened after the encounter with Strauss-Kahn. At first, she said that, after the attack, she cowered in a hallway until he left the room. Then she admitted that she had cleaned a nearby room, then returned to Strauss-Kahn's suite to finish off cleaning in there. Only then did she report to her supervisor that she had been attacked.

She also told investigators that her application for asylum included mention of a previous rape, but this was not the case. And she told the detectives that she had been subjected to genital mutilation, but again the details differed from what was in her asylum application.

Within a day of her encounter with Strauss-Kahn, Diallo phoned a man in prison and discussed the benefits of pursuing the charges against Strauss-Kahn. "Don't worry, this guy has a lot of money," she said. "I know what I'm doing."

The conversation was recorded. The recipient of the phone call had been arrested on charges of possessing 400 pounds of marijuana. He was among a number of individuals who made multiple cash deposits, totalling some $100,000, into the woman's bank account over the last two years. Investigators also learned that Diallo was paying hundreds of dollars every month in charges to five cell-phone companies. However, she insisted she had only one phone and said she knew nothing about the deposits except that they were made by a man she described as her fiancé and his friends.

When she had first been asked whether she had been a victim of other assaults, she said that she had been gang-raped in her own home by soldiers back in Guinea. Two weeks later she repeated the story with great emotion. But finally she admitted that it had never happened.

Strauss-Kahn was released from house arrest, then the charges against him were dropped. Though there had been evidence of sexual activity, there was no evidence that violence had been used. The victim had no marks or bruises. The only evidence against him was the accusations of the housekeeper, and she was an admitted liar.

Although Diallo continued to pursue a civil suit, Strauss-Kahn returned to Paris where friends and family rallied round.

"I don't believe for a single second the accusations of sexual assault by my husband," said his wife Anne Sinclair.

His previous wife, Brigitte Guillemette, insisted that violence was not part of his temperament and that it was "unthinkable and impossible" that he had raped a chambermaid. The Spanish writer Carmen Llera, a former lover, defended him in an open letter, declaring that "violence is not part of his culture" and denying that a book of poetry in which she wrote of a sadistic lover was about Strauss-Kahn. And Strauss-Kahn's biographer said that he was a "typical French lover, but he's not able to rape a woman".

Strauss-Kahn went on French television where, it was generally conceded, he was given an easy ride. Even Quatremer was kind. "He has been perfect," he said. "He sounded like someone who had committed a nine-minute, 'small' adultery."

However, there were demonstrators outside the studios who shouted, "Shame on you!" Most of them were women, and some carried signs saying, "When a woman says no, it's no!" Another read: "What's seduction for you?" A feminist group called *Le Barbe* – or The Beard – known for their ironic protests and wearing false beards, had called for demonstrations "in support of the Great White Men and their virile traditions".

Tristane Banon held off filing a legal complaint against Strauss-Kahn so that it could not be used in the New York case. But when he was released, she went ahead. Although Strauss-Kahn admitted trying to kiss Banon and that she had pushed him away, the prosecutors dismissed the case as there was no evidence of rape. The prosecutors admitted that they could have pursued charges on the lesser offence of sexual assault, but there was a statute of limitations on the charge and too much time had passed. Tristane dropped the charges.

*Le Journal du Dimanche*, a Sunday newspaper, then said that prostitutes working for the network that serviced senior police officers, lawyers and politicians had been flown to New York while Strauss-Kahn was there. *Le Figaro* also reported that Strauss-Kahn had met with prostitutes in a luxury hotel in Paris in 2010. One of the prostitutes claimed that she was paid €600 to attend an orgy with a "prominent political figure". *Le Figaro* said it was Strauss-Kahn.

This puts DSK in a new light. At least by choosing French girls, he was being patriotic this time. *Vive liberté, égalité, fraternité* – well, maybe not *fraternité* exactly in this case. However, it may not be enough to get Dominique Strauss-Kahn elected president – even in France.

## Jacob Zuma

Jacob Zuma became president of South Africa in 2009 after riding out a series of sex scandals. He is a polygamist who has six wives and twenty-two children. He brought his third first lady with him to dine with the queen in March 2010. By then he had divorced one wife, who went on to become Foreign Minister; another had committed suicide after twenty-four years of marriage, leaving a note to say life with Zuma had been "hell". But he was engaged to Gloria Bongekile Ngema who had already borne him a son and was pregnant with a second child.

This engagement caused a small ripple of scandal. Back in 2002, Zuma had paid the bride price of ten cattle for Princess Sebentile Dlamini, niece of the king of neighbouring Swaziland, but had not gone through with the marriage and has been married twice more since then. Fearing that he may no longer be interested in her, Dlamini has spent time in hospital for depression. Who can blame her?

He has a number of other children outside wedlock. There is Edward, whose mother is Minah Shongwe, the sister of Transvaal Deputy Judge President Jeremiah Shongwe. He was present at the marriage of his father to his fourth wife, Nompumelelo Ntuli, who already had two children by him, and is thought to be Zuma's heir. On the eve of his presidential address in February 2011, it emerged that he has two daughters, aged seven and twelve, with prominent Pietermaritzburg businesswoman Priscilla Nonkululeko Mhlongo.

There were also reports that he had a girl and a set of twins with a "coloured" woman from Johannesburg. Under the old apartheid classifications, "coloured" meant someone who was neither white nor black – that is, mixed race, Indian or Chinese. The girl, Bridget, lived with Zuma's fifth wife Tobeka Madiba, whom he married amid a media storm in 2010. The twins Duduzile and Duduzane have a reputation for their blinged-out lifestyle. Then there is his daughter Jabulile whose mother was a woman from Richard's Bay.

In January 2010, it was reported that Zuma had a love child with Sonono Khoza, daughter of South Africa's World Cup football chief Irvin Khoza, a family friend. Then it appeared that Zuma and Sonono might be married. The application for a birth certificate for their daughter Thandekile Matina Zuma has the answer "yes" in reply to the question: "Are the parents of the child married to each other?" Under "Nature of Marriage", the option "customary" was checked.

Meanwhile, the paternity of the son born to Nompumelelo Ntuli in August 2010 came into question. The child, Manqoba Kholwani, meaning "believe it", is said to have been born as the result of an alleged affair between thirty-five-year-old MaNtuli, as the fourth Mrs Zuma is known, and her bodyguard, Phinda Thomo.

Details were leaked in an anonymous letter to a local newspaper shortly before the 2010 World Cup in South Africa. It was said that Thomo, who was from Soweto, killed himself shortly after his alleged affair was discovered. The letter also claimed that the sixty-eight-year-old president and his wife had been estranged for some time before the birth of Manqoba Kholwani.

In April, MaNtuli's family presented Zuma with a white goat, which was then ritually slaughtered. This traditional ceremony was interpreted as MaNtuli atoning for "bad behaviour". It seemed there had been a row over Zuma's plans to take another wife. MaNtuli had earlier had two other children by Zuma. The president was said to have visited the mother and her new child before flying to Namibia for a regional summit. A presidential spokesman declined to comment on the birth. Nevertheless, the press ask how much Zuma's children cost the taxpayer and the opposition say that he is not setting a good example of safe sex in Aids-plagued South Africa.

In December 2005, Zuma was accused of raping a thirty-one-year-old woman at his home in Forest Town, Johannesburg. The alleged victim was from a prominent ANC family, the daughter of a comrade of Zuma's in the struggle against apartheid, who had since died. She was also an Aids activist who was known to be HIV positive. Zuma denied the rape charges and insisted that the sex was consensual. At the time, he had already been sacked as deputy president by Thabo Mbeki over charges of fraud and corruption, which were later dismissed, and his career was at its nadir.

The judge, Jeremiah Shongwe, grandfather of Zuma's son, had to excuse himself from the trial. When the case went ahead, up to a thousand people gathered outside the high court in Johannesburg. Most were Zuma supporters who sang and danced to pro-Zuma pop songs, and waved placards. One read: "You are the best JZ." Zuma himself sang the ANC anthem "*Lethu Mshini Wami*" – "Bring me my machine gun". There were also about fifty anti-rape protesters.

The Judge Willem van der Merwe allowed the defence to admit questions concerning the woman's sexual history, though her identity was not to be revealed. She had been diagnosed as HIV positive in 1999, but had not told Zuma until two years later. He had been a close friend of her father when they all lived in exile during the struggle against apartheid. She had known him since she was five and said she regarded him as an uncle and a father figure.

On 2 November 2005, she had stayed at his home. "Uncle said to me I must go and prepare for bed," the tearful woman told the hushed courtroom. "He said, 'Then I'll come and tuck you in.' I thought it was a bit strange."

Although one of his daughters was in the house, Zuma entered the bedroom and began to "massage" her shoulders. She said she told him "no", but he persisted.

"I said, 'No.' But he did not stop massaging me," she said. "At that point I saw that he was naked. I thought, Oh no, Uncle cannot be naked. He is on top of me and I am in his house. I thought, This can't be happening. And at that point I faced the reality that I was just about to be raped." She said he proceeded to rape her while holding her hands above her head.

The prosecution maintained that she did not put up any resistance to Zuma's advances because she was in a state of shock. She sobbed as she said she was too paralysed with fear to run away.

Although she had discussed the fact that she was HIV positive with him several times, he did not wear a condom.

The plaintiff said she waited for two days to report the alleged rape to police because she regarded Mr Zuma as "family" and had later come under pressure from various people. She said she had even been offered money to drop the case. "One said: 'Do you know what this will do to the ANC? It will rip apart the lives of people.' I felt very pressured."

Zuma responded in statement read by his lawyer, saying that the woman had consented to sex.

"My daughter was in the house," he said. "She could have left at any time."

"This is not a shy fifteen- or sixteen-year-old girl . . . She knows how to stand up for herself," said his defence lawyer.

During cross-examination, Zuma said that he had left the bedroom after having sex with the woman and taken a shower because this "would minimize the risk of contracting the disease [HIV]". Get a grip.

He also said that he was prepared to marry the woman who accused him of rape. Her aunts were discussing the possibility of marriage and a bride price as Zulu tradition dictates.

"Yes, if we had reached an agreement with that, I would have had my cows ready," Mr Zuma told the court. This was the traditional "*lobola*" whereby a would-be husband gives cattle to his intended bride's family.

Judge van der Merwe ruled that the state had failed to prove rape beyond reasonable doubt. "I find that consensual sex took place between the complainant and the accused," he said. He also criticized the complainant, saying she had not been a credible witness and citing defence witnesses who said she had previously brought false rape charges against them. Some had said she "needed help".

Delivering the judgment, he said: "It would be foolish for any man with a police guard at hand and his daughter not far away to surprise a sleeping woman and to start raping her without knowing whether she would shout the roof off."

Judge van der Merwe said "he would not even comment" on Mr Zuma's evidence that he had a shower after the intercourse to lessen his chances of contracting Aids. And he chided Zuma for engaging in unprotected sex with a woman who was a family friend, half his age, not his regular partner, and especially as he knew that she was HIV-positive. This was, he said, "totally unacceptable behaviour".

At a press conference the following day, Zuma apologized to the nation. He said he hoped that his trial would not be a setback for the campaigns against Aids and rape.

"I erred in having unprotected sex," he said. "I should have known better and should have acted more cautiously. I unconditionally apologize to all the people of our nation and I pledge to continue supporting the struggle against HIV and Aids and the struggle against gender-based violence."

At the African National Congress party conference in December 2007, Jacob Zuma was selected over Thabo Mbeki as president of the ANC. Despite further obstacles, he went on to become president of South Africa.

## Omar Bongo

President of the West African state of Gabon from 1967 until his death in office in 2009, Omar was implicated in a good old-fashioned sex scandal by a court case in Paris in April 1995. The court was told that Bongo was regularly supplied with prostitutes by the Italian couturier who made his made-to-measure suits.

The trial of Francesco Smalto, the Paris-based menswear designer, gave an insight into the ferocious competition in the fashion world to secure celebrity clients. It also painted a deeply unflattering portrait of Bongo. The court was told that Smalto hired the prostitutes and sent them to Gabon. But they were terrified of having sex with Bongo, because he refused to wear a condom. Bongo was not in court to defend himself, but his Parisian lawyer and doctor denied the charges on his behalf.

The Paris police had been investigating a deluxe call-girl ring when Smalto got caught in their net. Part of the ring was a model agency run by a young woman named Laure Moerman. She supplied Smalto with models for his collection. Several of the models said that they were sent to Gabon's capital Libreville with Smalto's collections of suits. Their job was to help the Gabonese president out of his clothes.

The presiding judge read out the testimony of a girl named Monica who had been on one of the trips to Libreville.

"It went very badly that evening," she said. "Bongo didn't want to wear a condom and, as he had a friend who had died of Aids, I refused to make love to him."

Another girl, Chantal, testified that she had been told that the going rate for sex with Bongo was £1,200 with a condom and £6,000 without.

Although these prices may seem a little over the top, money meant little to Bongo. He was one of the richest men in Africa. When the society jeweller Chaumet ran into financial difficulties, it was discovered that Bongo owed them £500,000.

Initially, Smalto had denied all knowledge of the girls' allegations. But then he told the court that Bongo was his best customer. He spent £300,000 a year on suits and other clothes and Smalto had been frightened of losing him to a rival.

"We knew that President Bongo was sensitive to a feminine presence," Smalto told the court. "That is why we sent a girl on every trip. I suspected that he kept her to sleep with, but I wasn't sure."

The transcript of the recording of a telephone conversation between two prostitutes named Ariane and Sarah was read out.

"Marika telephoned me, she had to go to Libreville. I told her that's dramatic. His [Bongo's] friend died of the thing," said Ariane.

"Aids? That's disgusting," said Sarah.

"Yes, the worst is, a great couturier proposed it," Ariane replied.

Smalto, who had been known as "the king of tailors and tailor to kings", was ruined. Bongo went elsewhere to buy his suits.

Nine years later, Bongo was embroiled in another sex scandal. In February 2004, the *New York Times* reported that Peru was investigating claims that a beauty pageant contestant was lured to Gabon to become the lover of the sixty-seven-year-old president. According to the Peruvian Foreign Ministry, twenty-two-year-old Ivette Santa Maria, then Miss Peru, was invited to Gabon ostensibly to be a hostess for a pageant there. Ms Santa Maria said that she was taken to the presidential palace just hours after she arrived in the country. When the president joined her, "he pressed a button and some sliding doors opened, revealing a large bed".

She said, "I told him I was not a prostitute, that I was Miss Peru."

She fled and guards offered to drive her to a hotel. But without money to pay the bill, she was stranded in Gabon for twelve days until international women's groups rode to her rescue.

Of course, these scandals did not hurt Bongo at the polls. In 1968, he had outlawed all opposition parties and used the country's oil revenues to buy himself political allies.

## Juan and Eva Perón

Thanks to Andrew Lloyd Webber and Tim Rice and their musical *Evita*, the whole world got to know that Argentina's most famous first lady had been a prostitute in her youth. But Messers Lloyd Webber and Rice neglected to inform their audiences of a greater scandal – her husband, Juan Domingo Perón, was eventually kicked out of office for being a paedophile.

Evita was born Maria Eva Duarte in the small town of Los Toldos in 1919. She was the daughter of wealthy local landowner Juan Duarte and his mistress of fifteen-years' standing Juanita Ibarguren. Eva was just seven when her father died. Her mother was left to make ends meet by running an *amoblados* or "love hotel".

Growing up in a dusty town in the pampas, her prospects were not good. At the age of fourteen, she slept with the small-time tango singer José Armani to get a ride 150 miles to Buenos Aires. She would later claim her first lover was singing star Agustin Magaldi, as in the musical.

Arriving in Buenos Aires, Evita had little option but to start at the bottom. She posed for pornographic pictures and worked as a prostitute. She had the looks to be an actress so, at the age of fifteen, she became the mistress of Emilio Kartulovic, publisher of the movie magazine *Sintonia*, for his contacts she needed. Then she moved on to the impresario Rafael Firtuso, owner of the Liceo Theatre. He cast her in one of his productions and she was sent out on a provincial tour in a play called *The Mortal Kiss*. Sponsored by the Argentine Prophylactic League, it was a morality tale about the evils of promiscuity – hardly typecasting.

Back in Buenos Aires, Eva landed a number of small parts in movies. At night she would entertain wealthy businessmen. Then she got her big break on the radio and quickly became queen of the soaps.

In June 1943, a number of ambitious officers, including Juan Perón, staged a military coup. Always ambitious, Evita began bedding the Minister of Communications, Colonel Anibal Imbert, who moved her into a smart apartment off the fashionable Avenida Alvear.

An earthquake destroyed the town of San Juan in January 1944 and Eva persuaded him to stage a benefit for the victims to be broadcast nationwide. Naturally, Argentine's leading soap star would be guest of honour. Juan Perón, the rising strongman of the new regime, arrived with the movie star Libertad Lamarque on his arm. But when Libertad stood up to sing, Eva slipped into the chair she had vacated beside him. The forty-eight-year-old Perón already had a reputation for liking young girls. Evita was already twenty-four, but she was younger than Lamarque. Thanks to her profession, she knew how to please a man and easily seduced him. A few days later, she kicked out Perón's teenage mistress and moved into his apartment.

In 1939, Perón had been military attaché in Rome and had travelled extensively throughout Germany, Hungary, Austria, Spain and Portugal. He was convinced that Fascism would work in Argentina and was planning a new coup with a few like-minded officers.

Evita convinced Perón that the traditional source of popular power in Argentina was the gauchos. Once the proud independently minded cowboys on the pampas, they had now migrated to the shanty towns around the cities in search of work. Then Minister of Labour, Perón was in the position to mobilize their support. He introduced a minimum wage, paid holidays, sick leave and a Christmas bonus.

His growing popularity among the poor *descamisados*, or "shirtless ones", was soon seen as a threat to moneyed interests, who staged a coup of their own. Perón was arrested, but Eva quickly rallied the labour unions. The *descamisados* took to the streets in protest. Perón was released. That night, he addressed a crowd of 300,000 from the balcony of the presidential palace. A few days later, he married Evita.

Elected president, Perón used his powers to cover up the details of Eva's past. Nude photographs of her were collected and destroyed. The regime invested a good deal in her popularity. Although she dressed in jewels and furs, she was portrayed as a woman of the people. In propaganda posters, she was portrayed as the Virgin Mary, the personification of Perónist beauty. Apparently, she worked tirelessly for the people, her only reward being a kiss on the forehead by Juan. Somehow the furs, jewels and bulging Swiss bank account were overlooked.

Not everyone was fooled. The writer and leading opponent of the regime, Jorge Luis Borges said: "Perón's wife was a common prostitute. She had a brothel near Junín. And it must have embittered him, no? I mean, if a girl is a whore in a large city that doesn't mean too much, but in a small town on the pampas, everybody knows everybody else."

One day, she was riding in an official car with an elderly Italian admiral when the crowd began taunting her. She said to the admiral, "Do you hear that? They are calling me a whore."

"I quite understand," he said. "I haven't been to sea for fifteen years and they still call me an admiral."

The Perón regime used torture and strong-arm methods to suppress political opponents. Evita kept a collection of rebel leaders' testicles in a glass jar on her desk to intimidate those who came to visit her. Otherwise, she maintained her position in the regime by using her womanly wiles on her colleagues who were exclusively men. However, Evita had not entirely turned her back on her past. She did try to legalize prostitution and regulate the red-light districts.

In 1947, Evita made a trip to Italy where she visited Aristotle Onassis in his villa on the Italian Riviera. She made love to him and, afterwards, made him an omelette as he wrote out a cheque for $10,000 for one of her charities. He remarked later that it was the most expensive omelette he had ever eaten.

She then visited Rome where she was greeted by crowds giving the straight-armed Fascist salute outlawed since the end of World War II. The police made arrests.

Evita died of cancer at the age of thirty-three. Florists in Buenos Aires ran out of flowers and eight people were crushed to death, and two thousand injured, in the mourning throngs. Her working-class followers tried to have her canonized. Sadly, her husband could not live up to the virtuous image he had created for her. After the state funeral, Juan Perón found his taste for teenage girls undiminished. He began to take an interest in the Union of Secondary School Students. It had branches in every school and young girl recruits were sent to luxurious "recreational centres" overseen by high-ranking government officials. There, medical teams were on hand to cope with unplanned pregnancies and sexually transmitted diseases.

Perón had his own private recreational centre, where he could watch teenage girls playing basketball or swimming. One of them piqued a special interest. Her name was Nélida "Nelly" Rivas. The daughter of a worker in a sweet factory, she was just thirteen. One day at the recreational centre, she was told that she had been picked to have lunch with the president. It was the first of many. Soon she moved out of her parents' small apartment where she slept on a sofa at the end of their bed and into the love nest built in the basement of one of Perón's villas, which had bearskin rugs on the floor and mirrored walls.

While the relationship was primarily sexual, he also spent time on her education. He even planned to send her on an educational trip to Europe, but she said she did not want to leave him. "The very thought of leaving the residence brought me to the brink of madness," she recalled later.

As the economy faltered and his repressive regime grew increasingly unpopular, stories about Perón's thirteen-year-old mistress appeared in the gossip columns. Asked about her age, the fifty-nine-year-old Perón said he was "not superstitious". Despite his wit, his supporters deserted him in droves. It seems he had besmirched the image of the saintly Evita. After a coup, Perón fled for his life, leaving Nelly behind. He sought refuge on a Paraguayan gunboat provided by Paraguayan strongman Alfredo Stroessner. Before it took him into exile in Venezuela, he wrote one last note to Nelly.

"My dear baby girl," it said, "I miss you every day, as I do my little dogs ... Many kisses and many desires. Until I see you soon, Papi."

A military court tried Perón in absentia for paedophilia and their lurid correspondence was published. He was convicted and stripped of his rank for "conduct unworthy of an officer and a gentleman".

In conclusion, the judge said: "It is superfluous to stress the horror of the court at the proof of such a crime committed by one who always claimed that the only privileged people in the country were the children."

While Perón moved on to Panama, where he copped off with Argentine nightclub singer María Estela Martínez, known as "Isabel", Nelly was sent to a reformatory for eight months, then went into exile with her parents in Montevideo. Evita's remains, which had been on display in the headquarters of the CGT labour union, were sent to Italy where they were buried under a false name.

Perón moved on to Spain where he married Isabel. In 1971, there was another coup in Argentina and, in a gesture of reconciliation, Evita's remains were returned to Perón in Spain.

In 1973, Perón returned to Argentina to run in the presidential elections with his third wife as his running mate. They were elected with sixty-two per cent of the vote, but Perón died the following year. His widow succeeded him, but she was no Evita. In a last-ditch attempt to cash in on her legacy, she had Evita's remains flown home from Spain and interred next to her husband in a crypt in the presidential palace.

But for many, this only seemed to confirm Isabel's illegitimacy. In 1976, the Air Force seized power. Isabel was held under house arrest for five years before being banished back to Spain, where she died in 1985.

## Eliza Lynch and Francisco Solano López

Eva Perón was not the first prostitute to be a first lady in South America. In the 1860s an Irish courtesan served as the consort of Francisco Solano López, one of the most scandalous dictators even that benighted continent has ever seen. He went to war with Argentina, Brazil and Uruguay in an attempt to fulfil his promise to make her the Empress of South America.

Born in Asunción, the capital of Paraguay, in 1827, Francisco Solano López was the eldest son of the Perpetual Dictator, Carlos Antonio López. He was not a pretty picture. The US ambassador to Asunción described him as:

... short and stout, always inclined to corpulence. He dressed grotesquely, but his costumes were always expensive and elaborately finished. His eyes, when he was pleased, had a mild expression; but when he was enraged the pupils seemed to dilate till it did not appear to be that of a human being, but rather a wild beast goaded to madness. He had, however, a gross animal look that was repulsive when his face was in repose. His forehead was narrow and his head small, with the rear organs largely developed. His teeth were very much decayed, and so many of the front ones were gone as to render his articulation somewhat difficult and indistinct. He apparently took no pains to keep them clean, and those which remained were unwholesome in appearance, and nearly as dark as the cigar that he had almost constantly between them. His face was rather flat, and his nose and his hair indicated more of the Negro than the Indian. His cheeks had a fullness that extended to the jowl, giving him a sort of bulldog expression.

Not exactly Brad Pitt, but that did not bother Francisco. He would simply grab any woman he wanted and jail her father if she did not comply.

Francisco wanted the beautiful young Pancha Garmendia, known as the "jewel of Asunción". He could not jail her father as he had already been executed by Carlos López's predecessor, El Supremo, the First Perpetual Dictator of Paraguay. So Francisco jailed her brothers instead. But still she resisted, so he kept her in chains to be beaten and raped daily until her death some twenty years later.

Next his attention turned to Carmencita Cordal. She refused him on the grounds that she was engaged to be married to Carlos Decoud, the son of one of the leading families of Paraguay. The night before their wedding, Carlos's naked and mutilated body was hurled through the window of Carmencita's home. Understandably, she went loopy and spent the rest of her life in widow's weeds, picking flowers by moonlight and praying at deserted shrines.

Paraguay's wealthy landowners took fright. Anyone with money and a passport began heading out of the country. To save the situation, Carlos López sent Francisco to Europe to buy a navy. Paraguay hardly needed one. It is landlocked.

He bought one paddle steamer in England, but the rest of the money was put to good use in Paris on, as the American ambassador put it, "his natural licentious propensities, and . . . the vices of that gay city".

Francisco fancied to make himself the Napoleon of South America and was eager to meet the great man's nephew Napoleon III, who was then on the throne of France. He was presented at court, but when he kissed the Empress Eugénie's hand she was so revolted that she vomited. The Emperor apologized, explaining his wife was pregnant. She wasn't.

A lot of the navy money Francisco had been entrusted with was spent on courtesans. One of the most famous *grande horizontales* at the time was Eliza Lynch. Born in County Cork in 1835, her family had fled to France in 1845 to escape the potato famine. At fifteen, she married an officer in the French Army who took her to North Africa, where she was raped by her husband's commanding officer. A career officer, her husband stood by and let this happen.

She was rescued by a dashing young Russian aristocrat. He killed her assailant in a duel and took her to Paris. They set up home together in the then up-and-coming Boulevard Saint Germain. But the Crimean War had just started. He had already killed one Frenchman, so he took off home to fight.

Eliza now had a large mansion to maintain and in the Paris of the Second Empire there was only one career path open to her and she was well qualified for it. An Argentine journalist wrote of her:

> She was tall with a flexible and delicate figure with beautiful and seductive curves. Her skin was alabaster. Her eyes were of a blue that seems borrowed from the very hues of heaven and had an expression of ineffable sweetness in whose depths the light of Cupid was enthroned. Her beautiful lips were indescribably expressive of the voluptuous, moistened by an ethereal dew that God must have provided to lull the fires within her, a mouth that was like a cup of delight at the banqueting table of ardent passion. Her hands were small with long fingers, the nails perfectly formed and delicately polished. She was, evidently, one of those women who make the care of their appearance a religion.

Added to that Eliza had a quick wit, a flair for languages and an eye for money. She had gaming tables set up outside her boudoir so that her gentlemen callers could lose their money while they awaited her attentions.

Francisco was spraying money around Paris like champagne. When he turned up at Eliza's establishment, she knew him for a mark and whisked him straight into the bedroom. This was a new experience for Francisco. He had never had a lover who did not put up a struggle before. In the morning, he offered to make her the Empress of South America.

They set off on a shopping trip around Europe. On their way, they visited the battlefields of the Crimea, where Francisco could pick up tips on modern warfare and, perhaps, Eliza could see her Russian lover. In Rome, Eliza held a "wickedly obscene" dinner party for the Pope. They also dropped in on the notoriously promiscuous Queen Isabella II of Spain.

Then, laden with trunks full of jewellery and expensive clothing, Eliza and Francisco set sail for South America. Unsure of the reception that awaited them in Asunción, Francisco and Eliza broke their trip at Buenos Aires. Back in Paraguay, Carlos had already heard that his son was heading home with "*una ramera Irlandesa*" – an Irish prostitute – but he was getting old and needed his son and heir back in the country.

Francisco and Eliza began the 1,000-mile trip up the Paraná and Paraguay rivers. By the time they arrived in Asunción, she was pregnant. Francisco's mother and sisters shunned her. But the beautiful Eliza, wearing the latest décolleté fashions from Paris, caused a sensation.

In Asunción, Francisco had other interests. He maintained his former lover and their two children in his town house, and took as many other lovers as he could handle. Eliza realized she could not stop this, so she took charge. She selected his new lovers for him. As a Catholic, she could not marry him herself, so she would make damn sure that he would marry no one else. No other woman would be allowed to challenge her position.

Francisco's seduction technique had not improved. When the daughter of Pedro Burgos, a magistrate from Luque, refused him, Francisco said he would confiscate her father's property. It was an empty threat as Burgos was a friend of Francisco's father, who was still in power. So Eliza intervened. Once deflowered, there was no danger that Burgos's daughter would marry Francisco. So she persuaded Burgos to give her up, on the promise that he would be well rewarded when Francisco came to power. He never got to cash in as Francisco had Burgos summarily executed when he took over.

By manipulating his mistresses, Eliza controlled Francisco. She persuaded him to begin a building programme to transform Asunción from a shanty town to an imperial capital. They built an opera house, but the architect did not know how to do roofs and the opera house remained open to the elements until 1955. But the centrepiece of the emerging city was a replica of Napoleon's tomb at Les Invalides in Paris. This was to be Francisco's own mausoleum.

When Eliza gave birth to a healthy son, Francisco was so delighted that he ordered a 100-gun-salute. The noise caused eleven buildings in downtown Asunción to collapse, including five newly built under Francisco's urban development plan. And one of the guns, which had not been cleaned properly, backfired, killing half the battery and injuring the rest.

To secure their new son's place in his father's affections, Eliza wanted the child baptized in Asunción's Catedral de la Encarnacion. Francisco's mother and sister objected, and Carlos banned it. And the Bishop of Paraguay, who was Carlos's brother, threatened to excommunicate any priest who performed the ceremony. But Eliza was not to be thwarted. She found a corrupt priest named Father Palacios to baptize the boy, promising to make him Bishop of Paraguay when Francisco succeeded to the presidency.

When the new National Theatre was opened, Carlos and his wife were ushered into the "royal box". This was a small box to the left of the stage, while Eliza and Francisco occupied a large box in the centre of auditorium.

The ladies of Asunción naturally sided with Carlos's wife and daughters, and refused to attend Eliza's salons. But they could not stop their husbands attending, lured there by Eliza's low-cut gowns and magnificent figure. However, Francisco was still determined that the ladies of Asunción, particularly his mother and sisters, accept his consort. He had organized an agricultural colony for French immigrants upstream in the Rio de la Plata region of Paraguay called New Bordeaux. There was to be an official visit there. While the diplomatic corps would travel there on horseback, the ladies would go by boat. They could hardly refuse. Madame Lynch was made official hostess on-board.

As the womenfolk embarked, they pointedly ignored Eliza. Once they set off, a huge buffet was laid out. Eliza tried to officiate, but the other women turned their back on her and would not let her near the table. So she ordered the captain to moor the boat in the middle of the stream and had all the food and wine thrown overboard. The women of Asunción were left there in the tropical heat without food or drink for the next ten hours.

When Carlos López died, Francisco took over and ordered that Madame Lynch should be accorded the same privileges as those usually enjoyed by the wife of a head of state. Good to her word, Eliza made Father Palacios Bishop of Paraguay. Now he passed on vital intelligence gleaned in the confessional. Soon half the population of Asunción were in jail or in exile for opposing Francisco.

The British ambassador called Eliza "the Paraguayan Pompadour". She began hosting glittering balls, which the ladies of Asunción had to attend. Francisco continued in his old ways, maintaining several houses where he entertained prostitutes. But as head of state, he felt that he should make a marriage suitable to his new status. He set his cap at Princess

Isabella of Brazil. But Eliza was not going to sit still for this. She demanded that Francisco legitimize their children. When Princess Isabella heard this, she decided to marry the Comte d'Eu, one of the French royal family instead.

To celebrate the first anniversary of Francisco López's accession to power, Eliza organized a carnival where, as one observer put it, the population of Asunción "actively engaged in raising the birth rate".

Eliza had ambitions of her own. Not content to be the First Lady of Paraguay, she reminded Francisco that he had promised to make her the Empress of South America. She inveigled him into war with Argentina, Brazil and Uruguay simultaneously and organized a victory ball, where the wealthy ladies of Asunción were expected to hand over their jewellery to support the war effort. She caused more scandal by throwing open the palace doors to the city's prostitutes, insisting that "all classes mingle as one on so festive an occasion". The victory was, of course, the first of a long series of defeats.

While Francisco was away at the front, Eliza served as regent. Then she was seen riding at the head of the cavalry and manning the defences. The war dragged on for six years. All the men in the country were called up, leaving the women to plough the fields. Not only were they both surrounded and hopelessly outnumbered, but Francisco turned every rout into an even greater disaster by summarily shooting his own men for cowardice. Eventually, it was said, there was not a man left alive over the age of nine. A truce was offered on the proviso that Francisco went into exile in Europe. He tortured and killed anyone thought to be in favour of it, including his two brothers.

If the odds were not stacked against him enough already, Francisco turned on Paraguay's foreign residents. Britain, America, France and Italy all sent gunboats to blockade the only river route in and out of the country. As the armies of the Triple Alliance advanced, they were forced to evacuate Asunción.

Francisco took his mother and sisters and imprisoned them in a bullock cart. His sisters and mother, though over seventy, were regularly flogged, while the jewel of Asunción, Pancha Garmendia, still in chains, was dragged along behind.

Eventually, they were cornered in the remote north-east of the country. Francisco was cut down by the Brazilian cavalry. Eliza was caught fleeing through the jungle in a ball gown. A young Brazilian officer took pity on her and smuggled her out of the country. She headed for London where 4,000 ounces of gold were waiting for her on deposit in the Bank of England. It had been smuggled out by the American and Italian ambassadors. The former American ambassador to Paraguay was often seen at her side, handling her business affairs.

Eliza returned to Paris to live in some style. When she died in 1886, she was buried in Père Lachaise Cemetery. Then one night in 1961, she was disinterred and taken back to Paraguay where she now lies in the largest marble mausoleum on the southern continent, a fitting resting place for the Empress of South America.

## Karl Marx

OK, so the founder of modern Communism lived in London for half his life. But he was refused British nationality, on the grounds that he had been disloyal to the king of Prussia. Nevertheless, he remained a foreigner and this book badly needs some political balance. After all, it is a relief to know that Marx did not spend his entire life scratching away in the Reading Room of the British Museum – which is a mere hop, step and a jump from where this book is being written.

In 1851, Marx faced a scandal. While his wife Jenny was pregnant, he managed to knock up Helene "Lenchen" Demuth, the maid they had brought with them from Germany. Jenny had been away in Holland at the time, trying to borrow some money from an uncle to support her feckless husband.

It would never have happened otherwise. The three of them shared a bedroom in a small apartment in Dean Street in London's Soho and Jenny was fiercely jealous.

On the birth certificate, the child was given the name Henry Frederick Demuth. But the space for the father's name and occupation were left blank. The child was swiftly fostered in London's East End. Marx made no attempt to see the boy, or make provision for him lest it gave substance to the rumours that were flying. To avert any scandal tainting the great man, the co-author of the Communist Manifesto and Marx's patron Friedrich Engels pretended the child was his, only confessing the truth on his deathbed in 1895, twelve years after the death of Marx.

Living in such close proximity, Jenny must have known what was happening, but kept quiet about it for the good of the cause.

Freddy Demuth spent his entire adult life in the London borough of Hackney. He worked as a lathe-operator in a number of East End factories until his death in 1929. A stalwart of the Amalgamated Engineering Union and a founding member of the Hackney Labour Party, he was remembered as a quiet man who did not talk about his family.

The truth only came out in 1962, though some dyed-in-the-wool Marxists claim that the documentary evidence was forged by Nazi agents in an effort to discredit socialism.

## Sophie Dawes

Barefooted winkle-picker from the Isle of Wight, Sophie Dawes made it big in – or, should that be, with – foreign parts and her irresistible rise was punctuated with scandal. Born in St Helens in 1792, she was the youngest daughter of a local oyster-catcher, whose sideline as a smuggler kept the family in comparative comfort. But when he died, they were reduced to winkle-picking on Bembridge Beach before going to the workhouse at Parkhurst.

Sophie ran away to Portsmouth. Then, to make the most of her physical charms, she moved to London. She got a job as an assistant in a milliner's shop, but was dismissed for having an affair with a young water-carrier. After selling oranges in Covent Garden, she took to the stage and became the mistress of a wealthy gentleman from Turnham Green. When he tired of her, she went to work in a brothel in Piccadilly. There she attracted the attention of Monsieur Guy, the manservant of an exiled French nobleman, Louis-Henri-Joseph, the Duc de Bourbon. She became his willing mistress and even allowed him to use her as a stake in a game of cards with the Duke of Kent. The Duc became so enamoured of her that he spent huge sums on having her taught French, Greek, Latin, music, dancing and deportment.

When Napoleon was exiled to Elba in 1814, the Duc returned to Paris. Sophie followed but found the Palais Bourbon and the family estates at Montmorency, Guise, Enghiem and Chantilly were closed to her as long as the Duc's father, the Prince de Condé, lived. For the next four years, she lived in lodgings in Paris, rarely seeing her lover.

Then in 1818 her patience was rewarded. The Duc's father died and he became Prince de Condé. She could now enter Bourbon's household, but not as his official mistress as she was a mere commoner. Instead, she would pose as his illegitimate daughter and, for the sake of appearances, she was married off to Adrien de Feuchères, an officer in Louis XVIII's Guards. But as mistress of the Bourbon estates, Madame de Feuchères was known as the Queen of Chantilly.

Now twenty-six, Sophie dominated the sixty-year-old prince, bringing her nephew, a meat-packer from London, over to be his equerry. She took a score of lovers, including the prince's own hairdresser. Finally, this all grew too much for her husband who horsewhipped and divorced her, causing a huge public scandal. Everywhere she went Sophie faced boos and catcalls.

The ageing prince's health began to deteriorate. Sophie feared that he might die without including her in his will. So she struck a deal with the impoverished Orleans family. If she could get the childless Prince de Condé to leave his wealth to the Duc de Aumale – the Duc de Orleans's penniless son – they would provide her with a substantial allowance. Eventually, she badgered the prince into settling eighty million francs on the Duc de Aumale.

However, in 1830, the Bourbon king, Charles X, was forced into exile and Louis-Philippe, Duc de Orleans, became king of France, with the Duc de Aumale as Dauphin. As the Duc de Aumale did not need the money any more, the Prince de Condé decided to change his will in favour of the Duc de Bordeaux, the exiled king's grandson. Louis-Philippe told Sophie to stop him at all costs.

On the night of 27 August 1830, at Sophie's behest, her current lover, a sergeant in the gendarmes, crept into the prince's apartment and smothered him while he slept. Then, he tied two handkerchiefs round the corpse's neck and hung it from the crossbar of the window to make it look like suicide.

An inquiry into the prince's death found that he hardly had the strength to walk, let alone reach up to the crossbar to attach the makeshift noose. Besides, the noose was not tight enough to cause strangulation. However, Louis-Philippe brought pressure to bear and Sophie escaped the guillotine.

However, this second scandal forced her to leave France with her nephew. He died soon after. It was rumoured he had been poisoned because he knew too much. But Sophie had him buried in St Helens under a magnificent memorial that says it was "Erected by his aunt, Madame La Barrone de Feuchères".

Sophie grew old and fat. She gave much of her fortune to the church and charities. When she died in 1840, she left £10,000 to her much-wronged husband Adrien de Feuchères. He was too proud to accept a penny of it and passed the money on to her niece and namesake Sophie Thavaron.

## Adolf Hitler

World War II and the Holocaust could have been prevented if Adolf Hitler had gone to jail over a sex scandal in Munich in 1931, resulting from the death of his niece Geli Raubal.

He got to know Geli in 1927 when he took on her widowed mother, Hitler's half-sister Angela, as a housekeeper at his mountain retreat in Bavaria. Geli was just nineteen at the time and idolized Uncle Adolf who was then thirty-eight. She called him "Uncle Alf". To get Geli away from her mother's watchful eye, Hitler moved her to his apartment in Munich under the pretext of Geli studying medicine there. She had little interest in medicine and was bored by politics. He would not let her go out dancing with people her own age and, once, when he saw her out on the street with a fellow student, he threatened to beat her with the whip he was carrying. He also lectured her on the dangers of sexual intercourse in the most graphic detail.

As a young man, Hitler had given friends similar lectures after taking them to the Spittelberggasse, then Vienna's red-light district. Due to the virulent anti-Semitism in Austria at that time, many young Jewish girls were forced into prostitution, sitting half-naked in the windows. It is believed that Hitler contracted syphilis in the Spittelberggasse.

Hitler stopped Geli going out with fellow Nazi Party member Otto Strasser. After that, he kept her locked up at night.

"He locks me up every time I say no," she told Strasser.

At one time, Hitler accused her of being a whore and had her mother Angela take her to a gynaecologist. When the doctor confirmed that Geli was still a virgin, he bought her an expensive ring – but still kept her under lock and key. Angela grew concerned about Hitler's intentions towards her daughter and asked him to promise that he would not seduce her. In fact, far more awful things were going on.

Otto Strasser fled Germany after this brother Gregor was murdered on the "Night of the Long Knives", where Hitler finished off his political opponents. He ended up in Canada where he was interviewed by the psychoanalyst Dr Walter C. Langer, who was preparing a psychological profile of Hitler for America's Office of Strategic Services. Being a Freudian, Langer focused particularly on Hitler's sex life. His report was circulated to Roosevelt and Churchill, and praised by British foreign secretary Lord Halifax.

Strasser told Langer what Geli had told him about her relationship with Hitler.

"Hitler made her undress," he said. "He would then lie on the floor. She would have to squat over his face where he could examine her at close quarters and this made him very excited . . .When the excitement reached its peak, he demanded that she urinate on him and that gave him his sexual pleasure. Geli said the whole performance was extremely disgusting to her and it gave her no gratification."

It was not just Geli telling him this. Strasser had heard similar stories from Henriette, daughter of Hitler's official photographer Heinrich Hoffman, but he had dismissed them as hysterical ravings. Geli told a girlfriend that Hitler was "a monster . . . you would never believe the things he makes me do". The chambermaids who had to clean Geli's bedroom also complained about the "very strange and unspeakable" things that had taken place there.

In 1929, pornographic sketches Hitler had made of Geli fell into the hands of their landlady's son. Father Bernhard Stempfle, a rabid anti-Semite and a friend of Hitler's, managed to buy them back. He, too, perished in the Night of the Long Knives.

With Geli safely locked up at night, Hitler was free to go out on the town. He spent time at the studios of Heinrich Hoffman, a hangout for homosexuals. Hoffman made pornographic films, which Hitler watched there. He also noted the Führer's unhealthy interest in his sixteen-year-old daughter.

During Hitler's absences, Emil Maurice, founder member of the SS, started seeing Geli. When Hitler discovered that

Geli had allowed Maurice to make love to her, he was beside himself with anger. Condemning Maurice as a "filthy Jew", he forbade her to have anything to do with any other man.

Other Nazi Party leaders were also growing uneasy about Hitler's relationship with his niece. The party was on the verge of a major breakthrough and a scandal would have wrecked Hitler's chance of seizing power. At the same time, Geli, now twenty-three, was becoming increasingly frustrated after Hitler had refused to let her go to Vienna to study music. The situation took on a special urgency when Geli discovered she was pregnant. It is not thought that the child was Hitler's. Pornographic drawings in one of his last letters to her indicate that he was impotent. Magda Goebbels later tried to get her own back on her philandering husband, propaganda minister Josef, by bedding Hitler, but also found he could not rise to the occasion.

The child may have been Emil Maurice's, though she had also slept with the young Nazi assigned to guard her. Or worse, Hitler's nephew, Liverpool-born William Patrick Hitler, claimed that the father was "a young Jewish art teacher in Linz".

On the night of 18 September 1931, Hitler and Geli had a terrible row. Hitler was leaving to attend a rally in Hamburg. Neighbours claimed to have heard Geli shouting to Hitler from their second-floor balcony as he was getting into his car. Hitler shouted back: "No. For the last time, no." Geli shut herself away in her bedroom. Next morning servants broke open the door and found her body.

The first detective on the scene, Heinrich Muller, rose to become head of the Gestapo while Wilhelm Gürtner, the Bavarian Minister of Justice, who hurriedly called off the investigation, became Reich Minister of Justice. There was not even an inquest.

The official story put out was that Geli had committed suicide because she was worried her voice was not good enough to be a singer. Hitler claimed that he was ninety miles away in Nuremburg when he heard of Geli's death. He took out a writ against the anti-Nazi *Munchener Post*, which reported that Geli's nose had been broken and other injuries had been sustained in a struggle.

There were other inconsistencies in the story. Three different people claimed to have broken down the bedroom door. While neighbours claim to have overheard their parting conversation, no one reported hearing a shot. There was no indication that Geli was depressed. She was halfway through writing a letter to a girlfriend when she died – indeed, she was halfway through the word "*und*", German for "and". The sentence read: "When I come to Vienna – hopefully soon – we'll drive together to Semmering an—"

Rigor mortis had set in and the police doctor estimated that she had died the previous evening. The bullet had entered above the heart, passed through her lung and lodged in her lower back at hip level. This meant the gun had to be pointing downwards and the hand holding it had to be higher than her heart, a very awkward way to commit suicide. The pistol used was Hitler's.

Her body was taken down the back stairs of the flats, sealed in a lead coffin and smuggled out of the country. Geli was given a Catholic burial in her native Austria, even though to bury a suicide in hallowed ground was against Church rules. The priest, Father Johann Pant, wrote to a French newspaper in 1939: "They pretended she committed suicide. From the fact I gave her a Christian burial you can draw your own conclusions."

Journalist Fritz Gerlich investigated Geli's murder. He claimed that instead of leaving for Hamburg that Friday, Hitler had dined with Geli in a restaurant and that Hitler, who seldom touched alcohol, drank beer. When they went back to the apartment, there was a row and he shot her. According to Otto Strasser, the public prosecutor wanted to charge Hitler with murder, but was overruled. He fled the country when Hitler came to power. Gerlich was murdered for his pains. So was the owner of the restaurant where he said they had their last meal together.

Gregor Strasser said that he had to stop Hitler committing suicide after he had shot Geli. He and his lawyer, Voss, who kept Strasser's private papers, both perished.

Hitler needed permission from the Austrian government to enter the country. It was granted, provided he did not engage in any political activity. The Austrian Nazi Party was ordered to do nothing when Hitler slipped over the border one night. The cemetery where Geli was buried was opened specially for him. He spent time alone there, returning to Germany before dawn. Later he commissioned a life-size bust of Geli. He wept when it was presented to him. He kept it swathed in flowers and he shut himself away every year on the anniversary of her death.

"Geli's death had such a devastating effect on Hitler it changed his relationship to everyone else," said his deputy, Hermann Göring.

If Geli's death had, indeed, been suicide, it was not the first time one of his lovers had topped themselves. Susi Liptauer hanged herself after a night spent with Hitler. He had wanted to move in with Mitzi Reiter, twenty years his junior, but she was so appalled by his cruelty she tried to kill herself.

Nineteen-year-old movie star Renate Müller spent a memorable evening with the Führer at the Reich Chancellery after he came to power. He began the date with gloating descriptions of how the Gestapo wrung confessions from their victims, boasting his men were more cruel and effective than medieval torturers. This was not a turn-on, but Renate had already reconciled herself to the fact that she was expected to sleep with the Reich Chancellor. But she was in for a shock. When they went into the bedroom and undressed, he threw himself on the floor and begged her to kick him.

"I am filthy and unclean," he whimpered. "Beat me! Beat me!"

She begged him to get up, but he was insistent. Eventually when she did kick him, he became more aroused. The whole thing sickened her. But this was not the worst of it, she told movie director Alfred Zeisler. There was more, things she could not bring herself to talk about. Renate died soon after, after falling from the window of her hotel room in Berlin.

Visiting star of the silent movies Linda Basquette tried to discourage the Führer's advances with a quick kick in the groin. It had the opposite effect. She eventually quenched his ardour by saying she was part Jewish.

Unity Mitford also tried to commit suicide after Hitler gave her the biggest brush-off in modern times by going to war with her homeland. Eva Braun, Hitler's long-term mistress who eventually became his wife, committed suicide with him in the bunker in 1945, but she had attempted suicide before, during their relationship. They had met in Hoffman's studio and became an item soon after Geli's death. Her diaries reveal that she both adored Hitler and was tormented by him. She did not go into the details of their sexual relationship, only saying obscurely: "He needs me for special reasons. It can't be otherwise."

On 1 November 1932, the twenty-year-old Eva shot herself through the neck, but narrowly missed an artery. Hitler was delighted, crowing to Hoffman that Eva had tried to kill herself for love of him. On 29 May 1935, suspecting he was seeing other women, she took an overdose of sleeping tablets. Her sister came round, found her unconscious and called a doctor.

Hitler introduced her to a doctor of his own, Dr Theo Morrell, a specialist in sexually transmitted diseases. Eva asked Dr Morrell to give Hitler something to boost his sexual potency. He gave the Führer a shot of Orchikrin – emulsified bull's testicles. It does not seem to have done the trick and he did not try it again.

At Berchtesgaden, Hitler's Bavarian hideaway, he liked to get her to strip off, saying: "It's too warm for clothes" – though it was not too warm for him to keep his uniform on. She would swim and sunbathe nude for his delectation. Sometimes he would help her undress with trembling fingers.

He would take nude photographs of her too, always from a low angle, saying that he did not want anyone to recognize her if they fell into the wrong hands. Hitler's commando chief Otto Skorzeny said that Eva told him that Hitler "doesn't even bother to take his boots off, and sometimes we don't get into bed. We stretch out on the floor. On the floor, he is very erotic."

According to her medical records, her vagina was too narrow for normal sex. She underwent painful surgery to have it widened. Afterwards, her gynaecologist died in a mysterious car accident. The operation did not seem to make much difference though. Her diaries continue to say: "He only needs me for certain purposes . . . This is idiotic."

The Nazi regime was riddled with sex scandals. Goebbels used his control of the theatre and cinema to keep his bed full of young actresses. Hitler ridiculed Göring, saying that he had become so fat because a bullet in the groin in World War I had left him impotent. It was said that Göring's daughter looked like Mussolini after the Italian dictator had come to stay. Though it was Hitler, not Göring who had taken the bullet in the groin during World War I, according to Magda Goebbels.

Certainly there were some irregularities down there. According to the Soviet autopsy report, Hitler did really only have one ball, though the corpse had been dowsed in petrol and was badly burned. It could not be determined whether he had been born that way or whether a testicle had been removed surgically, not an uncommon practice when syphilis reaches its third and final phase.

If some of the sex scandals concerning Hitler had come out at the time, one of the greatest catastrophes of all time might have been averted. However, some comfort may be drawn from a little footnote in history. At the 1936 Berlin Olympics, the movie-maker Leni Riefenstahl, who herself had at the very least danced naked for Hitler, filmed Hitler embracing Nordic beauty Tilly Fleischer after she won the gold medal for throwing the javelin. It is said that they had an eight-month affair, but Hitler dropped her after Tilly fell pregnant.

She married Dr Fritz Hoser, one of Hitler's aides, and gave birth to a daughter named Gisela. When she grew up she married the son of a French rabbi who had been murdered in Hitler's death camps. Eventually, she converted to Judaism herself. So it may be that Hitler's only offspring is a Jew.

# 5

## Sporting Feats

### Tiger Woods

In 1997, Tiger Woods became the first golfer of African-American descent to win the Masters Tournament at Augusta, Georgia. Four years later he became the first player to win consecutively the four major tournaments in golf – the Masters, the US Open, the British Open and the PGA Championship. For seven successive years, he remained the world's top earner in sport with earnings from winnings and endorsements of $90.5 million in 2010, despite a ten per cent fall off in his income.

Not only was Woods a world-famous sportsman, he led an exemplary home life. At the 2001 Open he was introduced to the Swedish beauty Elin Nordegren. A former model, she was then the nanny to the children of Swedish golfer Jesper Parnevik. Elin was the daughter of a well-to-do Swedish family. Her father was a prominent politician who rose to become Sweden's migration and asylum minister.

Woods had a well-known penchant for blondes and asked her out. She said no, but he persisted. Romance blossomed and in 2004 they had a $1.5-million wedding in the Sandy Lanes resort on Barbados. She was a regular fixture at matches until 2007 when she gave birth to a daughter. A son followed two years later. The only cloud in the sky was the appearance of nude photographs purporting to be of Elin from her modelling days. These were eventually shown to be fakes. However, the Irish magazine *The Dubliner* published one, saying that it was her. She sued for libel and won.

Everything was riding high in 2009 when Woods returned to the circuit after an eight-month layoff following knee surgery. Much to everyone's relief, he was back on form and was racking up the awards – when suddenly it all went terribly wrong.

On 25 November 2009, the *National Enquirer* published a story claiming that Woods had an extramarital affair with thirty-four-year-old New York party girl Rachel Uchitel at the Australian Masters. Rachel promptly denied this and Woods might have got away with it. After all the supermarket tabloid is not known for its reliability and her name had already been linked to another married celebrity, the actor David Boreanaz, star of the Fox show *Bones* – an affair she later admitted.

But by then the solids had hit the air conditioning for Tiger. Two days after the *Enquirer* story, he drove his SUV into a fire hydrant and a tree outside his Florida home. He was taken to hospital, but released after being treated for minor facial lacerations. The curious thing about the accident was that his wife had broken the back window of the car with a golf club. There was speculation that she had broken it to get him out, believing him to be trapped. On the other hand, had it been broken when he was fleeing from a golf club-wielding Valkyrie?

Cited for a traffic violation, Woods paid a $164 ticket, but avoided speaking to the police. Two days after the crash, he issued a statement saying that the incident was:

. . . obviously embarrassing to my family and me. I'm human and I'm not perfect. I will certainly make sure this doesn't happen again. This is a private matter and I want to keep it that way. Although I understand there is curiosity, the many false, unfounded and malicious rumours that are currently circulating about my family and me are irresponsible. The only person responsible for the accident is me. My wife, Elin, acted courageously when she saw I was hurt and in trouble. She was the first person to help me. Any other assertion is absolutely false.

So that was the end of it then? Well, no. He then cancelled his appearance at the Chevron World Challenge, the golf tournament that Woods hosted, and said that he would not be touring again that year, citing the injuries he had suffered in the accident. But some suspected that all may not be well in the Woods's household. Meanwhile, the papers were full of pictures of Rachel Uchitel. Then his name was linked to twenty-seven-year-old Las Vegas nightclub executive Kalika Moquin when a "friend" told *Life & Style* magazine that they had "hooked up a bunch of times".

The "friend" also told the magazine: "Tiger told Kalika that married life isn't all it's built up to be" and that Woods "wasn't happy in his marriage or his home life and that there was just so much pressure on him".

When confronted, Moquin said, "It's not appropriate for me to comment one way or the other. At this time, I'm just choosing to focus on my job."

Then San Diego cocktail waitress Jaimee Grubbs told the celebrity gossip magazine *US Weekly* that she had had a two-and-a-half-year affair with Tiger Woods, backing her claim with voice and text messages. One said: "Send me something very naughty. Go to the bathroom and take [a picture]. I will wear you out."

Another, more recent, said: "Hey it's Tiger, I need you to do me a huge favour. Can you please take your name off your phone? My wife went through my phone and may be calling you. So if you can, please take your name off that. Just have it as a number on the voicemail. You got to do this for me. Huge. Quickly. Bye."

After over twenty alleged encounters, she went on television to say that he was "horrible in bed", while she praised George

Clooney whom she also claimed to have had an affair with. By then evidence had emerged that Rachel Uchitel had indeed been in Australia during the Open.

"To see that he was inviting another girl to Australia, it hurts," said Jaimee. "I'm still bitter about it."

She reportedly got $150,000 from *US Weekly* for the story. A former reality TV star, it seemed she wanted a break into acting.

Woods responded with a second statement that, while admitting nothing, reads like a *mea culpa*. In it he said: "I have let my family down and I regret those transgressions with all of my heart. I have not been true to my values and the behaviour my family deserves. I am not without faults and I am far short of perfect. I am dealing with my behaviour and personal failings behind closed doors with my family. Those feelings should be shared by us alone."

He went on to rue the scrutiny of the tabloids and dismiss the idea that physical violence played any part in his car accident. He again begged for privacy and expressed his regrets at letting his family down, concluding: "I will strive to be a better person and the husband and father that my family deserves. For all of those who have supported me over the years, I offer my profound apology."

Plainly, Elin had him by the balls.

On 11 December, the high court in London granted Woods an injunction banning the publication of photographs or video showing him nude or having sex. His lawyers said: "This order is not to be taken as an admission that any such photographs exist."

You could have drawn your own conclusions. But you didn't have to. A week later, it emerged that twenty-six-year-old cocktail waitress Jamie Jungers did indeed have such pictures. During their eighteen-month relationship, she had snapped him naked with her mobile phone when he had passed out drunk in a hotel room. She told her family that she would take the pictures to the tabloids if she and Tiger broke up. Normally, he visited her in Las Vegas, but they also made love in his California home and it was alleged that he even wanted to fly her out to Florida for a romp there.

She claimed to have been in bed with him when he got the call saying that his father had died of cancer. She was engaged at the time. Later, her job description in the tabloid slipped from "cocktail waitress" to "former Vegas blackjack dealer, stripper and model" after she was arrested for driving under the influence, driving on a suspended registration and having no proof of insurance.

She claimed that he was cheap. "When we'd go out for dinner, he never left a tip or he'd ask for the meal to be complimentary because he was Tiger Woods," she said. "I just thought that was cheap and it always embarrassed me."

He never even bought her a gift, she said. "I didn't even get a birthday card."

But she claimed she was "in love" with Woods and enjoyed "wild and crazy sex" with him. She denied that he paid her for sex, saying they had a "boyfriend-girlfriend relationship". Nor was it a hole-in-the-wall affair.

"We went places together, people were taking our photographs in the nightclubs," she said. "When I went to see him at the MGM, I would have to check in under my name and say that I was there to see him, and Tiger would come down and get me."

There were more to come.

Mindy Lawton, a thirty-four-year-old waitress who lived on a trailer park in Orlando, said Woods had had an affair with her while his wife Elin was pregnant. And they went bareback as Tiger hates wearing a condom. She said he was "very well endowed . . . He had a very strong sex drive and knows his way around the bedroom. On a scale of ten I would give him twelve."

He may have known his way around the bedroom, but he also knew to steer clear of the bedroom – at least the marital bedroom – when he took her home, having her instead in the living room, in the shower, up against the wall in the hall, in the garage – and even in a church parking lot up against the side of the SUV he later crashed. She also said that he had a passion for the colour red, which he often wore at golf tournaments. But that was not the only place he enjoyed the colour.

"His favourite were my red panties with black lace," she said. "He had a thing about red and said he always wore it on Friday as that was his mother's favourite colour."

Apparently he liked to spice up their sex sessions with saucy underwear, she told the *News of the World*. And the sex was frantic.

"Sometimes I looked like a rag doll after we'd made love," she said. "He really did like it quite rough. He wanted to spank me and loved pulling my hair as we had sex. He also liked me to talk dirty to him, but hair-pulling was what really turned him on."

Only later did it dawn on her that he only wanted her for one thing!

"I realize now all he wanted me for was sex. The only time he would call was when he wanted it," said the poor disillusioned girl. "If it was early in the morning and Tiger was going away for a tournament he would call me up for quick, urgent sex and I was happy to oblige . . . He had an urge and I satisfied it. There was very little emotion from his side although I fell for him."

It was a thrill to be with such a famous man, a star she had seen on TV. In the end, though, she was bitter.

"All Tiger cared about was getting me into bed," she told the *News of the World*. "Tiger just used me as his sex toy. I thought I meant something to him, but all he cared about was lust. He is a selfish, heartless man."

Brute.

Mindy had already seen Tiger out with his wife before they

began their affair. He brought her to the pancake house where Mindy worked. It did not trouble her when Tiger asked her out as he looked so miserable when he was with Elin. They did not talk or hold hands.

"There was no affection there," she said.

So Mindy went out for an innocent drink with him. Around 3 a.m. he took her home. Then he cuddled up to her on the sofa and started kissing her.

"He started to strip off my clothes and I took off his," she said. "We were sitting on a brown sofa and within seconds we were both naked. As a sportsman he is in great shape, but he is also very well endowed. He kept on complimenting me on my figure and kissed me all over."

He was, she said, "very dominant". He knew what he wanted and what he was doing. By the time they finished "we both had big smiles on our faces".

But when his wife had the baby, Mindy was dumped. She said she was not surprised that there were other women.

"He had such a big sex drive and wanted it fulfilled," she said. She was just giving him what his wife wasn't.

But her understanding only went so far.

"I want his wife to know what a cheat he has been," she said. It was her duty to speak out. "He does not care for her otherwise he would not be having sex with me and these other women. I am so glad that I am no longer involved with him. He is just another cheating husband who has been caught out."

And how.

Then there was the thirty-one-year-old one-time aspiring model Cori Rist, whom he met in a Manhattan nightclub. A friend told the *New York Daily News*: "They went on to another party. One thing led to another and, pretty soon, Tiger was flying her out to hook up with him on tour."

However, with Cori, Tiger was uncharacteristically discreet. Tiger would usually get a large suite at a hotel, then he would get someone else to book Cori into an adjacent room. The trouble was he never wanted to leave the room in case someone saw them together.

After six months of this, Cori started to get tired of being cooped up. She felt like a bird in a gilded cage. However, she continued seeing him for another two years – though just as a "friend", she said.

Cori was married with a child at the time. When initially confronted, she said, "No comment . . . Not at this time." But then she went on TV to spill all. She said she thought she was the only "other woman" in his life and burst into tears when she told of how she discovered he was lying to her.

"I'd wake up sometimes in the night in hotels with him and hear him text messaging," she sobbed. "I'd lie there and realize he was having a conversation, so I suspected there were others."

Now she had come forward to expose him as a serial love cheat – and to respond to claims that he had paid her for sex.

"He has a way to make you believe that he is a very honest and good man," she said. "But I realized the things he was telling me were false. I'm not like most of these girls. I'm a mum and I try to set the right example by my son."

She then apologized to Woods's wife Elin: 'I'm just sorry for her pain. One day I will have to look my son in the face and explain all this.'

Asked how she felt when she learned she was just one of many mistresses, she said, "It's disappointing, because I think that we all would like to think we were special. I don't know how he had time to have so many women in his life."

There was porn star Holly Sampson who played the title role in the *Emmanuelle 2000* series, though she had begun her career in more hard-core movies under various aliases. She went on the adult website NaughtyAmerica.com, topless in a kitchen with two other women and spoke frankly about the services she provided at a "bachelor party" for Tiger Woods.

"He picked me to go into the room with him … he's the perfect gentleman," she said. "He would probably die if he knew I was telling this on the internet but that's OK, I don't care. It was fun, it's not like it was any big mystery."

She said he was "really good" and "me and my girlfriend sort of tag-teamed him". She also said: "We had sex for about forty-five minutes – it was amazing. I don't think he stopped smiling the entire time."

Another woman in the video commented that Holly looks similar to Tiger Woods's wife Elin.

"I know! He likes blondes obviously," Sampson said.

She later claimed that she did not have sex with Tiger Woods while he was married. Obviously a woman of some standards then.

Porn star Veronica Siwik-Daniels – who, as Joslyn James, starred in *Big Breast Nurses* – was named as the woman who had given "years of faithful service to his virulent sexual appetite". She claimed that he was a control freak who fantasized about having violent sex with submissive women.

"There were certain things about our relationship that were not conventional," James told the *New York Daily News*. "There were a couple of situations when he was a bit more aggressive than usual."

According to the *Huffington Post* she claimed that he made her pregnant twice after regular unprotected sex – "the first pregnancy ended in a miscarriage, while she arranged an abortion during the second pregnancy".

But James got her own back. After he made a public apology for his behaviour, she said he was faking it. Then when he announced that he was ending his four-month break from golf to compete in the Masters, she posted his texts on the web.

One said: "I would love to have the ability to make you sore." It was sent at 3.32 p.m. on 28 August 2009, while Woods was competing in the Barclays golf tournament in Jersey City. Four minutes later, he sent another text, proposing a threesome "with you and another girl you trust".

The next was darker.

"I want to treat you rough. Throw you around, spank and slap you."

From there, they got a whole lot worse with Woods texting his desire to "choke" her. She did not post her replies, but he was sure that she would comply.

"Whatever I want," he texted. "You are mine."

In the final text, dated 4 October 2009, Woods flipped out on James for apparently acting recklessly in public.

"Don't . . . talk to me," his text said. "You almost just ruined my whole life. If my agent and these guys would have seen you there."

Hollywood madam Michelle Braun told the *New York Daily News* that Woods would spend more than $60,000 on expensive prostitutes.

"He was rarely with just one girl," Braun said. "He usually wanted more. He liked three-ways."

What's more he was very specific about the girls he wanted.

"He would request the college-cutie, girl-next-door look," said Braun.

She also said the girls marvelled at the golf champ's endurance.

"He could go for days," she said. "He'd pay a flat rate for an evening, but an evening would usually be extended. The girls would talk about his stamina."

All the girls thought Woods was a "real gentleman" and a good lover.

"He'd shower them with gifts," she added. "He was very polite and he was amazing in bed . . . very sensual and well endowed."

According to Braun, one of his favourites was Loredana Jolie, a blonde from Sicily who had modelled for *Playboy*.

"She's a stunning girl," said Braun. "He went out with her

four or five times. She took part in group sex. They met up in 2006 or early 2007. I'd say he paid $15,000 for her."

Braun claimed that among her other employees were Holly Sampson and Jamie Jungers, though Jamie denied it saying, "I have nothing to do with prostitution and never have, never will." However, Loredana Jolie made no bones about her profession in her tell-all book about Tiger Woods.

"As a lover and sexual partner he is largely endowed and safe sex with him was definitely champion status," she wrote. "When I was having my relationship with Tiger, I was like on the seventh cloud especially from a sexual perspective" – apparently confusing cloud nine with seventh heaven. "There is at least no doubt about the fact that Tiger was awesome in bed."

She also kicked over some other stones. "He liked to watch girl-on-girl, and the girls would occasionally join us." She also noted that his fantasies included other men. "I'd make him fantasize. I'd ask about if I had another guy. It kind of turned him on."

According to some websites, Jolie would even claim that Woods indulged in gay sex – as if he did not have enough to handle.

"He would engage in sex from 9 p.m. until the sun came up the next morning," Jolie told the *New York Post*. "But he wasn't a healthy guy. He couldn't sleep and would stay up all night. I am not really sure rehab for sex addiction will help him."

He was addicted to pills, she said. But it got worse – or, at least, more outlandish.

"Tiger's sexual fantasies were not normal," Jolie said. "He likes role-playing, he likes to be the guy in control and wearing a suit while there are girls performing girl-on-girl and guys entertaining guys. By that, I mean they would dance for each other like girls would do for a man. He'd have different girls all the time, entertaining, role-play, fetishes, stuff like that . . .

It seems that Tiger also had a British mistress. Forty-two-year-old mother Emma Rotherham is said to have gone ballistic when the *News of the World* reported that she had taken a $500,000 pay-off to keep quiet about the eighteen-month affair. One of Tiger's security team was said to have handed over the money in $100 bills stuffed in a sports bag. In return, she signed a confidentiality agreement.

A source close to Tiger told the Irish *News of the World*: "Emma was his most recent mistress. They had a very, very passionate relationship and she has dozens of text messages and emails from him. Some were even sent while Tiger was trying to patch things up with his wife Elin. If those came out they'd bury him. He absolutely adored Emma and loved the sex. So did she."

The newspaper said that they romped on his office sofa at least once a week and he begged for saucy photographs of her in stockings and suspenders. She sent them on her mobile phone. "She had a killer body and Tiger was smitten," the source said.

Emma had moved to Florida in 2006 after her youngest daughter had finished primary school in England. They met in Woods's favourite hunting ground for women, the Blue Martini in Orlando in May 2008. Her tight black jumpsuit showed off her fabulous figure, which immediately caught Woods's roving eye.

"Tiger could not keep his eyes off her butt," the newspaper's source said. "Everyone in the room knew what was going to happen sooner or later."

He sat next to her most of the evening. Tiger loved her posh English accent and they exchanged phone numbers. A few days later, Woods contacted Emma by text and she agreed to meet at his office.

According to the newspaper's source, nothing much happened on the first date, just some kissing and fondling. But on her third visit they had sex on the couch. "She said it was 'awesome'."

Emma made no secret about their affair and boasted about her famous lover. Although she lived eighty miles away in Isleworth, Florida, she was always on call. But usually she had to fit him in early in the morning, before golf practice.

"They were at it all the time. Emma said Tiger was a great lover. But he never wore a condom, and she didn't take any precautions."

While Elin was pregnant with his son, Woods arranged for Emma to fly out to Michigan where he was competing in the Buick Open. She stayed in the same hotel as him, in a room reserved for his personal doctor. It was just down the corridor from Woods's room so she could sneak along there for sex. They took drugs to make the sex more intense and were at it all night. She said the sex was "mind-blowing". He went out to win the tournament the next day.

But he became jealous and controlling. When she was not with him, she would have to email him a photograph of what she was wearing out that night. He would then text back telling her to change if he thought the outfit was too revealing. But she would go ahead and wear the outfit anyway.

Once he suggested that she came back with him to his Florida house when Elin was visiting her family in Sweden. She refused.

Emma also believed that she was Woods's only mistress – until the car crash. She texted Woods, who replied: "Don't contact me. Elin is going through everything."

Then when the Irish *News of the World* found out about her, she called Woods, who said he would "sort it out".

He had a lot on his plate at the time, but told her not to worry. A black Mercedes with tinted windows picked her up and whisked her two hundred miles down the coast to Naples, Florida, where she had been booked into the Ritz-Carlton Hotel. The room had been paid for and she was handed an envelope containing $32,000 "spending money". She was told not to come out of the room in case the media were after her.

However, she was worried about her teenage daughter, so she got Woods on the phone and told him that she would never talk about their relationship. She was then moved to a rented villa on the Bay Park golf resort where it was easier for him to contact her. It was then that the $500,000 and the confidentiality pact turned up. His security team also wanted her mobile phone with the texts from Woods in it, but she refused to hand it over.

After that, she tried to contact him again, but he did not return her calls.

Once news of the pay-off came out, they faced a new problem. Emma faced a tax probe over the $500,000. Under US law a gift of such a large amount of cash has to be declared. Woods would also have to make a declaration to the tax authorities.

Emma was not the only lucky lady. Woods wired anywhere from $5,000 to $10,000 a month to several busty blondes, according to MSNBC. One lucky lady reportedly was on Tiger's tab to the tune of up to $20,000 a month, the network reported.

"The money comes via a wire transfer," another woman told MSNBC. "There's no contract about it, there's no discussion about what it's for, but it's implied that it's in exchange for keeping quiet about his affair."

MSNBC cited as their sources "several women who were involved with the golfer" but did not identify any of them. These payments could also cause problems.

"The IRS regulations require that someone gifting in excess of $13,000 per year file a gift tax return," said John Fisher, a Pennsylvania-based tax attorney.

Woods was still trying to save his five-year marriage at the time. As well as admitting his "transgressions" at a press conference, on 30 December 2009 he checked into Pine Grove Behavioral Health and Addiction Services clinic in Mississippi for therapy for his sex addiction. He then had to face "disclosure day" when he would have to tell his wife about every infidelity. By some accounts, Emma was Woods's nineteenth mistress. But not all have come forward. One has married since and wishes to remain anonymous. Others have run to lawyers to protect them, while the *Enquirer* claimed that he had had as many as 120 affairs behind his wife's back.

As part of the therapy, he had to list all the women he had had sex with. According to the supermarket tabloid, he left off the name of twenty-one-year-old Raychel Coudriet, the daughter of a neighbour he had known since she was fourteen.

Elin learnt of the dalliance while he was having dinner with friends following his golf comeback at the US Masters.

"She was screaming so loudly that everyone at the table could hear what she was saying," said the *Enquirer*.

Woods's estranged wife was quoted as saying: "This is the worst betrayal ever. I can't believe you had sex with that girl in our own neighbourhood. That's it – I'm divorcing you!"

It was alleged that the seduction took place just yards from where his wife was tending their newborn baby.

The break-up of his marriage and the worldwide coverage of his sex life put Tiger off his game and, despite flashes of form, he won nothing in 2010. In 2011, he was dogged by injury and fired his long-time caddy. Despite the revelations, Associated Press named him Athlete of the Decade. One could argue that he deserved it both on and off the golf course. Some sponsors backed away. But others saw a benefit as December 2009 saw a four thousand per cent jump in Google searches for Tiger.

"God bless Tiger. This week, we got a huge uplift," said Yahoo CEO Carol Bartz. She explained that the Tiger Woods sex scandal was more profitable online than even the death of Michael Jackson because it was easier to sell ads that appear alongside juicy content than funeral stories.

In August 2010, Woods's divorce was finalized. Elin received

$100 million in assets, though they could be worth five times that. But then, by 2009, Tiger Woods was the first athlete to earn over a billion dollars and his career is far from over both on the golf course and in the bedroom – sorry, in the shower, the garage or the church parking lot.

## David Beckham

Not that the marriage of David and Victoria Beckham has been entirely unbesmirched by scandal. On 4 April 2004, the *News of the World* reported that David Beckham had had an affair with his personal assistant Rebecca Loos. At the time Beckham had left Manchester United for Real Madrid and Dave was "a lonely man in a foreign country," the paper said.

While Ms Loos would not talk to the paper, the paper had managed to photograph them together in Madrid in September the previous year and reported that they had just kissed for the first time after playing a "sexy game of truth or dare". According to the newspaper, ninety minutes after the photograph had been taken he whisked her off to a suite at the Santa Mauro Hotel – "to the astonishment of his drivers and bodyguards".

A "friend" said, "As soon as they got in the room, Rebecca said he seemed a little nervous. He realized he was taking a very big step. He held Rebecca's head in his hands and kissed her passionately and said, 'I have wanted to be with you like this for so long.'

"It was a very powerful moment. He dimmed the lights and started taking his clothes off. Rebecca stripped off too and they stood naked in the middle of the room, kissing passionately."

Was the "friend" in the room at the time? How did they know this?

"David was a sensational lover – their sex was highly charged and explosive," they continued. "They made love for hours. He kept telling her, 'I know we shouldn't be doing this but I can't help it. I really want this to happen. It makes me so happy. I want you to stay with me all night long.'"

The evening had started innocently enough. Beckham and a group of friends had got merry on champagne and were playing truth or dare, when Rebecca asked if he had ever had sex on a plane. He said he had, but would not say who with. Beckham then dared Rebecca to go to the ladies' and walk through the restaurant with a strip of lavatory paper dangling from the back of her trousers. Not only did she do it, but she gave it a little wiggle in front of his table.

Then, according to the newspaper, after dropping off the other guests, they kissed and caressed all the way back to his suite.

"David was in a state of high arousal when they got into the bedroom at 4 a.m. and there was no going back," said the intrusive friend who seems to have installed a webcam. "She was lying on her tummy and he kissed her all over. She said David's stamina was extraordinary. She could feel his energy pulsating through her as he made love to her on the bed."

And that was not the end of it. The next night he was just as "passionate" but a little more "adventurous".

Victoria Beckham, a.k.a. Posh Spice, had been spending her time in England pursuing her music career. Somehow she got to hear of it and gave him "an earbashing". But the newspaper reported that the affair continued. After a party at the home of a Brazilian soccer star, Beckham texted Loos, asking her to come back to his hotel. She agreed.

"They didn't have full sex that night but decided to experiment, pleasuring each other in a variety of ways involving all manner of kissing and fondling," said the remarkably well-informed friend, presumably poring over the footage. There was one more meeting in another hotel in December. "It was least satisfying of all the meetings." Then Beckham broke off relations with the SFX Group, his former management company, where Rebecca worked.

Ms Loos was, of course, "heartbroken this story has come out but she knew it would eventually. Too many people have seen her texts and they've got into the wrong hands."

So why did she show them? And she should have been more careful with a name like hers. She must have known the tabloids were aching to call her a "Loos woman".

Beckham dismissed the allegations as "ludicrous". But corroboration came from Rebecca's brother John Charles, who told the *Daily Mail*: "She has confirmed to me she had an affair with David." Apparently, she feared being branded "a marriage wrecker" and denied taking £300,000 from the *News of the World* and wept when the story appeared.

The London *Evening Standard* said that David was going to face a grilling from his wife when he flew out to meet the family for a skiing holiday in Switzerland. According to the *Mail*, when they met up Posh had slapped Becks as he struggled to convince her that he had not been unfaithful – and he wept when he thought he might lose her. Pictures of the family cavorting in the snow were fetching £20,000 a time. The photographer Jason Fraser, who was said to have come across them by accident, was expected to make £250,000 out of them.

Pretty soon there was a blizzard of bimbos. Beckham had been seen with thirty Swedish models in a nightclub in Basle. He had kissed one and invited two to stay the night. A redhead called Helia claimed on Spanish TV that he had a liaison in a nightclub lavatory with an unnamed blonde. Another woman claimed to have had a threesome with David and Rebecca, even claiming she had photographs to prove it. Meanwhile Ms Loos claimed that she caught Beckham having "text sex" with twenty-six-year-old actress and model Esther Cañadas before she ditched him with the immortal line: "U R snding sex-txts 2 anthr girl. CYA." This convinced her to go public, a friend said. But she did not spill the beans to Piers Morgan, her second cousin, then editor of the *Daily Mirror*. Nevertheless, he remained loyal, banning Beckham from his chat show.

Twenty-three-year-old pneumatic Spanish model Nuria Bermudez – a.k.a "*Muchas Tetas*" which needs no translation – also claimed to have slept with Beckham. She was thought to have bedded at least half the Real Madrid team.

"I started getting texts and he'd tell me things such as: 'I am a real man and I'm going to show you what real men like me do,'" she said. "He invited me to his hotel room two or three nights after the first texts and we had sex."

She was touting her story around for £12,000, though she said that the texts had been erased when something went wrong with her SIM card. Meanwhile, Beckham's chauffeur Delfin Fernandez wanted £500,000 for his story, revealing that he had driven David to Esther Cañadas's apartment in a swish area of Madrid at least twice and he had entertained her at the Santa Mauro Hotel. Rebecca Loos choked back her tears and succumbed to the financial blandishments of the Sunday tabloids. Her bowdlerized texts were published, leaving the papers to puzzle out what they meant. Meanwhile, the *Sun* claimed that Loos was a bisexual who had nude romps with known lesbians. Former Wimbledon tennis champion Pat Cash said he was fifty per cent sure that he had bedded Rebecca Loos in Madrid.

"They all look the same after a while," he said.

Then Malaysian-born Sarah Marbeck came forward claiming to have bedded Becks after they met in Singapore.

She was ushered to his room at the Shangri-La Hotel by a bodyguard.

"It was a bit awkward at first," she said. "I sat in a chair and he sat on the bed. Then I said, 'Well, now what?' and without saying anything, he gently took my hand and led me to the bed. After a few seconds he started kissing me."

According to Ms Marbeck, who has modelled for Armani,

But he would only watch . . . He would also ask me to text him pictures of myself when we weren't together."

Julie Postle was a twenty-year-old cocktail waitress in the Roxy Nightclub in Orlando when Woods first started hitting on her, according to her ex-boyfriend Brian Kimborough, who was a barman there. He said that Tiger once chided her for calling her boyfriend from his Florida home.

"She was in his closet at 5 a.m. calling me," said Kimborough, "and he was in the background telling her to get off the phone." He added: "She said Tiger told her that his marriage was for publicity."

Theresa Rogers claimed that she was the mother of Tiger Woods's love child, though she was having an affair with a Serbian basketball player at the time the baby was born. Rogers claimed to have been his mistress both before and after his marriage. Some ten years older than Woods, she boasted that she "taught him everything he needed to know to be a great lover".

"Theresa was crazy about Tiger but she didn't want to feel like a bought woman, a paid escort," RadarOnline.com reported. "She just wanted to be the woman who schooled Tiger in the bedroom."

And the school fees were high. She asked for $2 million and hired Los Angeles celebrity lawyer Gloria Allred to negotiate the deal for her. It was reported that Allred had already got $3 million for Rachel Uchitel in return for her silence, and lesser sums for other mistresses.

Even very old girlfriends came out of the woodwork with kiss-and-tell stories. Woods's first girlfriend Diane Parr described how he ended their three-year relationship with a curt note sent from a California tournament. It said: "Please mail my necklace that I gave to you when you get back home. Don't show up at the tournament tomorrow because you are just not welcome."

She cried for two days. However, she said that six months later he wrote to apologize for his behaviour.

Gucci and Calvin Klein, they were soon both naked and having "perfect, really passionate" sex.

"I've no idea how long it lasted," she said. "When you're in bed with David Beckham you're not looking at the clock, believe me."

Then, she recalled, David said to her: "I know what we're doing is wrong, but I can't help it."

She also claimed to have traded explicit "sex texts" with him for over a year. In them, he referred to himself as "Peter Pan", her as "Tinkerbell" and Posh as "Wendy". "All I can think about is Tinkerbell . . . I can't be arsed talking to Wendy," he texted.

Her father, a former magistrate, was "devastated" by the news – a J. M. Barrie fan then.

Once he described how he wanted to make love to her on the bonnet of the Ferrari 550 that Victoria had bought for him. That's an awful lot of texting. It seems that David had a fantasy about the movie *Pretty Woman*, which was as well as the *Sun* revealed that Sarah was a £400-an-hour call girl who had signed up with the Boardroom Escorts Agency in Sydney, Australia, six months after her alleged second encounter with Beckham. The agency boss Graeme Edwards said she had been working as a prostitute in Singapore but, while she boasted about other famous men she had slept with, she never mentioned Beckham. He was also puzzled about the texts that had been published as, he said, she had lost two mobile phones since she had been in Australia. Another woman came forward to say that she and her boyfriend had a threesome with Ms Marbeck after a sporting event in Melbourne.

While New York rapper Damon Dash, who produced Posh's latest single, denied going to bed with her, Rebecca Loos went on television saying that she knew an intimate secret about Beckham's body, after Beckham's lawyers failed to silence her. She said that Beckham had "used her for sex" and she "felt like a whore" after accepting a reported £150,000 for the interview. The real problem for Posh was that Rebecca, daughter of a Dutch diplomat, was really posh.

But David knew the answer. He spent £1 million on diamonds for Victoria's thirtieth birthday and they were trying for another child. There was more trouble to come though. While innocently dispensing legal advice, *The Times* mentioned that a third woman, Celina Laurie, a "vicar's daughter", had also claimed to have sex with him. Apparently, she told a Danish tabloid that she had had a one-night stand with Beckham after meeting him in a nightclub in 2002.

"David answered the door wearing white Diesel boxer shorts," she told the *Sunday People*. "He had a fantastic body. I followed him through to the bedroom where he put his arms around me and kissed me ... He didn't throw me out afterwards, and he let me stay until he got up a bit before 8 a.m. He asked for my telephone number, and I gave it him. Unfortunately, he didn't give me his, and I haven't heard from him since."

She also revealed the "intimate secret" that Rebecca Loos had been holding back. David waxed. Oo, painful.

Still Posh and Becks said they would not split. But the allegations would not go away. Plenty of other women came forward saying that he had kissed them, or made some sort of advance. Worse. David Beckham turned down an appearance on *The Simpsons* after the show made jokes about the alleged affair.

The solution was obvious. Beckham would bid *adios* to the *senoritas* of Spain and head for the safety of Los Angeles where, according to the *Sun*, ravening packs of *Playboy* centrefolds lay in wait. He was going to a Galaxy far, far away – for a remake of Starlet Wars, perhaps. There were even stories that "text pest" Rebecca Loos intended to follow and the Beckham children were warned to keep the pet rabbits in the hutch, under guard.

As it was, the Beckhams had two more children and lived happily ever after.

## Ashley and Cheryl Cole

It all worked out so well for Posh and Becks. But Girls Aloud's Cheryl Cole's fairy-tale romance with Chelsea defender Ashley sank when they hit a reef on a similar rocky shore. She was working as a judge on *The X Factor* in Britain, before making her abortive debut on the American version of the show, when her marriage was hit by a sex scandal. Topless model Sonia Wild said she received nude photographs of the footballer sent to her mobile phone. Ashley said that he had not sent them. What had happened was, he had given the phone away, forgetting to delete the pictures first.

There had already been rumours that Ashley had been playing away games since their marriage. Eighteen months after the Coles' glitzy £500,000 magazine-deal marriage in July 2006, twenty-two-year-old hairdresser Aimee Walton told the *Sun* that she had had a wild night of drunken sex with our Ashley. Cole had been out on a binge with his mates, downing vodka cocktails and chatting up women. But he could not be bothered to chat up Aimee.

"The end of the night one of Ashley's mates just came up to me and said, 'Ashley wants you to go home with him,'" she said.

The soccer player was drunk and Aimee's friend offered to give him a lift home. He then vomited in the car. Aimee's friend was angry, but he said, "She should be privileged Ashley Cole was sick in her car."

When they arrived at his friend's place, he got Aimee into the bedroom.

"We started having sex but it wasn't long before he said he felt sick again," she said. "Then he just rolled over and vomited on the floor, all over the cream carpet. It was disgusting."

But she did not take it personally and it did not stop him scoring.

"He had some mouthwash," she said, "then jumped back into bed."

However, she forgot that football was a team game.

"We started having sex again but his mates piled into the room," she said. "After they left, we finally managed to get going again and tried several positions. Eventually, he finished and collapsed onto my chest. He was panting and clearly had had a good time."

Overall, Aimee was not terribly impressed.

"For a footballer, I didn't think he was in great shape," she said. But then: "He's wild – really rude in bed. He knew exactly what he was doing and was pretty good, despite not being very big."

Of course, Aimee was mortified in the morning, shocked that Ashley had broken his solemn marriage vows. "It was a big mistake and I regret it. I feel so sorry for Cheryl," she said. "Now I feel really guilty. She should know what he's really like."

Cole too was ashamed. "Please don't tell anyone," he said. "I'll get in so much trouble."

Naturally, Aimee respected that and the last thing to cross her mind was to contact the tabloids. It was, of course, an accident that she turned up on the front page of the *Sun*.

Two days later, the *Sunday Mirror* carried more cheating claims. Glamour model Brooke Healy claimed Cole had sex with her after a Christmas party just five months after his wedding. And she was then paid over £6,000 in cash to keep quiet about it. According to the newspaper, Ashley had already begged Cheryl's forgiveness and told her that he had been too drunk to have full sex with Aimee, but she warned him: "If you do anything like this again, it's all over."

But he seems to have been much more on the ball when it came to Brooke. She said that they met in the trendy club

Funky Buddha in London's Mayfair when the Chelsea players were having their Christmas night out in 2006.

Within minutes of walking into the swanky club, he told her he was taking her home that night. To avoid the paparazzi, they left the club separately and met up in a nearby casino. From there they headed for a spare bedroom at a friend's house.

"He grabbed my head and neck and pulled me towards him," she said. "He took my bra off. It was so hot and I was telling him not to pull my hair because I had extensions in. He was laughing and saying, 'I'm used to it with Cheryl.'"

She said he told her that he did not need to wear a condom because his club, Chelsea, gave the players check-ups and he was clean.

"I'd had quite a lot to drink so I took a gamble. Luckily, I didn't get pregnant – but for weeks I was worried I might be," she said. "After we'd had sex we both fell asleep and he put his arm around me which I hate."

In the morning, Cole was "stand-offish" and "a bit cold".

"I felt a bit hurt," she said.

He offered her £300 to get a cab home. Naturally, she declined.

But a few weeks later, she said a friend of Ashley's approached her and got her to sign a piece of paper saying that she had not slept with Ashley Cole and that she would not go to the papers with the story. He offered her £7,000 in cash, but she could only fit £300 in the purse that she had brought with her that night.

They arranged another meeting where a relative turned up with another £6,300. Like Aimee, Brooke said she was sorry for Cheryl's sake. "I feel bad for her because she married somebody who isn't faithful," she said.

Brooke's name has also been linked to other soccer players Darren Bent, Jermaine Pennant and Carlton Cole.

"Why date other men if I can date a Premiership star?" she said.

Another woman turned up at the *Mirror* offices, saying that she had had sex with Ashley Cole. But it had been before he had started dating Cheryl. New Zealand-born actress Coralie Robinson also claimed she was unimpressed by his prowess in the bedroom. But as her name has been linked to Robbie Williams, Russell Brand, Shane Warne and Ziggy from *Big Brother*, he was up against some stiff competition. According to the *Mirror*, she was given £10,000 and asked to sign the document in return for destroying all text messages, telephone messages and notes relating to her relationship with Cole.

One clause said: "While I know A (Ashley Cole) as a friend, I have never at any time had a sexual relationship of any nature with him. Not withstanding the non-sexual nature of my relationship with A I will keep all matters passing between A and myself and all information regarding A as a result of such relationship in the strictest confidence."

Nevertheless, to help him buck his ideas up, she decided it was her duty to sell – sorry, tell – her story to the tabloids.

One almost feels sorry for Ashley at this point. Cheryl certainly did and they reconciled. Perhaps he was better when he was playing at home.

But there was more to come. Two years later, it was revealed that he had bedded thirty-year-old soccer-club secretary Vicki Gough. Their assignation occured when Chelsea were playing away at Hull, only months after his reconciliation with Cheryl. It was arranged in an amusing series of texts, which the *Sun* got their hands on.

At 1.12 p.m. on 27 October 2008 he sent a text saying: "Mayb ill get another room what do u think x."

At 2.58 p.m. he texted to say mission accomplished: "Room done i said its 4 my bro and girlfriend. I get there at 4 so ill get the key and sort it 4 u x."

Eight minutes later he was all fingers and thumbs when he texted: "Call me when ur home and ill text u address x."

At 4.45 p.m., Vicki got her orders: "Forest pines broughton near brigg north linconshire dn20 0aq room 15 call me when u get here and i throw key out my window x."

She persuaded him that throwing the keys out of the window would not be a good idea. Then she took the three-hour drive and checked into the room that had been booked by a Chelsea official.

On her way, she got another text from eager Ashley, saying: "Ok u can get room service if ur hungry bring some wine x."

One can almost hear him panting when he texted at 5.52 p.m.: "Ur sexy legs. Go to reception and pick up key if they ask anything say ur Boy is coming up after work x."

Once the ball was in the back of the net, he sneaked out of her room. Then at 6.23 a.m. he texted: "Thank u 4 coming up i had a great time x."

In all, she reckoned that she got over three hundred texts from Ashley Cole, some with nude pictures attached or shots of him standing in front of a mirror in a pair of white briefs. Later, he texted: "I beg u to keep this between us x. Please delete all texts I'll have no balls left."

Then news came that, on a US tour with the club, he had spent a sleepless night in Seattle. Ashley was celebrating their victory over the Seattle Sounders when he met twenty-eight-year-old Ann Corbitt, a friend said.

"Ann said she spent the night with Ashley and then left the next morning," said the confidante. "She never saw him or spoke to him after that. She is about as different to a trashy British glamour girl as you can get."

Nevertheless she was "thinking about selling her story". Once again it was alleged that an attempt was made to silence her. Then when he feared the story would come out, he phoned her in tears and pleaded: "I can't lose my wife over this. If I lose my wife, I don't want to live."

According to Ann: "When he rang me and cried I asked him, 'What's wrong with you? Why do you cheat? Why did you have sex with me behind your wife's back?' But he just replied that he didn't know. He admitted he'd cheated on her before and been exposed in the press. He was most vehement that I was the first person he'd cheated with . . . since the last time he got caught! I think he's got a problem."

So Ann decided to make a clean breast of it to the *News of the World*. Apparently, Ashley had employed the tried-and-tested trick of a texting a picture of himself in a pair of tiny briefs.

"He looked really skinny and was smoking a cigarette," she said. "I thought it was really gross. Just nasty."

The rest of his seduction technique was also up to par. Back at his hotel after the match, someone spilt beer on the floor, which splashed dirt on her leg.

"Ashley immediately grabbed it and licked the mess off," she said. "That really grossed me out."

After visiting a club, Ashley kicked two "trashy-looking blondes" out of the team bus to make room for her. Back at the hotel, he begged her to stay, "just to sleep", she said.

"But almost immediately after that we started fooling around," she said. "When I raised the issue of a condom, Ashley acted like he was really shocked. He told me he couldn't believe I'd asked. He said having a condom would suggest he was banking on sex. So we carried on like that for a bit, him trying it on and me stopping him, but, in the end, we did have unprotected sex. It's the only thing about the evening that I'm ashamed about."

Otherwise the evening was quite a success, according to Ann. The sex lasted three or four hours.

"I was very taken aback by how intimate he was and how needy he was," she said. "It was like having sex with a boyfriend, someone who loves you. Ashley took my clothes off and was incredibly attentive. He was a creative and adventurous lover. At the end, he was satisfied and so was I. He was aiming to please, not just out to satisfy himself."

Afterwards, he wanted to cuddle. But it was too hot, so she

pulled away. Then he wanted to hold hands. Next morning, she felt awkward, but Ashley wanted to fool around.

"So we had sex again," she said.

He begged her to stay, or come back again that night. Then he offered to have her smuggled out of the hotel the back way. So when she got home she Googled him and found, not only that he was married, but that he had cheated on his wife before.

Ann was mortified. She should have known better. After all the soccer star had been smoking. She even texted him and asked him to keep quiet about their one-night stand. Ashley called back, saying that no one had said that to him before. And, like a gentleman, he promised not to say a word.

But when a reporter got wind of the affair and visited Ann, she phoned Ashley. He begged her to deny everything, then called in Steve Atkins, head of communications at Chelsea, who innocently gave her advice on how to handle the press. But Ashley's constant calls began to annoy her. Then she heard about the pictures being sent to Sonia Wild and decided to come clean about the fling.

Then, to top it all, glamour model Alexandra Taylor said that he had bedded her just when he and Cheryl first started dating. Alexandra was at the bar in the Funky Buddha club when the footballer and the singer were cheek to cheek on the dance floor, but Cheryl had to leave early because of commitments the following day.

Minutes after Cheryl had left what was their first official night out, Ashley went over to Alexandra to chat her up. Then he invited her back to his place, which was in the same complex as Cheryl's apartment, to party. His friends ushered her past the photographers to a waiting car. Back at his flat, Ashley wasted no time.

"He was really hands-on and flirty when we got back there," she said. "We were both attracted to each other – it was really intense. After about fifteen minutes, he said, 'I'm going upstairs to lie down,' and as he went he gave me the eye to follow him."

Leaving the others downstairs she trotted off after him.

"When I got up there, Ashley was already undressed and under the covers, just wearing his boxers," she told the *Daily Mirror*. "We were both really drunk, started kissing – and one thing led to another. He was so off his face with drink, he could barely do the deed. It lasted about fifteen minutes and was really lousy."

Ashley really gets rotten reviews.

"I tried to get some conversation out of him afterwards but he just wanted to roll over and go to sleep. It was like he had got what he wanted and that was all he cared about."

He did not know what he was missing. Alexandra was a formidable conversationalist, or at least she was when she talked to the *Daily Mirror*.

The glamour model left the soccer star snoozing and got a cab home. She claimed that she did not know that Cheryl was only a matter of yards away while they were at it. Indeed, this had happened two days before the story broke that Cheryl and Ashley were an item. Although Ashley and Alexandra continued to see each other socially, she did not give him a return match.

One of his friends called up to asked her to keep quiet about their tryst, she said. She said nothing, fearing it would damage her modelling career.

"But now I wish I had gone public – or at least tried to let Cheryl know what her man was like," she told the *Mirror*. "I was shocked when they got engaged. He was cheating on Cheryl with me from day one but I wondered if she had managed to convince him to settle down. But it's obvious he never changed."

Within days of these revelations, Cheryl announced she was leaving her husband and began divorce proceedings. She then announced that she would not take a penny from him, making a clean break. However, she would continue to use his name.

Ashley barely missed a stride. By October 2011, the newspapers were reporting that he had pulled a pair of twins who had posed for *Playboy*. He got twenty-one-year-old Carla and Melissa Howe to parade outside their home to see which would get the chance to sleep with him. Melissa won and was whisked off to the Surrey home where Ashley had lived with Cheryl. Two days later, after a gig at the $O_2$, he went off with one of Rihanna's dancers. Nevertheless, after four dates, Cole begged Melissa to move in with him, according to the *People*. She declined the offer, for the moment.

"I don't want him to think I'm one of those girls who just jumps into bed," she said. "And it's a bit too soon to be moving in, to be honest. Ashley is really good-looking and has a good body. He seems like a really nice guy too. I think he is pretty besotted and things could get serious. But I'm only twenty-one and I'm making him wait."

She should have seized the opportunity while it was on offer. While in September 2010, a divorce was granted in under a minute, the transfer window is now closed. By January 2011, the papers were reporting that Cheryl still had the hots for Ash. In July, the *Sun* said Ashley was planning to ask Cheryl to marry him again with a wedding ring carrying a diamond so big "it is visible from space". Hope springs eternal.

## Boris Becker

German tennis champion Boris Becker denied having sex with Russian model Angela Ermakova in a broom cupboard in a Japanese restaurant in London.

"It actually happened on the stairs between the bathrooms," he later confessed. "It was an act that lasted five seconds. It was poom-pah-boom."

According to a friend, this was not Angela's recollection: "They were by the staircase on the third floor outside the restaurant and she told me that Boris just started to kiss and cuddle her. That's when they found a storeroom open and Boris ushered her in."

And it lasted more than five seconds.

"Angela told me he was like a man possessed. He tore off her clothes and took off his trousers as he kissed her all over. It was a really passionate lovemaking session."

Whether it took five seconds or fifty minutes, Ermakova fell pregnant. She was convinced that the child was Becker's, claiming that he was the only man she had had unprotected sex with at the time. So she phoned him in Germany. He was, apparently, cool. On a second phone call, Ermakova got to speak to Boris's wife Barbara and told her that she was having her husband's baby, but she said that fans were always ringing up with such claims.

Before they had married, Becker and his wife-to-be had already created a sensation by appearing nude on the cover of *Stern* magazine in a photograph taken by her father, the African-American photographer Harlen Feltus, as a protest against racism.

Barbara Becker headed for the US to sidestep a prenuptial agreement, which would have given her just a $2.5 million payoff. The divorce proceedings in Florida were broadcast back in Germany. Meanwhile Boris was romantically linked with German rap singer Sabrina Setlur, though he denied a love affair. The divorce from Barbara reportedly cost him $14.4 million, plus their condo on Fisher Island, Florida, and custody of their two children.

After they had split – and a DNA test – he admitted being the father of Ermakova's child, explaining that he had just lost at Wimbledon and had decided to quit the game. After he had announced his retirement, he was going to meet up for a drink with pals. But they cancelled and he found himself alone and depressed. And one thing led to another.

Ermakova went to court to obtain child support, asking for £3 million. According to the judge, Becker made "an entirely reasonable and indeed generous" settlement. The *Daily Telegraph* reckoned that his sex fling cost him £400,000 a second, but that did not include the divorce settlement.

# 6

## Dirty Democrats

### Andrew Jackson

While George Washington was not a member of a political party and did not think them necessary, Alexander Hamilton formed the Federalist Party, while Thomas Jefferson and his successor James Madison formed the Democratic-Republicans. The Federalists disbanded, then the Democratic-Republicans split, making Andrew Jackson the first Democrat president.

Although he was born in a log cabin rather than a Palladian villa, Andrew Jackson plainly sought to emulate his distinguished predecessors. As a young man with no income he managed to scrape together $300 to buy a "negro woman named Nancy, about eighteen or twenty years of age". It is difficult to see what a young bachelor would need a young female servant for. On the other hand, it is not difficult to see what a young bachelor would need a young female servant for.

Living in Salisbury, North Carolina, he had already earned himself something of a reputation among the ladies.

"He was such a rake that my husband would not let him in the house," said one matron.

He outraged the whole town by sending invitations to the Christmas ball to two notorious prostitutes, Mary Ball and her fun-loving daughter. But when he tried to mend his ways and get married, he plunged himself into a scandal that would dog him for the rest of his life.

Moving to Nashville, Tennessee, he lodged at the boarding house of Mrs John Donelson and fell for her daughter Rachel. She was an extremely devout young woman, but at the age of seventeen she had married a landowner from Kentucky named Captain Lewis Robards. However, he was given to fits of jealous rage, accusing her of adultery while he himself was having affairs. This sent her scuttling home to her mother.

When Robards heard that Jackson had designs on his wife, he turned up and there was a fight. Jackson and Rachel then fled into Natchez, now in Mississippi but then in Spanish territory. As was the custom on the frontier at the time, Rachel began calling herself Mrs Jackson.

Hearing of their "elopement", Robards filed for divorce on the grounds of his wife's desertion. Jackson and Rachel seized the opportunity to get married. But Robards had only filed for divorce. It had not been granted. Consequently, the marriage was bigamous and invalid. Robards was then granted a divorce on the grounds of adultery and, in 1794, the Jacksons married again, this time legally.

Although it had been an honest mistake, Rachel had been publicly branded an adulteress. In the bitter presidential election of 1828, the *Cincinnati Gazette* asked: "Ought a convicted adulteress and her paramour husband be placed in the highest offices of this free and Christian land?"

And one anti-Jackson pamphlet read: "Anyone approving of Andrew Jackson must therefore declare in favor of the philosophy that any man wanting anyone else's pretty wife had nothing to do but take his pistol in one hand and a horsewhip in the other and possess her."

While Rachel was branded a bigamist, Jackson was an adulterer, enemies maintained. Even Jackson's mother was considered fair game. As she had given birth shortly after his father had died, she was branded a "common prostitute".

While Jackson was out on the campaign trail, Rachel remained at their home, the Hermitage, just outside Nashville, to run the estate, so Jackson managed to shield her from the invective. However, after he won the election, she came across some of the campaign literature. A religious woman, she said, "I would rather be a door-keeper in the house of God than live in that palace in Washington."

Knowing that everyone now knew of her shame, she promptly died of a heart attack. Jackson blamed his opponent John Quincy Adams for Rachel's death and never forgave him.

Rachel was buried in the ball gown she had bought for the inauguration. Her epitaph read: "A being so gentle and so virtuous slander might wound, but could not dishonor."

A young niece named Emily Donelson took over the duties of First Lady, which would not have passed without comment these days. When she died in 1836, the role was taken by Sarah Yorke Jackson, the wife of Andrew Jackson Jr, a nephew the Jacksons had adopted as they had no children of their own.

Jackson's administration soon found itself mired in another sex scandal. It involved Peggy Eaton, the daughter of the keeper of a Washington tavern frequented by politicians. She was a game lass and was happy to dance with the customers and bounce upon their knees. Indeed, the distribution of her favours was the talk of Washington. However, when one young congressman from Tennessee, who had a lovely wife at home, got fresh she hit him with the fire tongs.

At the age of fifteen she planned to elope with an army officer, but her father put a stop to it. Then she married navy purser John Timberlake and had three children, one of whom died in infancy. But while her husband was away at sea, she began an affair with Senator John Henry Eaton, Jackson's old friend and campaign manager. Timberlake died in the Mediterranean. It was said that he either committed suicide or drank himself to death over the affair.

Eaton married Peggy and joined Jackson's Cabinet as Secretary of War. However, the other Washington wives would not accept her into their ranks. Their husbands were forced to take sides. Some used their political advantage to attack both Eaton and Jackson himself. Presidential hopeful Henry Clay made a Shakespearean quip at Peggy's expense: "Age cannot wither her, nor custom stale her infinite virginity."

Jackson believed that this type of malicious gossip had destroyed his wife, so he backed Eaton in what became known as the "Petticoat Affair". However, he was pitted against Floride Calhoun, wife of Vice President John C. Calhoun, who continued to snub Mrs Eaton, refusing to invite her to dinner parties where the other Washington wives would be present. The infighting became so intense that it was almost impossible for the government to conduct its regular business. But Jackson stood firm.

"I did not come here to make a Cabinet for the ladies of this place, but for the nation," he said.

At a formal Cabinet dinner, he seated Peggy next to him. For the occasion, she wore a plunging neckline, which further outraged the Washington wives. They walked out when she took to the dance floor.

Secretary of State Martin Van Buren, a widower freed from wifely pressures, offered a cure for the "Eaton malaria". He offered to resign, asking the rest of the Cabinet to do likewise. In exchange, Jackson named him ambassador to the Court of St James. But the appointment had to be ratified by the Senate. The vote there was tied. As vice president, Calhoun had the casting vote. He voted against. Clay saw this was an error, telling Calhoun that while he had destroyed an ambassador he had created a vice president.

Indeed, Jackson picked Van Buren as his running mate in the 1832 election, introducing the two-thirds rule in the nominating convention, giving no other contender a chance. The two-thirds rule stayed in place until 1936.

Peggy's scandalous life did not end there. When Eaton died, he left her a small fortune. At sixty-one, she married twenty-one-year-old Antonio Buchignani, her granddaughter's dancing teacher. Less than a year later, he eloped to Italy with all her money and her granddaughter. Peggy had to take work as a dressmaker to support herself. She died in 1879 and is buried in Oak Hill Cemetery next to John Eaton. At her funeral a large bouquet of white roses sent by the president and Mrs. Rutherford B. Hayes was placed on her grave.

## Martin Van Buren

Being a widower did not protect Martin Van Buren from sexual gossip. Rather it fuelled it. He enjoyed the company of beautiful women, inviting a good deal of speculation. His good friend Congressman Louis McLane of Delaware suspected him of "licentious" behaviour and filled his letters home with reports of Van Buren's alleged affairs.

His name was linked with Thomas Jefferson's granddaughter. At a ball, she asked the band to play "The Yellow-haired Laddie" – as a young man he was known for his golden locks. But gossips also had him married off to one of her sisters.

Washington insider Churchill C. Cambreleng linked his name to a "Mrs. O. L." Van Buren called him a rogue and admitted that the accusation had caused him a "peck of trouble". And when he became president Van Buren appointed Cambreleng minister to Russia to get rid of him.

Grande dame of the Washington scene, Harriet Butler accused Van Buren of being promiscuous with his affections with a number of ladies. Van Buren's response to her accusations was to write to her saying: "Nothing serves so well to season the perpetual dissipation of Sodom as an occasional letter from a kind-hearted and sensible female friend." Van Buren regularly wrote to women, sometimes to the consternation of their husbands. He claimed to enjoy their gossip.

There were other, more scurrilous rumours. Soon after arriving in Washington, Van Buren had moved into Peck's Hotel in Georgetown with Senator William Rufus DeVane King. There was talk that they were so close that he was "wedded to Mr King". He was also known for his colourful style of dress – orange silk cravats, yellow kid gloves, green dress coats, white ducks, velvet collars, fur hands, white-topped Moroccan boots and the extravagant use of lace.

All this might have invited more suspicion had it not been completely overshadowed by a sex scandal involving his vice president Richard Johnson. A Kentuckian, Johnson had taken as his mistress Julia Chinn, a slave girl he had inherited from his father. He was open about his relationship with Chinn and claimed her two daughters as his own. This cost him his seat in the Senate in 1829, though his district returned him to the House the following year.

When Julia died of cholera in 1833, he took another of the family's slaves as his mistress. And when she ran off with an Indian, he had her captured and sold. Her place in his bed was filled by her younger sister.

Johnson's scandalous private life was discussed in the press, on the hustings and even in Congress, where mention was made of "the vice-president's swarthy wife and dingy children". There was speculation that, if Van Buren should die, Johnson would move his "coloured family" into the White House. Such a thing, of course, could never happen.

On 22 August 1839, US Postmaster Amos Kendall wrote to Van Buren, protesting that the vice president was living with his third coloured mistress. Johnson was not nominated for a second term.

## James Buchanan

William Rufus DeVane King also made an appearance in the life of James Buchanan. After one of his first loves, the heiress Anne Coleman, died in mysterious circumstances, Buchanan remained a lifelong bachelor. Her father refused him permission to attend the funeral, fuelling the suspicion that she had committed suicide after he spurned her.

Although he frequently talked of his intention to get married, in Washington he fell under the thrall of Senator King. They were room-mates and friends for twenty-three years. It was noted that King's "fastidious habits and conspicuous intimacy with bachelor Buchanan gave rise to some cruel jibes".

Andrew Jackson called King "Miss Nancy". He was also known as Buchanan's "better half", "his wife" and "Aunt Fancy". And when King became vice president under Franklin Pierce, he was known as "Mrs Vice President". Buchanan's own postmaster Aaron V. Brown called King "Mrs B." and made smirking references to "Mr Buchanan and wife" and "Aunt Fancy . . . rigged out in her best clothes".

This was not confined to Washington insiders. The contemporary press also speculated about Buchanan and King's relationship. When they died, their relatives destroyed their correspondence. But some survived. In one letter, Buchanan wrote to King, after King left on a trip to France in 1844, saying: "I am now solitary and alone, having no companion in the house with me. I have gone a wooing to several gentlemen, but have not succeeded with any one of them."

Buchanan remains the only unmarried president of the United States, while King was the only unmarried vice president.

## Grover Cleveland

The twenty-second president of the United States survived two sex scandals, one on the hustings and one in office. In 1884, Cleveland ran against the Republican James G. Blaine who, while in Congress, had been accused of accepting

$100,000 in bribes from the railroads. Huge features about the origins of Blaine's wealth filled the Democrat newspapers and Cleveland's supporters took up the chant: "Blaine, Blaine, James G. Blaine, the continental liar from the state of Maine".

The Republicans countered with the charge that, ten years earlier, Cleveland had fathered an illegitimate child and chanted back: "Ma, ma, where's my pa?" To which the Democrats would riposte: "Gone to the White House, ha, ha, ha."

To dampen the scandal, Cleveland adopted the unprecedented ploy of telling the truth. It was true, he said, that he had once had an "illicit connection with a woman and a child had been born and given his name". But while he was governor of New York he had never entertained her "in a bad way" in the gubernatorial mansion in Albany.

In fact, the child probably was not even his. The boy's mother, Mrs Halpin, had been seeing other men, including Oscar Folsom, a partner in Cleveland's legal practice. He was a married man. Indeed, the child was named Oscar Folsom Cleveland after Cleveland, who was single, agreed to take the blame.

Mrs Halpin wanted marriage, but Cleveland only provided child support. Nevertheless, the more that came out about the Halpin affair, the more Cleveland appeared to have acted honourably. With paternity now on the agenda, the Democrats then discovered that Blaine's first child had been born just three months after his wedding. Cleveland refused to use this against his opponent, saying, "The other side can have the monopoly on all the dirt in this campaign."

This was politics, so the story leaked out anyway. Blaine claimed there had been a mix-up. There had been two wedding ceremonies – the first six months earlier. But he could produce no evidence to back this. Cleveland's audacious plan to tell the truth to the electorate seemed to have paid off handsomely.

Even so, the election was neck and neck and everything depended on New York, where Cleveland had earned the opposition of Tammany Hall. So Blaine sought to woo the Irish voters, boasting that his mother was a Catholic and his sister a mother superior. But then at a rally in New York City, a supporter condemned the Democrats as the party of "rum, Romanism and rebellion". This was seen as anti-Catholic and Cleveland won the state and the election.

It seems that the stout, balding Cleveland enjoyed the role of Lothario, or at least saw that there was some political advantage in it, as there was another lady who put a twinkle in his eye. In 1875, Oscar Folsom – the putative father of Cleveland's illegitimate son – had died in a coaching accident and Cleveland was appointed administrator of Folsom's estate. He looked after Folsom's widow and oversaw the upbringing of his ten-year-old daughter Frank – later known as Frances – whom he had known since she was a baby.

In August 1885, five months after he took office, the forty-nine-year-old President Cleveland proposed to the recently graduated Frances Folsom, who had just turned twenty-one. However, they did not announce their engagement until five days before their wedding, which took place in the White House on 2 June 1886. The twenty-seven-year difference in their age caused a sensation – especially as he had essentially been her guardian for ten years. The story circulated in the press that, when she was a child, he had bought her first baby carriage.

He weighed 260 pounds (nearly nineteen stone) and was bull-necked and physically unprepossessing. She was young, slim, doe-eyed and dainty. The newspapers wrote scandalous articles warning her of the dangers of intimate relations with a man of such bulk. Journalists followed them to their honeymoon cottage in Deer Park, Maryland, camping outside with telescopes to observe the cavorting couple.

More sexual scandal was to follow. In the 1888 election, Tammany Hall issued a pamphlet accusing Cleveland of bestial perversions during his youth in Buffalo and the brutal treatment of his young wife. Although he won the popular vote, the electoral college gave the presidency to his opponent Benjamin Harrison.

When Mrs Cleveland left the White House on 4 March 1889, she said to the staff: "Take good care of the furniture . . . for I want to find everything just as it is now when we come back again. We are coming back just four years from today."

They spent his time out of office refuting allegations of marital strife. The first two of their five children were produced before they returned to the White House in 1893. Two years later, Mrs Halpin surfaced again. She wrote to the president demanding money and threatening to rekindle the scandal by publishing her side of the story. Nothing came of it.

Until Cleveland had married, the role of First Lady had been played by his sister Rose, a spinster lady with a successful career as a teacher, novelist and literary critic. In 1889, she began a romantic friendship with Evangeline Simpson, a wealthy thirty-year-old. The two women exchanged a series of romantic letters. In one, Rose admitted: "I tremble at the thought of you," and "I dare not think of your arms." Simpson replied, calling Miss Cleveland "my Clevy, my Viking, my Everything". After Simpson's husband died, the women moved to Italy in 1910 and lived together until Miss Cleveland died in 1918.

## Woodrow Wilson

While steering his nation through the troubled waters of World War I and redrawing the map of Europe at the Versailles Conference of 1919, Woodrow Wilson skirted two major sex scandals. The first threatened to break as early as 1912, when he was seeking the nomination of the Democratic Party. His long-term mistress Mrs Mary Peck was seeking a divorce and it was rumoured that his name would be mentioned in the suit. It was even said that one of his love letters to Mrs Peck had been shown to the judge as evidence. Theodore Roosevelt, who was running for an unprecedented third term, suspected that he was using the Grover Cleveland ploy.

"You can't cast a man as Romeo when he looks and acts so much like an apothecary's clerk," said Roosevelt.

Despite being dyslexic, Wilson became an academic who translated erotic work, including a bedroom scene from Théophile Gautier's *Mademoiselle de Maupin*, which was based on the life of a celebrated lesbian opera star. In 1885, he had married Ellen Louise Axson, the daughter of a minister from Rome, Georgia. They had three daughters. But then in 1907, he met Mrs Peck, a sophisticated woman of the world.

Born Mary Allen in Grand Rapids, Michigan, in 1862, she married Thomas Harbach Hulbert in 1883. When he died six years later, she went to live in Rome in a scandalous ménage à trois with her father-in-law and his young woman companion whom he later adopted. After two years, she returned to the US to have an operation to correct damage caused in childbirth.

In 1890, she married Thomas Dowes Peck. He was mean and cruel. She fell into depression, but a sympathetic physician recommended that she visit Bermuda on her own. She took these solitary winter breaks away from her husband every year after 1892. In 1907, she met Woodrow Wilson who was taking his first holiday without his wife on the island. Their main topic of conversation – and mutual interest – was marital unhappiness.

They met again the following year. They walked along the beach together, read each other verse, and soon fell deeply in love. One of Wilson's unsent letters was addressed to "my precious one, my beloved Mary".

Wilson wrote home to his wife about Mrs Peck, but claimed they were just good friends. When he returned to Princeton, where he was a professor, there was a blazing row and Ellen refused to accompany him on a trip to Britain. Things seemed to have been smoothed over when he returned. Ellen

To dampen his ardour, they told him that Mrs Peck was circulating his love letters around town. This only inflamed him. He rushed around to Mrs Galt's house to spill the beans about his affair with Mrs Peck and beg her to forgive him. When she did, he sent out a press release, announcing their engagement.

Then on 9 October 1915, after their first official outing as a couple, they fell victim to an embarrassing typo. They had attended a social evening at a local theatre. In their report of the event, the *Washington Post* had intended to print "rather than paying attention to the play the president spent the evening entertaining Mrs Galt". What it actually printed was "rather than paying attention to the play the president spent the evening entering Mrs Galt".

Now the cat was out of the bag. Malicious rumours circulated that Wilson had been neglecting his wife's grave. It was said that he had been cheating with Mrs Galt before Ellen was dead – even that Mrs Galt had been behind a bizarre plot to murder the First Lady. The genteel ladies of America were outraged and the press turned hostile.

To limit the political damage, Wilson decided that they should get married as soon as possible. On 18 December 1915, they wed in her home in front of forty guests. Once Mrs Galt was installed, Mrs Peck was banned from the White House. Wilson seems to have paid her off. There is evidence that he gave her $15,000 not to reveal details of their extramarital affair. Although she fell on hard times, she refused an offer of $300,000 to tell all. It was only in 1933, nine years after Wilson died that she wrote her kiss-and-tell autobiography *The Story of Mrs Peck*.

The bad press about Mrs Galt continued after her marriage. When President Wilson fell ill after returning from the Versailles Peace Conference, she effectively took over the reigns of government for the remaining two years of his presidency. In her book *My Memoir*, she called this period her "stewardship". Others talked of the "Petticoat Government" and "Mrs

Wilson's Regency", while Wilson himself was derided as her "First Man".

## Franklin Delano Roosevelt

After the relatively scandal-free administrations of Calvin Coolidge and Herbert Hoover, who as a youth had a hot affair down under – that is, in Australia – FDR brought sexual shenanigans back to the White House. But he had established a pact with the press who never once mentioned that he was confined to a wheelchair. There were more important issues at stake – coping with the Great Depression and World War II.

As a young man, Roosevelt had a reputation as a womanizer, a drinker and a careless flirt. Nevertheless he married his po-faced cousin Eleanor, swearing eternal fidelity – a pledge he singularly failed to live up to.

During World War I, Roosevelt was assistant secretary of the navy, which meant that he stayed in Washington while Eleanor spent her time at their holiday home on the island of Campobello off the coast of Maine. This gave him all the time he needed to date other women.

In 1918, Eleanor found love letters between Roosevelt and Lucy Mercer, the social secretary she had hired four years earlier. After thirteen years of marriage and five children, she offered her errant husband a divorce.

"Don't be a goose," he replied.

Roosevelt's redoubtable mother Sara insisted that there be no divorce. The scandal would ruin her only son's political career. She told him that she would cut him off without a penny if he left Eleanor. Perhaps a bigger factor in Roosevelt's mind was that Lucy was a Catholic. So even if he had divorced Eleanor, Lucy would not have married him.

If the marriage was to continue, Eleanor insisted that he give up Lucy. Again Roosevelt promised. Again he lied and continued seeing Lucy until his death twenty-seven years later, often with the connivance of his eldest daughter. He was a great politician.

Sacked by Eleanor, Lucy needed a new job. Luckily, she found employment in the Navy Department in Washington and she lived nearby, which was handy for the secretary of the navy. That summer, Eleanor delayed her return to Campobello to keep an eye on them. Her fears were allayed when Roosevelt employed British diplomat Nigel Law as a beard so he could be seen out with Lucy without arousing suspicion.

Even Eleanor's cousin Alice Longworth was in on the secret. She would invite Roosevelt and Lucy to dinner. Roosevelt "deserved a good time," she said, "he was married to Eleanor."

According to Roosevelt's son James, Eleanor knew full well what was going on. She even had evidence that Lucy and her husband had checked in to a hotel in Virginia Beach together as man and wife. However, she maintained the pretence that she did not wish to know anything that her husband did not want to tell her.

In 1919, Roosevelt risked scandal again when he took on a new secretary, Marguerite "Missy" LeHand and promptly made her his mistress. Eleanor seems to have known about this too, but tolerated it as Miss LeHand was of a lower social class. Besides Eleanor's interests now lay elsewhere. After 1920, all her friends were of a Sapphic persuasion. Between the wars, lesbianism was all the rage among the upper classes.

By then Lucy had married wealthy sportsman Winthrop Rutherfurd who was twice her age. Roosevelt was shocked when he heard the news, but he did not stop seeing her. When he was president, the secret service gave the codename "Mrs Johnson", so she could visit him in the White House.

Roosevelt remained a flirt, a notorious bottom-pincher and knee-holder. Nor did he hide his light under a bushel. He even took Missy LeHand out on the campaign trail with him. Their affair went on for twenty years, with Missy playing hostess at the White House when Eleanor was away.

Vacationing on Campobello in 1921, Roosevelt went swimming and was struck down by polio. His legs were paralysed. While Missy LeHand oversaw his hydrotherapy, Eleanor was employed to keep his name centre stage in Democratic circles. Though shy, she quickly became an effective public speaker.

Roosevelt and Missy set up home together on a houseboat in Florida where they could be seen relaxing on deck in their night clothes. One guest called it a "negligee existence". Eleanor rarely visited. When she did, she came with one of her girlfriends. Roosevelt and Missy also had a cottage in Warm Springs, Georgia, where he established a foundation for the care of polio victims. Again, when Eleanor visited, she was the guest while her husband's mistress was the hostess. Missy also had a room in the family home at Hyde Park, upstate New York, and in Roosevelt's house in Manhattan. Later she lived in an apartment in the White House.

By 1923, Eleanor had set up home in Greenwich Village and in Val-Kill, not far from Hyde Park. But her interests there were not entirely Sapphic. In 1929, the forty-five-year-old Eleanor took up with thirty-two-year-old bodybuilder Earl Miller, who was a notorious womanizer. He was a New York State police sergeant whom her husband had assigned to her as a bodyguard. An Olympic athlete and former navy middleweight boxing champion, he taught her to ride, shoot and dive, and coached her at tennis. Some of her lesbian friends were distressed to see him manhandle her, especially when they were in their bathing costumes. Again there was nothing secret about the affair. He squired her around her public duties, but the press made nothing of it.

When Roosevelt became president in 1933, Eleanor talked of running away with Miller. That would have caused a scandal. However, Miller claimed that Missy had organized night shifts with him at Warm Springs, so he could come to her room. There was speculation that Roosevelt had sanctioned the affair to prevent Eleanor running away. The emergency was over when it was discovered that he was also playing around with one of the girls in the Executive Office. Missy was heartbroken and took to her bed and cried for three days. Eleanor took the whole thing in her stride. She even encouraged his romances and kept her hold over him through his three marriages, all of which ended in divorce.

Again the whole edifice teetered on the edge of a disastrous scandal when, on 13 January 1947, Ed Sullivan wrote in his column in the *New York Daily News* that a "navy commander's wife will rock the country if she names the co-respondent in her divorce action".

While Earl Miller denied having a physical relationship with Eleanor Roosevelt, saying he preferred "pretty young things", the aggrieved Mrs Miller threatened to name Mrs Roosevelt as co-respondent, rather than one of the "pretty young things" her wayward husband seemed incapable of resisting, because she was in possession of some of Mrs Roosevelt's letters and knew that threatening to publish them would be the most likely way to win herself a lucrative settlement out of court – as she did eventually. Eleanor's son James wrote of his mother's relationship with Miller: "I personally believe that they were more than friends." However, Miller hardly rates a mention in Eleanor's autobiography.

Throughout Roosevelt's long presidency, he and Eleanor played the perfect couple in public. Behind closed doors though it was a different story. Although Missy had a suite of her own in the White House, she was often seen in the president's room in her night clothes. Meanwhile, Eleanor was in the other wing with her cigar-chomping lesbian pal Lorena Hickok.

They had met in 1928 when Hickok, a reporter for the Associated Press, came to interview Eleanor. In her story, she eulogized her "lace-trimmed hostess gown" and her "long slender hands". From then on they were inseparable. She cooked up stories with Eleanor and built her public image.

In 1933, she quit her job, claiming she could no longer be objective about the Roosevelts, now they were about to enter the White House. Eleanor found her a job as chief investigator of the Federal Emergency Relief Administration. On the day of FDR's inauguration, Eleanor was seen wearing a sapphire ring Lorena – or "Hick darling", as she called her – had given her. Eleanor had also given Lorena one in what I suppose we can call an exchange of rings.

Lorena was no looker. Just five foot eight, she weighed two hundred pounds (over fourteen stone). As well as the cigars, she occasionally smoked a pipe and drank bourbon on the rocks like "one of the boys". On the other hand, Eleanor was hardly eye candy either.

In February 1934, *Time* magazine hinted at Hickok's inclinations, calling her a "rotund lady with a husky voice" who wore "baggy clothes". In letters, Eleanor spoke of "longing to kiss and hold" Lorena in her arms. "I can't kiss you, so I kiss your picture goodnight and good morning!" she wrote. "Goodnight, dear one. I want to put my arms around you and kiss you at the corner of your mouth. And in a little more than a week now – I shall."

There's more: "I wish I could lie down beside you tonight and take you in my arms"; "I ache to hold you close"; "Most clearly I remember your eyes with a kind of teasing smile in them, and the feeling of that soft spot just north-east of the corner of your mouth against my lips . . ." And this was just what slipped through. Hick would edit and retype Eleanor's letters and burn the originals in an effort to sanitize their affair.

The White House staff soon realized what was going on. The maid Lillian Parks remembered that Mrs Roosevelt and Hick would disappear for long sessions in Eleanor's bathroom, claiming that it was the "only place they could find privacy to do a press interview". On the other hand, they considered this "hardly the kind of thing one would do with an ordinary reporter, or even with an adult friend".

Roosevelt knew what was going on. He hated Hickok and was once heard to yell: "I want that woman kept out of this house." And he was the president of the United States.

On the other hand, he had his own live-in mistress. Also on hand was Crown Princess Marta of Norway, who took up residence at Roosevelt's invitation after her country was occupied. It is rumoured that she occupied him.

In January 1941, Hickok moved into the White House, living there until 1945. However, her relationship with Eleanor grew shaky when Hickok took up with the Honourable Marion Janet Harron, a United States tax court judge who was nineteen years younger than Eleanor.

Eleanor got her own back by starting an affair with the young Joseph P. Lash, who later found fame as her biographer. This outraged the president. Lash was a Socialist who had appeared before the House Un-American Activities Committee. He had a security file and the room they shared in the Blackstone Hotel was bugged by army intelligence. According to his FBI file, the tapes "indicated quite clearly that Mrs Roosevelt and Lash were engaged in sexual intercourse".

Eleanor was not best pleased to have been bugged, but the rumpus blew over. She and Hick kissed and made up. Eleanor continued to find jobs for Hick within the Democratic Party. Hick co-authored *Ladies of Courage* with Eleanor in 1954 and pumped out *The Story of Eleanor Roosevelt* in 1959. She lived in a cottage on the Roosevelt estate to be near to Eleanor. When she died there in 1968, she left half her papers to the FDR Library at Hyde Park. The rest went to the National Archives under the proviso that they be sealed for ten years after her death. When they were opened, they were found to contain 2,336 letters from Eleanor.

While Eleanor and Hick were tipping the velvet in one wing of the White House, Roosevelt was carrying on in his distinctive heterosexual way in the other. To the outrage of feminists everywhere, each year, on his birthday, he would hold a drinks party at the Cufflinks Club where he would appear dressed as a Roman emperor and his female guests were supposed to turn up as Vestal Virgins.

Despite this frenzied sexual activity within the walls of the White House, a sex scandal suddenly engulfed the administration from another quarter – Undersecretary of State Sumner Welles, who had been Roosevelt's trusted special envoy, first to Hitler and Mussolini, then to Churchill. In January 1941, J. Edgar Hoover outed Welles as a homosexual and produced a number of affidavits from two African-American porters on a Pullman train saying that Welles, while drunk, had propositioned them. Roosevelt stuck by Welles, but the matter leaked and Welles was forced to resign.

The man behind Welles's downfall was his rival in the State Department, William Bullitt. Roosevelt's son Eliot later wrote that his father believed that Bullitt had bribed the porters to make overtures to Welles. Bullitt was having an affair with Missy LeHand at the time. To get his own back, Roosevelt suggested that Bullit run for mayor of Philadelphia while secretly telling the local Democrat leaders there to "cut his throat".

Missy had a stroke and Roosevelt rewrote his will, leaving her half the income from his estate. In the end, she died before he did, so the money went to Eleanor.

Without Missy, Roosevelt was short of female company, so two unmarried cousins, Margaret Suckley and Laura Delano, became his "handmaidens". Margaret Suckley was told to burn his letters. Those that survive betray a certain intimacy.

"There is no reason why I should not tell you that I miss you very much – It was a week ago yesterday," Roosevelt wrote her after spending time with her at Hyde Park. "I have longed to have you with me," he wrote another time during a cruise to Panama.

"He told me once," she wrote in her diary soon after his death, "that there was no one else with whom he could be so completely himself." There was certainly plenty of speculation that their relationship was sexual.

accompanied her husband on a visit to the Pecks in Pittsfield, Massachusetts, and even invited Mrs Peck to come and stay with them in Princeton. When she arrived, it caused a tremendous stir.

In 1909, Wilson and Mrs Peck even discussed divorcing their partners so they could be together. Then he grew jealous when he heard that she had received an invitation from the governor of Bermuda, whose name had also been linked to her romantically. That winter he visited her at least six times, in and around New York. She had an apartment on East 27th Street, not far from where Wilson's father kept a mistress.

As it was, her divorce went off without anything leaking to the press. Once in office, Wilson took his family on holiday to Bermuda where Mrs Peck joined them. She also visited him in Washington, though Ellen or his cousin Helen Bones acted as chaperone. They continued to correspond and Mrs Peck visited him again after Ellen had died of kidney disease in August 1914. There was speculation that they may marry and he supported her financially. However, by then, he had met Mrs Edith Bolling Galt. She had been introduced to him by Helen Bones, who had taken over the role as official hostess at the White House and had invited Mrs Galt around for tea in March 1915.

Returning early from a game of golf, Wilson promptly invited Mrs Galt for dinner. He plied her with flowers daily and installed a private line between the White House and her Washington home. Within two months, they were engaged. It was said that, when he proposed, she was so shocked that she nearly fell out of bed.

It seems that they were, indeed, physically intimate before they were married during a clandestine vacation in New Hampshire. World War I was now raging in Europe. Although America was not yet involved, the last thing the country needed was a lovesick president. His Cabinet reminded him of the political damage he would do himself if he got married so soon after the death of his first wife.

Towards the end of his life, Lucy Mercer began to play a more prominent role again. She had always been there for him in the background at key moments in his life. She had been at the Democratic National Convention in 1936 when he made his acceptance speech and secretly attended all four inaugurations.

In 1941, Winthrop Rutherfurd had a stroke and she got back in touch with Roosevelt. He would have the Secret Service drive him out to Canal Road beyond Georgetown, where she would meet him. They also met at Hobcaw Barony, Bernard Baruch's estate in South Carolina when Roosevelt took a break there, and the story circulated that Roosevelt's railroad car was shunted into a siding near Rutherfurd's estate at Allamuchy, New Jersey. But the world was at war, so no hint of this assignation made the press.

After her husband died, Lucy began visiting the White House while Eleanor was away. She was also with him at the cottage in Warm Springs when he died. Margaret Suckley and Laura Delano were there too. But while they could stay on, to prevent a scandal, Lucy had to pack her bags and leave.

## John F. Kennedy

Jack Kennedy could not keep it in his pants and risked scandal throughout his career. Shortly before his inauguration, he slipped away to Palm Springs to spend two or three days with actress Angie Dickinson. A reporter from *Newsweek* barged into their holiday cottage and found them in bed. The Roosevelt press pact still applied and he promptly forgot everything he saw.

Dickinson is credited with saying her fling with the president was "the best twenty seconds of my life". Others testify that Kennedy was indeed more interested in the conquest than the consummation. However, ever since, Dickinson has maintained a dignified silence on the subject.

On another occasion, Kennedy flaunted his sex life in front of the American people. There was an audience of fifteen thousand people at Madison Square Garden – and a TV audience coast to coast – on 19 May 1962, when Marilyn Monroe, currently his mistress, seductively sang "Happy Birthday, Mr President" in a dress that left nothing to the imagination. It was made of a sheer, flesh-coloured fabric covered in 2,500 rhinestones with nothing underneath. Under the lights, the fabric seemed to disappear, leaving only the rhinestones. Veteran diplomat Adlai Stevenson described the dress as "skin and beads – only I did not see the beads".

President Kennedy hardly helped the situation when he came on stage afterwards and said: "I can now retire from politics after having had, ah, 'Happy Birthday' sung to me in such a sweet, wholesome way."

Although the press still operated an *omertà* when it came to presidential dalliances, the humorist Art Buchwald had already hinted at his affair with Monroe in his column in the *Washington Post*. When Kennedy was first elected, he wrote: "Who will be the next ambassador to Monroe? This is one of many problems which president-elect Kennedy will have to work on."

Later he urged the president to stand firm on the Monroe Doctrine.

"Obviously, you cannot leave Monroe adrift," he wrote. "There are too many greedy people eyeing her."

It was rumoured that Buchwald himself had been an ambassador to Monroe. She liked men of letters.

Kennedy was simply following in the footsteps of his father Joe who was a legendary sexual adventurer. With the money he made from bootlegging, Joe Kennedy went into the movie industry, purely so he could seduce ambitious starlets. He bought the biggest movie star of the day, Gloria Swanson, by setting up Gloria Productions, Inc. and financing her films. But he wanted more. One evening, he turned up at her Palm Beach Hotel.

"He just stood there, in his white flannels and his argyle sweater and his two-tone shoes, staring at me for a full minute or more," she said, "before he entered the room and closed the door behind him. He moved so quickly that his mouth was on mine before either of us could speak. With one hand, he held the back of my head, with the other he stroked my body and pulled at my kimono. He kept insisting in a drawn-out moan, 'No longer, no longer. Now.' He was like a roped horse, rough, arduous, raving to be free. After a hasty climax—" like father, like son "—he lay beside me, stroking my hair. Apart from his guilty, passionate moaning, he had still said nothing coherent."

He contrived to introduce Swanson to his wife Rose, said he wanted to have a baby with her and even visited Cardinal O'Connell to try to get the Church's permission to leave Rose and set up a second home with her. The affair ended when she discovered that all the expensive presents he had given her had been charged to her company.

As a boy, Jack Kennedy was well aware that his father was cavorting with actresses and showgirls. He often brought mistresses home with him. One even stayed for a month and joined in family activities. Later, when his father was ambassador to London, Jack would advise women guests to lock their doors at night as "the ambassador has a tendency to go wandering". In his sixties, Joe Kennedy made a play for Grace Kelly and, in his seventies, he was seen touching up a hooker that Dominican playboy Porfirio Rubirosa brought to a party.

Joe Kennedy was determined that his boys should be chips off the old block. Jack once came home from school to find his bed covered with girlie magazines showing naked women in the most explicit of poses. It was "Dad's idea of a joke," he told a friend.

At the age of seventeen, Jack lost his virginity to a hooker in Harlem. He went with his schoolfriend Lem Billings. She charged them $3 each. They were then terrified that they had caught an STD. But the panic passed. In May 1936, he wrote to Billings about an adventure he had had with his friend Smokey Wilde south of the Rio Grande: "Got a fuck and a suck in a Mexican hoar-housse [*sic*] for 65 cents, so am feeling very fit and clean. Smoke and I set out yesterday, went over the border and arrived at a fucking Mexican town. Met a girl there who is really the best thing I have ever seen but does not speak English. Am writing to her tonight to get a date with her because she wouldn't go out with me last time and it is really love at first sight. They have the best-looking girls in those towns. Anyways Smoke and I ended up in this two-bit hoar-house and they say that one guy in five years has gotten away without just the biggest juiciest load of clap – so Smoke is looking plenty pallid and even I occasionally think of it, so boys your roomie is carrying on in true 9 South style and is upholding the motto of 'always get your piece of arse in the most unhealthy place that can be found'."

This escapade did indeed result in a dose of clap. His next letter to Billings was signed "your gonnereick roomie". But his interests were not confined to prostitutes.

"Went down to the Cape with five guys from school," he wrote. "EM [Eddie Moore] got us some girls thru another guy – four of us had dates and one guy got fucked three times, another guy three times (the girl a virgin!) and myself twice – they were all on the football team and I think the coaches heard because they gave us one hell of a balling out. The guy who got the virgin just got a very sickening letter, letting [him know] how much she loved him etc and as he didn't use a safer he is very worried. One guy is up at the doctor's seeing if he has a dose and I feel none too secure myself. We are going down next week for a return performance, I think."

A new coach was brought in and clamped down on such behaviour. Kennedy complained: "I will have to wank plenty to 'tame' it down."

At Harvard, he spent much of his time chasing women, successfully it seems.

"I can not get tail as often and as free as I want, which is a step in the right direction," he boasted. In his letters, he also complains of how sore his cock was and how he "brands" co-eds with his "red-hot poker". He called his penis "Lay More", though renamed it "J. J." after he was circumcised in 1926. He liked casual sex with secretaries and air hostesses – no one who was going to make "intellectual or strong demands on him which he was not ready to fulfil," said a friend of his sister. He also courted high society girls. There was talk that he might get engaged to Charlotte McDonnell, the daughter of a Wall Street broker. But when her father heard about it, he called Kennedy a "moral roustabout" and forbade him seeing his daughter again.

Olive Crawley dropped him after he disappeared during a date at the Stork Club to seduce the hatcheck girl. He dumped Harriet "Flip" Price when she would not put out. While there was talk of marriage, Kennedy admitted that he was more interested in "slam, bam, thank you, ma'am". And he continued to sow his wild oats in Britain when his father was appointed ambassador there.

In the autumn of 1941, Kennedy joined the navy and was posted to the Office of Naval Intelligence. At the time he was having an affair with Ingrid Arvad, a Danish beauty queen whom Hitler had cited as a perfect example of Nordic beauty. As a journalist, she had interviewed Hitler and accompanied him to the Olympic Games in Berlin in 1936. There were even rumours that she was his lover. As a suspected Nazi spy, the FBI kept tabs on her. They bugged the couple and J. Edgar Hoover had tapes of them making love. Early in his political career, Kennedy bragged that when he got to Washington, he would get hold of those tapes. He never managed to.

As it was, Kennedy was seen as a security risk and sacked from Naval Intelligence. His superiors wanted him cashiered from the navy, but his father stepped in. Instead, he was sent on active duty in the Pacific where, as commander of a PT boat, he became a hero – though it was said at the time that he spent more time chasing models than enemy submarines.

At one point, Kennedy had even wanted to marry Ingrid and had taken her to the family compound at Hyannis Port. His father prohibited this because she was not a Catholic, but that did not stop him trying to seduce her himself. She went on to have an affair with British Member of Parliament Robert Boothby, the long-term lover of the wife of the prime minister Harold Macmillan who also enjoyed homosexual orgies laid on by East End gangster Ronald Kray.

In 1944, Kennedy met the twenty-four-year-old model Florence Prichett. She was a divorcee so there was no question of them marrying. Their affair went on for years. In his appointment book for 28 June 1947, she wrote: "Flo Prichett's birthday: SEND DIAMONDS."

That year, she married a forty-four-year-old stockbroker, who later became US ambassador to Cuba. In 1957 and 1958, in the run up to the Cuba revolution, Kennedy would go over to Havana to see her and amuse himself with the prostitutes in the Hotel Commodoro. Later, they had adjoining properties in Palm Beach. When he was president, he would often give his Secret Service men the slip so he could see women. On one occasion, he jumped over the fence to take a dip in Flo's pool. Growing increasingly frantic because they had lost the president yet again, the Secret Service called the FBI. They in turn called Palm Beach Police Chief Homer Large. He knew exactly where to find Kennedy. He was, he said, in Flo Prichett's swimming pool and "they weren't doing the Australian crawl".

After the war, Kennedy was briefly a journalist, though he appeared in the gossip columns more often than he contributed. As well as socialites, he dated a string of chorus girls.

During his campaign for Congress in 1946, he was caught in the act of congress on his desk with a young campaign worker. She later missed her period. Kennedy said: "Oh, shit." And skipped lightly onwards.

Kennedy used his sexual charisma to good effect in the election and he did not turn off the charm once in office. When he was running for a second term, Massachusetts Governor Paul Denver addressed a campaign meeting, saying: "I hear it being said that my young friend Jack Kennedy isn't working down there in Washington, that he's too fond of girls. Well, let me tell you, ladies and gentlemen, I've never heard it said of Jack Kennedy that he's too fond of boys."

In his book *The Dark Side of Camelot*, Pulitzer Prize-winning investigative journalist Seymour Hersh said that, around this time, Kennedy married Palm Beach socialite Durie Malcolm. At the time, the marriage was hinted at by the *New York World-Telegram*'s society writer Charles Ventura. Hersh quotes Charles Spalding, a retired New York stockbroker who had known Kennedy since World War II. It was "a high-school prank," said Spalding, that lasted "twenty-four hours. They went down and went through the motions. I remember saying to Jack, 'You must be nuts. You're running for president and you're running around getting married.'"

As early as 1947, Kennedy was being groomed for the White House by his father who "had a haemorrhage" when he heard about the marriage. Not only was Malcolm twice divorced, she was an Episcopalian. According to Spalding, Joe "demanded that it be taken care of. They were afraid the whole thing was going to come out."

Spalding said that Jack asked him to go and get the marriage papers from Florida.

"I went out there and removed the papers," said Spalding. He told Hersh that he got the documents with the help of a lawyer in Palm Beach. The marriage was officially never terminated. In other words, Kennedy later became a bigamist. But even if it had been terminated, Kennedy would have been something equally scandalous for a Catholic – a remarried divorcee.

After Kennedy became president, *Newsweek* got wind of the story, which had been circulating in small Republican journals across the country. Kennedy's friend Ben Bradlee, Washington bureau chief for *Newsweek*, personally vetoed the *Newsweek* article.

In 1951, Kennedy was dating Alicia Darr and, it is said, they got engaged and she fell pregnant by him. Joe was against the match. When he became president, she told the Italian magazine *Le Ore* about the affair. She was divorcing her husband, English actor Edmund Purdom at the time. Kennedy paid $500,000 to have the whole thing hushed up.

Kennedy continued taking absurd risks. At a benefit dinner, after defeating Henry Cabot Lodge in the Massachusetts senatorial race, he disappeared with his date to a closet and the guests had to wait to retrieve their coats until the new senator had finished his rutting. He liked to make love on the floor of his office and, on his desk, he kept a photograph of himself with several nude girls, taken on a yacht. The press were soon calling him the playboy senator.

Clearly, if he was going to run for president, Kennedy was going to have to have a wife. The pose, charm and sophistication of Jacqueline Bouvier fitted her for the position. She was also the daughter of John Vernou "Black Jack" Bouvier III, a notorious womanizer – so she would know what she was getting herself into.

On their first date, they were having sex in Kennedy's convertible in Arlington, Virginia when they were caught by the police. But the patrolman recognized the senator and let them finish their erotic engagement with no further interruptions. She was engaged to stockbroker John Husted at the time and quickly broke it off.

They married in September 1953. The beautiful "Jackie" perfectly complemented the handsome young senator and they became Washington's most glamorous couple. But the outward appearance of a respectable married life was not going to inhibit Kennedy's womanizing. With his best man George Smathers, a senator from Florida, he took a suite in the Carroll Arms Hotel in Washington where they could conduct their extramarital affairs.

"Jack liked to go over there and meet a couple of young secretaries," said Smathers. "He liked groups."

They would hold orgies there, even while legislation was passing. "That sort of thing was his favourite pastime," said Smathers.

He recalled one time when they had gone back to the suite with two women the phone rang telling Smathers he was wanted back at the Senate. He was halfway there when he realized that the Senate was not sitting. When he got back to the suite, he found Kennedy making love to both women.

"Jack felt he could walk on water so far as women were concerned," said Smathers. "There is no question about the fact that Jack had the most active libido of any man I've ever known. He was really unbelievable – absolutely incredible in that regard, and he got more so the longer he was married."

"I'm not through with a girl till I have had her three ways," Kennedy told another colleague. It is clear what he meant.

"No one was off limits to Jack. Not your wife, your mother, your sister," said Smathers.

Once Kennedy tried to seduce the distinguished historian Dr Margaret Coit.

"Do you do this to all the women you meet?" she asked.

"Good God, no," he said. "I don't have the strength."

Keeping everything safe and discreet and behind closed doors was not Kennedy's style. He would bring lovers along to receptions where Jackie was present, though he would sometimes use his brother-in-law, the English actor Peter Lawford as a beard. When Jackie was away in Europe, he would arrange "house parties" in Maine. To allay suspicions, he would arrange for a respectable older lady to drive him to church in the morning. This was supposed to put the press off the scent.

For years, Kennedy had suffered problems with his back and Addison's disease, a disorder of the adrenal glands. This meant he had to spend a lot of time in hospital, surrounded by nurses. A number of so-called "cousins" would visit. Playing along, Jackie hired Grace Kelly to be his night nurse, just to see his reaction when he opened his eyes. It was doubly delicious as Kennedy's father had thrown his hat into the same ring.

In 1956, he met Joan Lundberg, an attractive divorcee, and took her to Peter Lawford's Santa Monica beach house. They were lovers for three years. During that time, he picked up her bills and arranged an abortion when she got pregnant. She said he loved threesomes with him and two women, and he was a voyeur. To cap it all, they made love in Jackie's marital bed in Georgetown. They ended the affair when he won the Democratic nomination at the convention in Los Angeles in 1960.

One night in 1958, Florence and Leonard Kater were awoken by a man throwing pebbles at the window of their lodger Pamela Turnure, a twenty-year-old Georgetown debutante who was said to have looked like Jackie. The man they recognized as Senator Kennedy. Pam Turnure was his secretary and worked on his campaign. When Kennedy became a regular night-time visitor, the strait-laced couple were outraged. They planted a tape recorder in Pamela's rooms and photographed him going in and out, if you will pardon the expression. Then they took this evidence to every newspaper, magazine and TV station within reach. No one was interested.

Naively, they contacted Joe Kennedy and even complained to Cardinal Cushing, the Archbishop of Boston. When that did no good, they followed Kennedy around on the campaign trail holding up placards denouncing him as an adulterer. When that did not sway the voters, they ended up picketing the White House. But still the scandal would not break. Instead, they were persuaded to hand the pictures and tapes over to J. Edgar Hoover, head of the FBI.

Meanwhile, Kennedy had persuaded Jackie to take Pam Turnure on as her press secretary, though she had no previous experience in the field. Asked what it was like having his mistress working for his wife, Kennedy said: "Like living life on a high wire."

She moved from the Katers and moved in with Jackie's friend, the artist Mary Meyer, who knew of the affair. However, after a while Kennedy grew tired of Pam and started bedding Mary instead. During their lovemaking sessions in her studio, in the homes of friends and, later, in the White House, they experimented with marijuana and LSD. Peter Lawford also supplied them with cocaine and amyl nitrate poppers, which they tried out on two White House secretaries. Kennedy also used novocaine and cortisone to dull the pain in his back. Dr Max Jacobson – known as "Dr Feelgood" to his high-class clientele – travelled with Kennedy to give him his shots of amphetamine and steroids. He was struck off after one of his patients died.

Long before Kennedy reached the White House, his marriage was on the rocks. When Jackie gave birth to a stillborn child in 1956, Kennedy was cruising in the Mediterranean with George Smathers and a bevy of beautiful girls. Kennedy was reluctant to return to her bedside. It took Smathers three days to convince him that, if he did not fly home, he risked not only his marriage but also his political career. Jackie was so upset that, when she left hospital, she did not go home. Instead, she went to stay on her stepfather's estate. Things got worse when she heard that their fifteen-year-old babysitter, supplied by a veteran newsman, was pregnant, claiming Kennedy was the father. She was despatched to Puerto Rico for an abortion.

As always, Joe Kennedy stepped in to patch things up. He offered Jackie a financial settlement, provided that she did not leave Jack. She accepted, but she punished Jack by ruinous spending sprees and wild flirtations with the objective of making him jealous. She may even have had affairs of her own. Kennedy's secretary Evelyn Lincoln talked of a "dashing Italian count". There were rumours that she had succumbed to the owner of Fiat Gianni Agnelli, after Kennedy had flirted openly with his wife, and fallen for one of her security guards.

FBI chief J. Edgar Hoover was an old friend of Lyndon Johnson. They lived next door to each other in Washington. When Johnson ran against Kennedy for the nomination in 1960, he gave the pictures and tapes he had got from the Katers to Johnson, along with Kennedy's overstuffed FBI file. By that time Kennedy had moved his extramarital activities to the Mayflower Hotel, which the FBI called "Kennedy's personal playpen". Hoover also had "affidavits from two mulatto prostitutes in New York". It also contained a report from an FBI informant saying that he had seen Kennedy and Senator Estes Kefauver have sex with two women in front of him, then switch partners and do it again.

Kennedy continued to court scandal on the campaign trail. He hung out in Las Vegas with Frank Sinatra and the rat pack while they were filming *Ocean's 11*. According to an FBI report, "showgirls from all over town were running in and out of the senator's suite".

Then he began the most scandalous affair of his career. In February 1960, Sinatra introduced him to Judith Campbell, a wealthy divorcee Sinatra had picked up the previous year. Edward Kennedy also fancied her, but Jack got in first. The following month, Kennedy and Campbell spent four days together in the Plaza Hotel in New York. Then Sinatra introduced her to Sam Giancana, the boss of the Chicago crime syndicate that had originally been set up by Al Capone.

Campbell confessed that the president's persistent back pain eventually made their lovemaking rather perfunctory and one-dimensional. Writing in her memoir *My Story*, Campbell said Kennedy always lay on his back with her on top, and "the feeling that I was there to service him began to really trouble me".

In April, Jackie was pregnant with John Jr. and had gone to Florida for a vacation, so Judith could visit Jack in his Georgetown home. He asked her to put him in touch with Giancana. The Kennedy campaign needed fresh funds.

Judith had broken up with Sinatra because he had proposed a threesome with another woman. Kennedy suggested the same thing. One night in Peter Lawford's suite in the Beverly Hilton, he took her into the bedroom where she found another woman waiting.

"He assured me that the girl was safe and would never talk about it to a single soul," she said.

Kennedy tried to persuade her that she would enjoy it, but she tearfully rejected him. However, he won her back with flowers, phone calls and tickets to the convention. He promised that, if he lost, they would go away together, somewhere where they would never have to wear clothes. His marriage, he said, "had not worked out as they had hoped". That would have been a political bombshell, if it had ever come out. Jackie was one of Jack's greatest assets on the stump and he was having trouble keeping her on side. His relentless womanizing had sent her into a deep depression.

The Democratic convention in Los Angeles that summer was influenced by sex scandal. When Kennedy had won the nomination, much to Judith's chagrin, he had to pick a running mate. Lyndon Johnson came to him. He had read the FBI file Hoover had given him and knew about Kennedy's wartime affair with Ingrid Arvad. Johnson said, unless Kennedy put him on the ticket, he would not only destroy Kennedy's image as a clean-living family man, but also lose him the Jewish vote. World War II had only been over for fifteen years and sleeping with someone so closely involved with the Nazis was still sensitive.

Kennedy said, "I'm forty-three years old. I am not going to die in office, the vice-presidency does not mean a thing."

But Johnson was adamant. "I looked it up," he said. "One out of every four presidents has died in office. I'm a gamblin' man and this is the only chance I've got."

Johnson was proved terribly right.

Safe in the knowledge that his Democratic rival was not going to sink him, Kennedy felt free to party on in Peter Lawford's beach house. Dean Martin said that Lawford was Kennedy's pimp.

"The things that went on in that house were just mind-boggling," said Martin.

Lawford denied procuring for Kennedy. "I was Frank's pimp and Frank was Jack's," he said later. "It sounds terrible now, but then it was a lot of fun."

And knowledge of the goings-on in Santa Monica was not confined to a small circle. Even Lawford's widowed mother knew what was going on. "I find it difficult to place complete trust in a president of the United States, who always had his mind on his cock," she said.

Even the press commented on the statuesque green-eyed brunette Janet des Rosiers, who travelled with him on Kennedy's plane. She groomed and massaged the candidate in a private compartment. She had performed similar duties for his father, having been his mistress for nine years and practically living at Hyannis Port. She said she had been seduced by Joe when she was a twenty-four-year-old virgin.

He was not a religious man, she said. "He did not go to confession. Oh God! If a priest heard his confession."

J. Edgar Hoover was still desperate to thwart Kennedy. He gave the Republican candidate Richard Nixon a picture of Kennedy with an attractive brunette naked on a beach. But sex, or rather the lack of it, was about to be Nixon's undoing.

The 1960 election is famous for having the first televised debates between the two principal candidates. Those who heard the debates on the radio thought that Nixon had won;

those who saw them on TV thought Kennedy was the winner. Nixon was famous for his "five o'clock shadow". He looked tense and awkward, and perspired under the hot television lights. Kennedy appeared relaxed and totally in control.

The night before the first debate, Kennedy said to his aide Langdon Marvin: "Any girls lined up for tomorrow?"

Consequently, a beautiful prostitute was laid on. Marvin took the girl to Kennedy's room and stood guard outside. Fifteen minutes later, Kennedy came out grinning from ear to ear. The pre-show sex gave him a glow, which the cameras picked up. Before each subsequent debate, his aides made sure that a prostitute was provided.

During an election party in New Orleans, Kennedy had sex in a closet with the stripper Blaze Starr, the mistress of Louisiana Governor Earl Long while he waited outside. This was a professional courtesy both on his part and hers. Kennedy had already sampled the delights of Starr's great rival, the "Queen of Burlesque", stripper Tempest Storm.

Judith Campbell was invited to the inauguration, but declined. Angie Dickinson could not resist.

"From the moment I met him, I was hooked, like everyone else," she told a magazine. "He was the sexiest politician I ever met . . . He was the killer type, a handsome, charming man – the kind your mother hoped you wouldn't marry."

During the Inaugural Ball at the Statler Hilton, he left Jackie for half an hour for a private meeting with Angie Dickinson upstairs, then returned sheepishly with a copy of the *Washington Post* under his arm as if he had just popped out to buy a paper.

Later, he attended a private party with Frank Sinatra, Janet Leigh and Kim Novak. Then when he arrived at a party at the Georgetown home of columnist Joe Alsop, the first thing he asked was: "Where are the girls?"

The place was heaving with Hollywood starlets and other attractive young women, including the daughter of an ambassador who was clearly available. Peter Lawford lined up six candidates. Kennedy picked two of them and went to celebrate his inauguration in true presidential style.

One of Kennedy's duties in the White House was to read through the FBI files of everyone in his administration. He enjoyed this at first as it told him which secretaries were available. But gradually he became repelled by the extent of the FBI's snooping.

"I'd like to see what they have got on me," he said, before refusing to read any more files.

Judith Campbell visited the White House more than twenty times. She was smuggled in and out by a Secret Service agent. They also met in Palm Springs, where he would go to search out fresh meat. Campbell also recalled sitting in a hotel bathroom while Kennedy and Giancana discussed the assassination of Fidel Castro – the Mafia's attempt on Castro's life is thought to have backfired and led to Kennedy's own assassination.

Mary Meyer would also visit the White House, bringing joints. On one occasion, Kennedy smoked three joints, but refused a fourth, saying: "Suppose the Russians drop a bomb."

But at formal dinners, Jackie would be one step ahead of Jack. She would seat one of his mistresses either side of him, so he would have no access to fresh talent. But it was a hopeless task. His long-serving White House secretary Evelyn Lincoln said: "Kennedy didn't chase women. The women chased Kennedy." And he did not mind getting caught, she admitted. Kennedy was "a ladies' man".

Male colleagues would send over attractive female volunteers. One compliant columnist sent over a *Playboy* centrefold.

"Got your message," Kennedy replied in a note. "Both of them."

"It was a revolving door over there," said one staffer. "A woman had to fight to get on line."

"We're a bunch of virgins, married virgins," said Fred Dutton, secretary to the Cabinet, "and he's like a God, fucking anybody he wants to any time he feels like it."

The White House kennel keeper Traphes Bryant recalled nude swimming parties in the White House pool. At one, there was a sudden warning that Jackie, who had been on her way out to Virginia, had forgotten something and was coming back. Everyone scrambled. But once she had gone the nude party resumed.

Bryant also recalled that, one day when he was making a routine trip to the basement, the doors of the elevator opened and a naked office girl came flying out so fast that she almost knocked him down. She stopped just long enough to ask where the president was. On another occasion, two presidential aides had urgent business with the president. They knocked on the door of the Lincoln bedroom. Kennedy let them in. There was a young woman in the bed. He slumped down in a chair, read the classified telegrams they had brought, issued his orders, ushered them out, then went back to what he had been doing.

There was a strict code of silence about these goings-on. Any mention of them, particularly to Jackie, was considered disloyal, if not downright unpatriotic.

"That's just the way Jack is; it doesn't matter," said the wife of one of Kennedy's older male friends. "Everyone at court knows it. No one minds, of course, unless they're jealous of the ones he chooses – or they feel bad for Jackie."

But even the nude parties began to pall. At one, Kennedy was seen slumped in a chair reading the syndicated columnist Walter Lippmann. On another occasion, he phoned a friend, saying that he was in the Oval Office with two naked girls, but all he was doing was reading the *Wall Street Journal*.

"Am I getting too old?" he lamented.

It must have been an off day. Usually the sheer number of women passing through gave the Secret Service a headache. They were supposed to give everyone a security check, though it was easy to see the girls coming to the pool parties were not carrying any concealed weapons. On the other hand, they weren't carrying an ID either. The Secret Service gave Kennedy the code name "Lancer" – ostensibly for its associations with Camelot.

The household staff had to search the presidential suite for hairpins, lipsticks and other incriminating evidence. They cursed his preference for blondes. Telltale hairs got everywhere. If he had slept with brunettes like Jackie it would have been much easier to cover his tracks. And sometimes things went massively awry. Jackie once found a pair of panties stuffed in a pillowcase. Carrying them disdainfully between forefinger and thumb, she delivered them to the president and said: "Would you shop around and see who these belong to. They're not my size."

But, thanks to Joe Kennedy, divorce was not to be countenanced. When a friend of Kennedy's said he was thinking about getting a divorce, Kennedy said: "Try it the way I am doing it."

Somewhat aghast, the friend replied: "I go home five nights a week. You're in this Arabian Nights never-never land of the White House. Some nights you don't go home at all."

After some thought, Kennedy called a couple of days later and said, "You're right. If I had to go home three nights a week, I'd go up the wall."

There were two mistresses Jackie definitely knew about. When showing Italian journalists through the White House, she opened a door to an office. There were two attractive blonde secretaries inside.

"Those two are my husband's lovers," she said.

They were Priscilla Weiss and Jill Cowan, former college room-mates who had joined the Kennedy campaign, then got jobs at the White House, ostensibly working for Kennedy's press secretary Pierre Salinger and Evelyn Lincoln. They were full of fun and often dressed alike. The Secret Service code-named them "Fiddle" and "Faddle". They were on call twenty-four hours a day and took it in turns to accompany him everywhere he went. Washington insiders had long come to the same conclusion as Mrs Kennedy.

*Dirty Democrats*

Kennedy's need for sex was a pathological condition. At a summit meeting on Bermuda in 1961, Kennedy asked a shocked sixty-seven-year-old Harold Macmillan: "I wonder how it is for you, Harold? If I don't have a woman for three days, I get terrible headaches."

He complained to others that he could not sleep properly unless he had had sex first.

Sex became the currency of diplomacy. When he visited the president, the French ambassador Hervé Alphand was often accompanied by two young women, said to be his nieces, though they seem to have been no relation at all. This was to counter the British who had installed Kennedy's old friend David Ormsby-Gore as their ambassador to Washington, at the president's request. He supplied Kennedy with embargoed Cuban cigars and was so close to the family it is said that he had an affair with Jackie after the assassination of JFK.

During the Cuban missile crisis, when the world stood on the brink of nuclear annihilation, Kennedy, who was on speed at the time, asked Robert McNamara, the secretary of defense, about a secretary in the Pentagon, saying: "Get me her name and number. We may avert war tonight."

And there were always the movie stars. His affair with Marilyn Monroe began in 1959, before he was president. They used Peter Lawford's beach house for their assignations. Lawford took pictures of them naked together while she performed oral sex on him in the bathtub. On the night of his acceptance speech at the 1960 convention they attended a skinny-dipping party at Lawford's house. Still, he was shocked when he put his hand up her dress in a restaurant that night and found she was wearing no underwear.

Hollywood insiders knew of the affair. They also trysted in Bing Crosby's estate in Palm Springs and in the Beverly Hilton. She even called her masseur to settle an argument about anatomy and put Kennedy on the phone to prove the point. Before the inauguration, her publicist Michael Selsman was told about the relationship. His job was to keep her private life out of the press.

"It wasn't hard in those days," he said. "It was a different era. Today it would be impossible to keep anything resembling that a secret."

Selsman's colleague Patricia Newcomb said that she knew her client "had been with the president. It never occurred to me to talk about it. I couldn't do it."

Kennedy and Monroe had to be a little more discreet on the East Coast, though he took her to Hyannis Port. She also took a ride on Air Force One. But their main arena of amorous activity was the Carlyle Hotel in New York, where she was smuggled in surreptitiously, wearing sunglasses and a black wig. As newspaper reporters staked out the lobby of the Carlyle, the Secret Service found another way in via an underground tunnel from another hotel. Agents would have to steer the president of the United States around steam pipes with a flashlight and map so that he could spend a blissful half-hour with Marilyn or his latest playmate. But this was a better option than letting him get away with his usual trick – simply giving them the slip, leaving behind the army officer with the nuclear football containing the codes to authorize a nuclear strike strapped to his wrist. If the Soviet Union had launched an attack while Kennedy was in the sack, America would have been defenceless.

But even creeping through underground tunnels did not keep them safe from the predations of J. Edgar Hoover. He had Peter Lawford's beach house bugged. The FBI soon had more tapes of Kennedy making love. Hoover had overheard Bobby Kennedy, who was then attorney general and Hoover's boss, threatening to sack him. With the Marilyn tapes his job was safe. Hoover even kept a nude photograph of Marilyn in a basement, along with other cheesecake pictures, to counter the oft-repeated rumour that he was gay.

There were other guests at the Carlyle Hotel. Lawford brought high-priced New York call girl Leslie Devereux there for Kennedy, who enjoyed the professional touch. She was not told who the client was to be and was shocked to discover it was the president. She returned there on four other occasions, though she initially found their lovemaking rather prosaic.

"I'd been with a number of powerful politicians and the one thing they always liked was mild S and M," she said. "So we did a little of that. I tied his hands and feet to the bedposts, blindfolded him and teased him first with a feather and then with my fingernails. He seemed to enjoy it."

Devereux also visited Washington where she spent fifteen minutes in a small room off the Oval Office. Kennedy knew that this was where his Republican predecessor Warren Harding had made love to his mistress Nan Britton. He had once told Blaze Starr about it. On her second visit, they repaired to the Lincoln bedroom. She questioned the propriety of making out in Lincoln's bed. He said that if you made a wish in Lincoln's bed, it always came true. As he had to be careful with his back, he lay back and she climbed on top.

"See," he said. "It never fails."

Marilyn Monroe was fatally addicted to alcohol and pills, and became dangerously mentally unstable. At one point during the 1960 election campaign, Marilyn was on a binge with liquor and pills, and Kennedy had to send Charles Spalding to Los Angeles to make sure she did not speak out of turn. On another occasion, Smathers had to send a mutual friend to "talk to Marilyn Monroe about putting a bridle on herself and on her mouth and not talking too much, because it was getting to be a story around the country".

"She devised all sorts of madcap fantasies with herself in the starring role," said Lawford. "She would have his children. She would take Jackie's place as First Lady."

When no divorce seemed to be on the horizon, Monroe began calling Kennedy's private apartment in the White House. When Jackie answered, she would hand the phone to her husband and go on about her business.

Jackie was not at Kennedy's birthday in Madison Square Gardens in 1962. She was a "surprise contestant" at a horse show in Virginia. Afterwards, the press was full of speculation about Kennedy and Monroe. Jack called on the inspector general of the Peace Corps William Haddad, a former reporter on the *New York Post*, and asked him to "see the editors. Tell them you are speaking for me and that it's not true."

But Kennedy knew it was time to put an end to the affair. He told Marilyn bluntly: "You're not really First Lady material."

Then Marilyn turned up unexpectedly in Washington. Kennedy, Smathers and a few others took her on a motorboat trip down the Potomac. They did not get back until 11.30 at night. Marilyn did not stay at the White House, but Jackie knew all about it. At a White House ball, she told Smathers: "Don't think I am naive about what you and Jack are doing with all those pretty girls, like Marilyn, sailing on the Potomac under the moonlight."

With the affair over, there was renewed danger that she may go to the press. A scandal had to be avoided at all costs, so Kennedy sent his brother Bobby to reason with her. According to Peter Lawford, she took it pretty hard. Bobby felt for her. They met the following day and spent the afternoon walking along the beach.

"It wasn't Bobby's intention, but that evening they became lovers and spent the night in our guest bedroom," said Lawford. "Almost immediately the affair got very heavy ... Now Marilyn was calling the Justice Department instead of the White House."

Bobby's personal assistant Angie Novello had long conversations with Marilyn whenever Bobby was not around. Pretty soon Marilyn announced that she was in love with Bobby and he had promised to marry her.

"It was as if she could no longer tell the difference between Bobby and Jack," said Lawford.

Fearing for his own position, Bobby suddenly went into reverse, which hardly helped Marilyn's state of mind.

"She went up the wall," said Lawford. "'They treat everyone like that,' she said. 'They use you and then they dispose of you like so much rubbish.'"

Within a couple of months Marilyn was dead from an overdose of drugs. There have been numerous theories about how this happened. The latest is that Kennedy, Lawford and others goaded her into attempting suicide then, instead of saving her at the last minute, left her to die.

There was no satisfying Jack's appetite for blonde movie stars. He got Lawford to arrange an introduction to Jayne Mansfield. With her forty-two-inch bust and her eighteen-inch waist, she was even more spectacularly built than Monroe. At the time, she was still married to bodybuilder and actor Mickey Hargitay, but they were on the road to the divorce courts.

According to Lawford, they met at least three times. On one occasion she was visibly pregnant. She said she found him cold. A week after an assignation in Palm Springs, she was having drinks with her press agent when Kennedy called. An argument broke out and she hung up on him after shouting: "Look, you'll only be president for eight years, but I'll be a movie star for life."

His name was also linked with Marlene Dietrich, though she was sixty-one at the time.

In 1963, Kennedy risked being sucked into the Profumo affair. There were other prostitutes at the sex parties Keeler had attended. Two of them – a Chinese-American named Suzy Chang and Maria Novotny, a bleach-blonde Czech born in London – had also worked as high-class prostitutes in New York and had serviced Kennedy when he was a senator.

The president turned to Bobby to keep a lid on the scandal. J. Edgar Hoover contacted the FBI's legal attaché in London and told him to "stay on top of this case and ... keep the Bureau fully and promptly informed of all developments with particular emphasis on any allegation that US nationals are or have been involved in any way". The CIA was given similar instructions. The deputy chief of station Cleveland Cram said he spent the next "three or four" weeks at MI5 headquarters going through the Profumo files.

"It was lots of fun," he said.

At the time, he had no doubt that they were trying to find out whether "one of the Kennedys" was linked to the Profumo girls. He noted that a special request had come from the president himself. They needed to know whether anything was about to be made public on the grounds that "forewarned is fore-armed."

On 23 June, Kennedy made his "*Ich bin ein Berliner*" speech in Berlin. After a visit to Ireland, he had to stop off and visit Harold Macmillan, whose government was on its last legs because of the Profumo scandal. England was the last place Kennedy wanted to be.

Meanwhile, back in the US, the *New York Journal–American*, a Hearst newspaper, reported that: "One of the biggest names in American politics – a man who holds a very high elective office – has been injected into Britain's vice-security scandal." The reporters, James D. Horan and Dom Frasca, quoted Maria Novotny saying that the connection involved "a beautiful Chinese-American girl now in London", adding that the "highest authorities" had "identified her as Suzy Chang".

The story – which ran on the front page under the three-deck headline HIGH US AIDE IMPLICATED IN V-GIRL SCANDAL – was pulled after the first edition. Horan, who died in the eighties, told his sons that the story had been spiked due to pressure from Bobby Kennedy.

Bobby then called Warren Rogers, Washington correspondent for *Look* magazine, and told him to get on the phone to his fellow reporters to find out if anyone knew who the man mentioned in the *Journal–American* story was.

While Bobby was trying to cope with the scandal, brother Jack had gone to see the Pope. On his way home, he had arranged to visit a villa on Lake Como where Gianni Agnelli's wife Marella would be waiting.

Bobby Kennedy summoned Horan and Frasca to the Justice Department and demanded to know who the high official involved in the Profumo scandal was. FBI liaison officer Courtney Evans, who was taking notes at the meeting, said that Horan and Frasca were reluctant to answer, but eventually admitted: "It was the president of the United States."

Their source of the story was Peter Earle, a reporter on the *News of the World* in London. The Sunday paper had signed up Maria Novotny for her story, which Earle had been assigned to write. The attorney general then berated them for writing a story about the president of the United States "without any further check being made to get to the truth of the matter". But Frasca said he had "other sources of a confidential nature".

In 1987, Anthony Summers was researching his book *Official and Confidential*, a biography of J. Edgar Hoover, and tracked down Suzy Chang, then living under another name on Long Island. She said, "We'd meet in the 21 Club. Everyone saw me eating with him. I think he was a nice guy, very charming." He asked for sex. She said yes. "What else am I going to say?"

Maria Novotny had been arrested for prostitution in New York in 1961. She died in 1970, leaving the manuscript of an unpublished autobiography. In it, she claimed that Peter Lawford had recruited her to have group sex with Jack Kennedy a few weeks before his inauguration, and she and another prostitute had pretended to be a doctor and nurse, while the president-elect was their willing patient.

Kennedy had another affair with security implications. At the Quorum Club, an exclusive watering hole in the Carroll Arms Hotel where Suzy Chang and Maria Novotny had both worked, he asked to be introduced to Ellen Rometsch. Born in Kleinitz in 1936, at the end of World War II, she found herself in East Germany. She joined the Communist Party Youth Group. In 1955, she fled to West Germany. Her first marriage ended in divorce. Then she married Rolf Rometsch who, in 1961, was posted to Washington as air attaché. Ellen began hanging out at the Quorum Club.

Bobby Baker, an aide to Lyndon Johnson who ran the Quorum Club, made the introduction. According to Burton Hersh in *Bobby and J. Edgar*, after Jack's first date with Ellen, the president phoned Baker to rave: "That was the best blow job I ever had in my life." Baker said the couple had several other sexual sessions. Ellen, he noted, was equally gratified during these encounters, telling Baker: "Jack was as good as it got with the oral sex. He really was a satisfier . . . made me happy."

In July 1963, the FBI picked up Ellen and questioned her about her background. They quickly concluded she was a Communist spy. According to historian Michael Bechloss, Hoover told Bobby: "We have information that not only your brother, the president, but others in Washington have been involved with a woman whom we suspect as a Soviet intelligence agent, someone who is linked to East German intelligence."

Hoover even told Courtney Evans that she had worked for Walter Ulbricht, the Communist leader of East Germany. Bobby Kennedy promptly had her deported.

President Kennedy told J. Edgar Hoover that he was "personally interested in having this story killed". However, the *Des Moines Register* carried a story claiming that the FBI had "established that the beautiful brunette had been attending parties with congressional leaders and some prominent New Frontiersmen from the executive branch of Government . . . The possibility that her activity might be connected with espionage was of some concern, because of the high rank of her male companions."

Information about Ellen Rometsch was also leaked to John Williams, a leading Republican senator who was investigating the activities of Bobby Baker. Sensing danger, Bobby Kennedy sent aide LaVerne Duffy to West Germany, where, in exchange for a great deal of money, he got Rometsch to sign a statement formally denying that she had slept with important people in Washington.

It was then a matter of quashing any Senate investigation. Bobby had the Senate leaders in. It was easy to persuade the Democrats to keep shtum. But only J. Edgar Hoover had the necessary firepower in his files to shut up the Republicans. President Kennedy cut a deal with him. He agreed to bail out the president only on two conditions – that Kennedy would never fire him and that the FBI could escalate its bugging of Martin Luther King.

Kennedy acceded and Hoover showed Senate leaders the FBI files he had on dozens of senators. He explained that if the Senate exposed the president's sex life, no one would be safe. The same day the Senate leaders announced there would be no investigation into Ellen Rometsch. Soon after, Kennedy said to Ben Bradlee: "Boy, the dirt he has on those senators, you wouldn't believe it."

Later, when Kennedy was asked why he did not fire Hoover, he said, "You don't fire God."

In August 1963, Jackie was rushed to hospital and gave birth to a boy six weeks premature. The child died after a couple of hours. In October, she flew to Athens to take a cruise on the yacht of Greek shipping magnate Artistotle Onassis. The trip had been organized by Jackie's sister, "Princess" Lee Radziwall – though her husband the Polish Prince Stanislaw Radziwill had become just plain Mr when he had taken British citizenship in 1951. Onassis's long-term mistress, the opera singer Maria Callas, was not on-board as she had just discovered that Onassis had taken Lee as his lover. It used to amuse Onassis to be seen out together with both of them, until Callas discovered that he had bought Lee an expensive diamond bracelet.

Bobby Kennedy was outraged when he heard about the affair. But Onassis, who had already had several run-ins with the attorney general, knew about the Kennedy brothers' involvement with Marilyn Monroe and said, "Bobby, you and Jack fuck your movie queen and I'll fuck my princess."

Everyone was amazed when Jackie accepted Onassis's invitation. Her motivation seems to have been revenge for her husband's philandering. Onassis had already expressed an interest in the president's wife.

"There's something provocative about that lady. She's got a carnal soul," he told a friend.

According to Evelyn Lincoln, Onassis and Jackie became lovers on that cruise. However, the trip brought her bad press and, when she returned, she agreed to travel with her husband to Texas where he was killed the following month.

It has also been alleged that Bobby Kennedy had sex with Jackie. According to David Heyman, Jackie's biographer, their shared grief led to a long affair. When Bobby became a New York senator, Jackie moved to New York. When she had a house-warming party at her new apartment on Fifth Avenue, Bobby seemed very much the man of the house. At other times, they were seen returning there late at night. Neighbours said they also saw them leaving together in the morning. Tongues wagged and Jackie discreetly asked her Secret Service guard to stand down at 11 p.m.

This may have been some cause of jealousy. Onassis's biographer Peter Evans told the *Daily Mail* that Onassis paid for Robert Kennedy's assassination. Jackie married Onassis four months after Bobby's death.

Then there was the curious death of Mary Meyer. On 12 October 1964, eleven months after the death of JFK and two weeks after the report of the Warren Commission into his death was made public, Mary was shot dead as she walked along the towpath of the Chesapeake and Ohio Canal in Georgetown. There was a bullet in the back of her head, another in her heart. Both had been shot from close range. A black man was seen standing over the corpse.

An African-American named Raymond Crump was arrested nearby. No gun was found and no link was established between him and the murder. Nevertheless he went on trial. No mention of Mary's involvement with Kennedy was made in court and that information was withheld from the defence. Crump was acquitted and the crime remains unsolved.

Although Jack and Bobby Kennedy managed to keep the lid on the presidential sex scandals during their lifetime, after they were dead it began to come out. Even forty years later, bimbos were still coming out of the woodwork. In 2003, Marion "Mimi" Beardsley admitted that she had had an affair with John F. Kennedy when she was a teenage White House intern. At the age of nineteen, she was one of a harem of young girls hired by the press office principally to be at the president's disposal. She was flown around the country on Air Force planes so that she was on hand for JFK on his travels.

"From June 1962 to November 1963, I was involved in a sexual relationship with President Kennedy," she said when the *New York Daily News* tracked her down. "For the last forty-one years, it is a subject that I have not discussed."

In the meantime, she told no one, not even her immediate family. Marion Beardsley had gone to the same exclusive school as Jackie Kennedy and was editor of the college paper when she came to the White House in 1961 to write a profile of the First Lady. Mrs Kennedy was too busy to see her, but the president did meet her on this visit. Apparently, he had more leisure time than Mrs Kennedy.

On the president's instructions, the White House press office hired Ms Beardsley despite her evident lack of qualifications.

"Mimi had no skills. She couldn't type," said former press aide Barbara Gamarekian. "She could answer the phone and she could handle messages and things, but she was not really a great asset to us."

However, she did have her role as one of a group of girls who were invited to pool parties and went on presidential trips.

"We all went on trips one time or another, but Mimi, who obviously couldn't perform any function at all, made all the trips," Mrs Gamarekian said.

In the Bahamas in 1962, Mimi was spotted by aides hiding in one of the cars waiting to take the president to the airport after the summit with Harold Macmillan where they discussed the deployment of British Polaris nuclear missiles. According to Mrs Gamarekian, "they walked over and looked in the car and there seated on the floor was Mimi". The aides said nothing and neither did the press. At that time, Mrs Gamarekian said, "this is the sort of thing that legitimate newspaper people don't write about or don't even make any implications about. It was kind of a big joke."

With Jack and Bobby both dead, their younger brother Senator Edward Kennedy had his hands full, keeping up the proud family tradition of drinking and womanizing. Garry Wills, author of *The Kennedy Imprisonment* said: "Ted Kennedy was born and bred to act like the last of the Regency rakes: to be a boor when it pleases him, to take what he wants, to treat women as score markers in the game of sexual sport and to revel in high stakes risks."

But while his brothers had gotten away with it during their lifetime, Ted did not. Although the press was prepared to hush up a certain amount of drunken philandering, after the death of young campaign worker Mary Jo Kopechne at Chappaquiddick nothing could be done to suppress the scandal.

On the night of 18 July 1969, Ted Kennedy was on Chappaquiddick Island in Massachusetts, where he was giving a party for the Boiler Room Girls, a group of young women who had worked on Bobby's presidential campaign the previous year. Ted Kennedy was driving home from the party when he veered off a bridge and into a deep tidal channel. Mary Jo was in the back seat and, while he claimed he was just giving her a lift back to her hotel, it was widely believed that he was hoping to have sex with her. Kennedy swam ashore to save himself, but left Mary Jo to drown.

It was nine hours before he reported the accident. In the meantime, he walked back to his motel, complained to the manager about a noisy party, took a shower, went to sleep, ordered the newspapers when he woke up and spoke to a friend and two lawyers before finally calling the police. Divers later estimated that if he had reported the accident immediately, they would have had time to save Mary Jo. She had not drowned straight away, but had survived in an air pocket inside the car for several hours, finally asphyxiating when the oxygen gave out.

But Kennedy was on home turf. It is thought that if he had not been in Massachusetts and his name had not been Kennedy he would have been charged with homicide. As it was he pleaded guilty to leaving the scene of an accident and was given a two-year suspended sentence. Kennedy lawyers arranged for him to pay £55,000 to the Kopechne family from his own pocket with a further £30,000 from his insurance. Mary Jo's mother later said, "I don't think he ever said he was sorry." But he was sorry though. The incident scuppered his chances of ever becoming president.

But it did not stop him drinking and womanizing. His wife Joan, left at home in Boston to raise three kids, seemed to accept that was what Kennedy women had to put up with. But gradually his philandering drove her to drink and, in 1981, they announced that they were getting a divorce. When the divorce was granted the following year, he staggered from sex scandal to sex scandal, with the lurid details spelled out in the supermarket tabloids.

One sixteen-year-old said that she had been propositioned by Kennedy from the back seat of his limousine on Capitol Hill. She testified that he leant from the window, waved a wine bottle and asked whether she or the friend she was with wanted to join him. And in Washington's La Brasserie restaurant, he once threw a waitress over a table in a private room and tried to have sex with her.

However, the *New York Times* and *Washington Post* gave him an easy time because he had somehow held on to his political clout and his legislative skills. He won re-election after re-election and was credited by the Left for an unrivalled body of liberal legislation.

In 1991, Ted Kennedy was embroiled in another sex scandal, which, this time, hit the front pages, when his thirty-year-old nephew William Kennedy Smith was accused of a date rape. The Kennedy men had gathered at the family's winter beach house in Palm Beach, Florida. On the evening of Good Friday, 29 March 1991, Ted Kennedy had taken his son Patrick and Smith to the Au Bar, a trendy nightspot, to hunt for women. Smith met twenty-nine-year-old Patricia Bowman and another young woman at the bar. They returned to the beach house with the Kennedys. Ted Kennedy was lounging around in his boxer shorts, while Smith coaxed Bowman down to the beach for a swim. They then had sex on the lawn. He said it was consensual, though "rough"; she said it was rape.

The trial was televised and went into every detail, including where she had bought her panties and the number of grains of sand found in them after the encounter. However, the testimony of three other women who claimed Smith had sexually assaulted them, though they had not complained to the police, was ruled inadmissible.

On the witness stand, Ted Kennedy was masterful. He later apologized to his constituents, saying: "I recognize my own shortcomings – the faults in the conduct of my private life. I realize that I alone am responsible for them, and I am the one who must confront them."

Kennedy Smith was acquitted. In 2004, another woman in Chicago, his personal assistant at the Center for International Rehabilitation he had founded, accused him of sexual assault. A judge dismissed a civil lawsuit she took against him. However, he settled with another employee out of court. Sadly, this has had none of the style of Marilyn Monroe singing, "Happy Birthday, Mr President."

## Lyndon Baines Johnson

LBJ was Kennedy's successor and his sexual rival. He once famously said: "I had more women by accident than he had on purpose." A poor boy from Texas, Johnson was always extremely competitive. And he had an easier time keeping the lid on scandal. He was not dogged with Kennedy's good looks. But he had maintained a string of mistresses throughout his life. With a head like a potato, who would have guessed it? The truth only came to light in 1987, nearly fifteen years after he died, when his illegitimate son Steven Brown filed suit against Johnson's widow for his inheritance.

Throughout his life though, Johnson was rarely discreet. While at college, he bragged about his sexual conquests, giving detailed descriptions of his partners' anatomy and blow-by-blow accounts of the action in the crudest terms. He was also inordinately fond of exposing himself, whipping out his large penis, which he called "Jumbo", at the slightest excuse. Once, when flying out of Thailand during the Vietnam War, an unwary journalist asked him how he had enjoyed Bangkok. Cue the presidential penis. No friend of the highfaluting Brits, who would not back him in the war, he would interview the British ambassador while on the john.

As a young man, Johnson had decided early on to marry for money. He dated Carol Davis, the daughter of a rich businessman, and bragged that, when they went out, she picked up the tab. Then he dated Kitty Clyde Ross, daughter of the richest man in Johnson City. After that, he ruthlessly pursued Lady Bird Taylor, the daughter of a wealthy businessman who owned 15,000 acres of cotton fields and two general stores. When she turned him down, he issued an ultimatum. Either she married him or he would never see her again. Reluctantly, she accepted.

In 1938, when he was a freshman congressman, Johnson met Alice Glass, the live-in lover of local press baron Charles E. Marsh. He owned a dozen newspapers in Texas and could make or break Johnson at any time. Nevertheless, Johnson took Alice as his lover. She moulded the crude country boy and put a shine on him, improving his diction, brushing up his manners and introducing him to poetry and classical music. She was the love of his life. They even discussed marriage, but divorce in those days would have spelt the end of his political career.

They continued their affair through the late 1930s to the early 1940s, under the noses of Marsh and Mrs Johnson. At Alice's behest, Marsh even facilitated land deals that made Johnson independently wealthy. However, it was plain that Lady Bird knew what was going on. Alice's sister Mary Louise said: "The thing I never understood was how she stood it. Lyndon would leave her on weekends, weekend after weekend, just leave her home. I wouldn't have stood for it for a minute. We were all together a lot – Lyndon, Lady Bird and Charles and Alice. And Lady Bird never said a word. She showed nothing, nothing at all."

But while others were sniggering behind her back, Lady Bird went on to become First Lady. She bore his two daughters and she seems to have loved him. Jackie Kennedy once observed: "Lady Bird would crawl on broken glass down Pennsylvania Avenue for Lyndon."

Marsh eventually tumbled. One night, while drunk, he confronted Johnson. But, by then, Johnson was too powerful to pull down. The affair continued and nothing more was said. It only ended in 1967, when Johnson and Alice fell out over the Vietnam War. She burned his love letters, then married Marsh – then divorced him.

Not that Johnson was faithful to his mistress. In Washington, his aide Bobby Baker ran the Quorum Club so there was a continuous stream of new women to entertain him. He always had an eye for pretty women.

Once in the Oval Office, he followed in the Kennedy tradition. White House Press Secretary George Reedy said: "He may have been 'just a country boy from the central hills of Texas', but he had many of the instincts of a Turkish sultan in Istanbul."

He was constantly seeking to extend what the White House staff referred to as his "harem". One highly qualified woman was denied a position on his staff when Johnson said, "She's got everything but good looks."

Johnson was shameless about it. "I put high marks on good looks," he said. "I can't stand a woman who looks like a cow that's gonna sit on her own udder."

When he spotted an attractive journalist at a press conference, he told her: "You're the prettiest thing I ever saw." The next day she had a job on his staff. The rest of the press corps called him the "Lochinvar of the Pedernales" – Johnson's valley homestead.

He hired six pretty secretaries and had five of them. One had sex with him on the desk in the Oval Office. Another was caught sitting on his lap and claimed that she had tripped over a rug. And it wasn't just in the Oval Office. He also had sex with them on Air Force One and *Sequoia*, the presidential yacht.

Johnson's approach was straightforward. When one female staffer had to stay overnight at Johnson's ranch after working late with him, she awoke in the middle of the night to find a naked man climbing into bed with her.

"Move over," he said. "This is your president."

And he encouraged others to do likewise. When a congresswoman was giving a member of the administration problems over an education bill, he instructed an aide to "tell him to spend the afternoon in bed with her and she'll support any goddamn bill he wants".

This was, of course, before the word "sexist" entered the American language.

He encouraged good relations with the press and had regular sex sessions in the Oval Office with a woman reporter from the *Washington Star.* Towards the end of his administration, gossip also circulated that he was having an affair with a blonde graduate student from Harvard named Doris Kearns, who had famously written a "Dump Johnson" article for *The New Republic*, because he spent so much time alone with her. Later, she was the first woman journalist to enter the Boston Red Sox locker room.

A lifelong liberal, Johnson was proud that he, as a southerner, got to sign into law all the sixties Civil Rights legislation. He showed a similar lack of prejudice in his sex life when he bedded a beautiful black girl named Geraldine "Gerri" Whittington. He saw her working in a government office, and requested that his "special assistant" Jack Valenti get her home phone number. Johnson called her unannounced one evening, and asked that she come in that night for an interview. According to audiotapes of Johnson's phone calls, Whittington at first thought the call was a joke, but realized that he was all too serious. She got the position.

Lady Bird knew about her husband's philandering. According to one Secret Service agent, she even caught him having sex with a secretary on the couch in the Oval Office. She accepted this stoically. "That's just one side of him," she said.

Years later she explained: "You have to understand, my husband loved people. All people. And half the people in the world are women. You don't think I could have kept my husband away from half the people."

Despite all this frenzied heterosexual activity, the only scandal that hit his administration was a homosexual one. On 7 October 1964, a month before the election, Johnson's White House Chief of Staff Walter Jenkins was arrested in the restroom of the YMA for "disorderly conduct" with a sixty-year-old man. Then it came out that, five years earlier, he had been arrested in the same place, doing the same thing. During the ensuing scandal, one kindly journalist enquired whether he was suffering from overwork or was it "combat fatigue". And a helpful Republican suggested that Johnson change his campaign slogan from "All the way with LBJ" to "Either way with LBJ".

The extent of Johnson's philandering only became clear in 1987, when Steven Brown stepped into the limelight with a $10.5-million suit and demanding to change his name to Johnson. Standing at six feet four, he certainly looked like his putative father. In February 1987, his mother had had a heart attack. Fearing she was going to die, she confessed all and told him about his parentage.

His mother, Madeleine Brown, had married a soda jerk when she was very young. He was later confined to a mental hospital but, being a Catholic, she did not divorce him. In 1948, when she was twenty-three she met the youthful congressman at a reception at his radio station in Austin. Three weeks later, they met again at a party in the Driskill Hotel.

"He looked at me like I was an ice-cream cone on a hot day," she told *People* magazine. "And he said after a while, 'Well, I'll see you up in my apartment.' He had a certain amount of roughness about him, and maybe that's what I liked, you know. He commanded. I've been told that every woman needs to act like a whore in bed and I guess that's what I did."

According to Madeleine, Johnson was an aggressive lover, highly sexed and liked to play games in bed.

"He was a little kinky and I loved every second of it," she said. "So did he. We spent our time doing, not talking. Once, after he was through, he went to the window and opened it and bellowed like a bull, yelling, 'My God, I love Texas in the morning.'"

She used the phrase in the title of her memoir *Texas in the Morning: The Love Story of Madeleine Brown and President Lyndon Johnson.*

They never discussed politics. The affair was only about sex. She was his bit on the side, never to be publicly acknowledged.

"He told me from the beginning," she said. "'You see nothing, you hear nothing, you say nothing."

They communicated via Jesse Kellam, the manager of the radio station in Austin and a close friend of Johnson's. When Johnson was returning from Washington, Kellam would call Madeleine. She would fly in from Dallas. Met at the airport by the radio station's mobile news unit, she would be taken to the Driskill and smuggled up to his suite.

An ambitious politician, Johnson was a busy man. It would all be over in half an hour. Only once did he dawdle and stay three hours. Madeleine believed that Lady Bird knew about the affair from the early sixties. Nevertheless, Madeleine had her own ambitions to be First Lady.

"Sometimes, when I'd hint around, he'd just say, "Today's today, tomorrow's tomorrow.' That was his favourite answer. I guess it could have meant anything. I like to think it meant someday I'd be in the White House. I would have been like Nancy Reagan. I wouldn't have stood it if he had other women."

As it was, she did. Though she was upset and unhappy about it, the hit-and-run nature of their relationship meant he had plenty of time to dally elsewhere. In spring 1950, she fell pregnant. Johnson, by then a senator, went incandescent with rage. He called her "dumb Dora" and thrust the entire blame onto her. But when he calmed down, he said he would look after her and the child, leaving his attorney, Jerome Ragsdale, to tie up the details.

Steven was born in December 1950. As Madeleine was still married, she put her husband's name on the birth certificate. Ragsdale bought her a large house with a live-in maid and picked up all the expenses, though Madeleine continued to work as a media buyer for an advertising agency in Dallas. Work colleagues were amazed when she turned up in an expensive mink coat. She explained: "I got my mink the same way minks get minks."

There were other gifts and flowers between the snatched interludes in hotels in Austin, Houston and San Antonio, all arranged by Kellam. After the death of her husband, Kellam even arranged a marriage of convenience, though she never lived with her new husband.

On 21 November 1963 – the day before Kennedy's assassination – she claimed Johnson told her: "After tomorrow those SOBs will never embarrass me again."

Brown believed that a plot to kill JFK had been hatched at the 1960 Democratic Convention, when Johnson lost the nomination to Kennedy.

"When they met in California, Joe Kennedy, John Kennedy's father, and [oil tycoon] H. L. Hunt met three days prior to the election – they finally cut a deal according to John Currington [an aide to H. L. Hunt] and H. L. finally agreed that Lyndon would go as the vice president," she said. "This came from the horse's mouth way back in 1960 – when H. L. came back to Dallas I was walking . . . with him . . . and he made the remark, 'We may have lost a battle but we're going to win a war,' and then the day of the assassination he said, 'Well, we won the war.'"

As president, Johnson still found time to fly down to Austin for sessions in the Driskill Hotel. Then in 1967, Madeleine had a car accident, badly scarring her face, and she feared that she would never see her lover again. By that time, he was deeply unpopular across the country because of the Vietnam War and was terrified that his illicit affair would be found out. Kellam constantly reminded her to be a "good girl" and keep quiet.

After he left office in 1969, Johnson was attending a parade in honour of the Apollo 11 astronauts in Houston and arranged to meet her there. They met in a room in the Shamrock Hotel.

She was shocked how tired and old he looked. While the Secret Service agent waited outside, for once, they talked.

"We talked for almost two hours," she said. "I cried. We kissed. But we didn't even try to make love."

She thought that he did not have much longer to live and urged him to recognize Steven as his son.

"I can't do that," said Johnson. "I've got the girls to think about."

They got to know about it in the end.


## Gary Hart

A rash young senator from Colorado named Gary Hart blew the moratorium on the presidential sex lives that had existed since Franklin Roosevelt. After that, it was open season.

Rumours that he was having an extramarital affair surfaced when he declared his candidacy for president in April 1987 – he was a clear front-runner for the Democratic nomination in 1988. A few weeks later, on 3 May 1987, in an interview in the *New York Times*, he issued a challenge to the press corps.

"Follow me around," he dared them. "I don't care. I'm serious. If anybody wants to put a tail on me, go ahead. They'll be very bored."

Reporters from the *Miami Herald* took him at his word. They had already spotted a young woman leaving Hart's town house in Washington, DC, who they identified as twenty-nine-year-old model Donna Rice. The same day Hart's dare appeared in the *New York Times*, the *Miami Herald* burst his bubble by printing the Donna Rice story.

The following day, Rice herself poured petrol on the fire, volunteering that she had been on vacation with Hart in Bimini the previous month, on-board a boat called, wouldn't you know it, *Monkey Business*. A picture emerged of Hart wearing a "Monkey Business" T-shirt with Donna Rice sitting on his lap, though it was not published in the *National Enquirer* until Hart's candidacy was cold in its grave.

But the scandal was not confined to the tabloids. The *Washington Post* decided that as Hart's private behaviour raised broader questions about his honesty and judgement and, as he had declared that he held himself to a high moral standard, his sex life was fair game.

At a press conference in New Hampshire, *Washington Post* reporter Paul Taylor asked him directly: "Have you ever committed adultery?"

"I'm not going to get into a theological definition of what constitutes adultery," Hart replied.

Then he tried penitence. "I made a mistake in my personal life," he admitted on the TV. "I've also insisted, as I think I have a right to, that my mistakes in my personal life be put against the mistakes of this administration – selling arms to terrorists, lying to Congress, shredding documents."

But it would not wash. It was all over. On 8 May, Hart dropped out of the race. In a press conference, he railed at the media. There are even theories that it was a honey trap.

"I said that I bend, but I don't break," he said defiantly, "and believe me, I'm not broken."

Afterwards, he received a letter from Richard Nixon saying that he had "handled a very difficult situation uncommonly well". He was dancing on Hart's grave.

On 15 June, Donna's friend Lynn Armandt, owner of the Too Hot Miami bikini boutique, told all to *People* magazine. She and Donna had met Hart at a party given by rock singer Don Henley in Aspen. She had made up a foursome on *Monkey Business* with Rice, Hart and Hart's fundraiser William Broadhurst.

"It was absolutely clear that she had slept with Gary," she said. "She's not one to detail [sexual adventures], but she said she had a wonderful time with him . . . that he was very gentle and romantic."

Lynn was also in Washington when Donna was staying in Hart's town house and they found themselves besieged by reporters from the *Miami Herald*.

Hart re-entered the race in December 1987, with an unofficial slogan, which said, "My heart is for Bush, but my bush is for Hart." He was murdered at the polls and withdrew a second time.

## Bill Clinton

Slick Willie proved himself the master of the sex scandal. Even though he had served five terms as governor of Arkansas, he was unknown nationally until the New Hampshire primary in February 1992, when the supermarket checkout scandal sheet *The Star* ran the banner headline, DEMS FRONT-RUNNER BILL CLINTON CHEATED WITH MISS AMERICA'. This rocketed him to fame.

*The Star* went on to name five women whom Clinton was alleged to have slept with, including Miss America and *Playboy* centrefold Elizabeth Ward Gracen. The information came from a lawsuit filed by a disgruntled former state employee named Larry Nichols, linking Clinton to the five named women and making the unsubstantiated charge that he had been fired as part of an attempted cover-up involving a secret fund used to facilitate Clinton's trysts.

Clinton fought the suit and, when asked by a local TV station in New Hampshire whether he had ever committed adultery, he replied with a twinkle in his eye: "If I had, I wouldn't tell you."

But Hillary held the line. She told the crowd that their marriage was strong.

*The Star* hit back with MY 12-YEAR AFFAIR WITH BILL CLINTON. The subtitle was "Mistress Tells All, the Secret Love Tapes that Prove It."

This time it wheeled out former Little Rock nightclub singer, Gennifer Flowers. Clinton's campaign manager David

Wilhelm immediately dubbed her the "smoking bimbo". Though it was widely reported that he denied having an affair with Flowers, Clinton, a master of words, merely said, "That allegation is false." So it was only an eleven-and-a-half-year affair then?

In an interview Flowers said, "We made love everywhere, on the floor, in bed, in the kitchen, on the cabinet, the sink. I called his testicles 'the boys' and he called my breasts 'the girls'."

She also said that he once tried to have sex with her in the men's room in the governor's mansion while Hillary was entertaining on the lawn outside. He even used his jogging as cover – he jogged over to her apartment, made love to her and jogged home. That way, him being sweaty did not arouse Hillary's suspicions.

"I admired his stamina," Flowers said, "being able to make love with such enthusiasm after running. I used to tease him about running back much slower."

He even got her a job on the state payroll.

Naturally the media loved such tales. In a press conference in 1992, one reporter brought the house down by asking Flowers, "Did the governor use a condom?"

By then the British tabloids were offering $500,000 for the next kiss and tell on Clinton. The story was not going to go away. Instead Clinton exploited it. He managed to secure an interview on CBS's *60 Minutes* right after the Super Bowl. It was airtime you could not pay for. The slot guaranteed a huge audience, feeling good after watching the game and, more than likely, full of beer.

With Hillary, the dutiful wife, sitting alongside him, Clinton was asked wide-eyed: "Who is Gennifer Flowers and why is she saying these things?"

Using well-rehearsed lines, Clinton admitted that there had been problems in his marriage. Flowers was only "a friendly acquaintance", but he acknowledged unspecified "wrongdoing" and "causing pain in my marriage". When asked whether that meant that he had committed adultery, Hillary answered coolly, "People who have been married a long time know what it means."

The producer of *60 Minutes* Don Hewitt, kneeling off camera near Clinton, twice prompted him to admit adultery. Clinton did not take the bait.

It was a riveting performance. In one fell swoop, the two of them blew every other candidate out of the water. Hillary made only one slight slip when she said that she was not there just to "stand by my man like Tammy Wynette". She later apologized to Tammy when the spin doctors feared they risked losing the country-and-western vote.

Hewitt quickly realized what they had done.

"The last time I had something as important was the Nixon–Kennedy debate, and I like to think we helped create a president," he said. "I'd like to think we'll do it again."

On the flight back to Arkansas, Clinton was ebullient if a bit edgy. But when they got home and watched the broadcast with daughter Chelsea, he was furious. The segment was much shorter than he had been led to believe, and he thought the best bits had been cut out. He was so incensed that he did not sleep that night. He was even madder when he woke up.

"It was a screw job," he said. "They lied about how long it was going to be. They lied about what was going to be discussed. They lied about what the ending would be. It couldn't have been worse if they had drawn black Xs through our faces."

But the polls soon showed that eighty-two per cent of people thought enough had been said about Clinton's private life – and now everyone knew who Bill Clinton was.

Other scandals surfaced. He was accused of dodging the draft and smoking marijuana. His response to that was the highly implausible: "I did not inhale."

It was an aide of Democratic rival Bob Kerrey, who had won the Medal of Honor and lost part of his leg in Vietnam, who spiked the press corps' guns over the draft dodging charge. On

Valentine's Day, Bill Shore dashed off some timely verse for the baby-boomers in the press pack: "Roses are red, violets are blue/Clinton dodged the draft and most of you did too."

Paul Tsongas won the New Hampshire primary. Clinton came second and promptly dubbed himself the "Comeback Kid". After that, there was no stopping him. He was fireproofed against any further sexual allegations. Asked by TV talk-show host Phil Donahue whether his sexual peccadilloes were a thing of the past, he said: "I've told you the only facts I think you're entitled to know. Have I had any problems with my marriage? Yes. Are we in good shape now? Yes."

Nevertheless, four months before the election, Clinton campaign aide Betsey Wright told the *Washington Post* that she was on full-time alert to quell potential "bimbo eruptions". And she had her work cut out for her. In July 1992, former Miss Arkansas Sally Perdue claimed to have had an affair with Clinton in 1983, when she was a radio-show host in Little Rock. She said that the governor of Arkansas would cavort around her apartment in her nightie. After the affair was over, she claimed a Democratic Party official had promised her a $40,000 job if she "behaved like a good girl". And if she did not? She said that a Democratic Party staffer told her that "they knew that I went jogging by myself and he couldn't guarantee what would happen to my pretty little legs".

Other stories were circulating. Rock 'n' roll groupie Connie Hamzy claimed that she had had a brush with Clinton back in Little Rock. She told *Penthouse* magazine that an Arkansas state trooper had approached her on behalf of the governor as she lay sunbathing by a hotel swimming pool in a scanty bikini. She claimed that she and Clinton had looked for "a place where they could have some privacy for an assignation, but couldn't find one". She also boasted that she had fondled the future president. Clinton's story was different. He said Hamzy had approached him in a hotel lobby, flipped down her bikini top, and asked him, "What do you think of these?" Clinton's senior political adviser George Stephanopoulos secured affidavits from three staffers who had been with Clinton, telling the same story. That corked the Hamzy eruption for the time being.

Bill Clinton won the election, but almost as soon as he entered the White House journalist David Brock began unearthing "Troopergate". Soon after the inauguration, Brock received an unsolicited tip that a number of Arkansas state troopers who had been assigned to the governor were considering coming forward to tell everything they knew about the Clintons, including extensive first-hand knowledge of Clinton's philandering. Two of them, Larry Patterson and Roger Perry, were eventually persuaded to go on the record. As a result, in January 1994, *American Spectator* published "His Cheatin' Heart". They were aggrieved.

"We lied for him and helped him cheat on his wife, and he treated us like dogs," Patterson said. When one of the troopers asked Clinton to sign some photographs for his family after the election, he said the president-elect snapped: "I don't have time for that shit."

Clinton also assured Patterson that he would get him a lateral transfer within the state police before leaving office, but he never found the time to make the call. They confirmed that Clinton had had an affair with Gennifer Flowers. It lasted several years. She called the governor's mansion regularly, asking for "Bill". If Hillary was not at home, he would take the call. But if Hillary was there, the troopers were told to tell her that he would call back. A little later, he would come down to the troopers' guardhouse and disappear into a back room where he could use a line that Hillary could not intercept from inside the residence. This became his regular method of handling calls from women.

Patterson often drove Clinton to the Quapaw Towers in Little Rock, where Flowers lived. He would wait in the parking lot for up to two hours for Clinton's return. According to Patterson, everywhere they went, even a private party, the troopers would go in with him, except a woman's house. Patterson thought that this was because he had begun his relationship with Flowers long before he acknowledged his philandering to the troopers. He even had a cover story. He would tell them that he was visiting Maurice Smith, director of the state highway department, who lived in the same building, though it was late at night and a damned unsociable hour to call.

In an interview with Brock, Gennifer Flowers said that, initially, Clinton had come in through the lobby and taken the lift to her apartment on the second floor. But gossip spread, so when she saw the governor's Lincoln turn up, she went down to the first floor and propped the fire exit open with a newspaper so that he could enter the building without being seen.

Gradually, Clinton loosened up in front of the men. Once, after a particular satisfactory encounter, Clinton praised Flowers's oral accomplishments with the memorable phrase, she "could suck a tennis ball through a garden hose". High oratory indeed.

Patterson and Perry also heard Clinton organizing a job for Flowers when he was planning to run for president. She lost the job when she did not turn up to work three days running after her story first broke in *The Star*. In the weeks running up to *The Star* interview, they knew something was up. She began calling several times a day. They feared that she may be trying to tape the calls, so when she introduced herself as "Gennifer Flowers", Perry would say "Gennifer Fowler?" as if he did not know who she was. According to Patterson, Hillary had the phone logs destroyed. But it was too late. Flowers had already taped their calls.

Meanwhile Clinton was alternately worried and angry. In the back of his Lincoln, he was heard to say: "What does that whore think she's going to do to me?" And he dismissed Flowers as a "fucking slut". Clinton had believed that Flowers would stick by him.

"If they ever hit you with it just say 'no' and go on," he was heard to say on Flowers's tapes. He would be free and clear on the womanizing issue so long as "they don't have pictures".

Far from his infidelity being confined to the early part of his marriage, for at least a decade, Clinton had been continually having extramarital affairs, often more than one at a time, along with numerous one-night stands. According to the state troopers, these clandestine sexual encounters occurred even after the presidential election and continued during the president-elect's final days in Little Rock.

The troopers said that, while on duty, they were regularly instructed by Clinton to approach women and get their telephone numbers for the governor. They would organize hotel rooms and scout parking lots and other meeting places for sex. They had to drive him in state vehicles to rendezvous points and guard him during these sexual encounters. Clinton would also borrow their state cars so he could slip away and visit women unnoticed. The troopers also had to deliver gifts from Clinton to various women. And some of them, like Flowers, got jobs with the state.

There were dozens of women – some married with children, but all, apparently, willing. There were no indications that he used drink or drugs to seduce them. The troopers would even have to sneak women into the governor's mansion while Hillary and Chelsea were sleeping, then mount a "Hillary watch". It was also their job to keep tabs on Hillary as she went about her business, lie to her about her husband's whereabouts and generally aid the cover-up. Hillary knew what they were up to and cold-shouldered them, keeping the details of her schedule to herself, which made their job doubly difficult.

The general impression was that Hillary was more concerned about his political fortunes than he was.

"I remember one time when Bill had been quoted in the morning paper saying something she didn't like," Patterson said. "I came into the mansion and he was standing at the top of the stairs and she was standing at the bottom screaming. She has a garbage mouth on her, and she was calling him motherfucker, cocksucker and everything else. I went into the kitchen, and the cook, Miss Emma, turned to me and said, 'The devil's in that woman.'"

On another occasion, in the early morning of Labor Day in 1991, she was just leaving the governor's mansion. It was early and the flag was not flying, so she did a U-turn and sped back, squealing to a halt in a cloud of dust.

"Where is the goddamn fucking flag?" she screamed. "I want the goddamn fucking flag up every fucking morning at fucking sunrise."

Hillary liked to humiliate the troopers. She would refer to their guns as "phallic symbols" and send them to fetch her sanitary napkins. But this is understandable. Hillary was frustrated. She certainly was not getting her share. Listening to the audio monitor at the rear porch of the main house, Patterson said he heard Hillary tell Bill in an argument: "I need to be fucked more than twice a year."

She would also complain bitterly when he lingered over an attractive woman at a public event, a common occurrence by all accounts.

"Come on Bill, put your dick up," she was heard to say. "You can't fuck her here."

On the other hand, it was common knowledge among the staff of the governor's mansion that Hillary was having an affair with her legal partner Vince Foster. Whenever Clinton was out of town, he would turn up to see Hillary, staying until the early hours. They would also spend time alone together in a mountain cabin in Heber Springs, maintained by the law firm they both worked for. On several occasions they were seen embracing and French kissing. Patterson also saw him squeeze her butt on his way to the men's room in a French restaurant one day. He winked and made an "OK" sign at Patterson. On his way back, when Hillary's female companion was not looking, he squeezed her breast and made the same "OK" sign. Meanwhile, Hillary cooed, "Oh Vince."

When Clinton became president, a job was found for Foster on the White House staff. He was later found dead in mysterious circumstances in Fort Marcy Park, though subsequent investigations have concluded that he committed suicide.

Clinton was not above being the kettle calling the pot black. During the 1990 gubernatorial race, he asked Patterson to locate a woman who it was rumoured had had an illegitimate child by one of his opponents in the primary. Although it was illegal for state troopers to take part in political campaigns, Patterson said: "Clinton told me to go to the Holiday Inn at the airport, find the woman, and offer her money or a job to sign a statement [about the illegitimate child]." Patterson followed Clinton's instructions and offered the illegal bribe, but the woman declined the offer and never came forward.

Soon after Brock's first interview with the troopers, Perry and two others who wished to remain off the record received telephone calls from their former supervisor on the governor's security detail, Captain Raymond L. "Buddy" Young, whom President Clinton had then appointed to head a regional Federal Emergency Management Agency office in Texas. Perry said Young told him that he was aware that they were thinking of going public. According to Perry, Young told him: "I represent the president of the United States. Why do you want to destroy him over this? You don't know anything anyway . . . This is not a threat, but I wanted you to know that your own actions could bring about dire consequences."

Patterson said Young sent him a handwritten note expressing concern for his health. That, apparently, was not a threat either.

Young confirmed that he had been in contact with Perry and Patterson, but denied making threats. However, another two state troopers had been given jobs at a company in Little Rock that Young part owned.

According to Patterson, Young told him that he had been assigned to deal with the women.

"If one more came out, they knew Gennifer would be credible," said Patterson. "He said they could weather the storm on one, but not two. He told me he went to Texas to talk to Elizabeth Ward."

Young denied this. But if he was to keep the lid on the other women, he had his hands full. Clinton's long-term mistresses since 1987, in addition to Gennifer Flowers, included a staffer in Clinton's office; an Arkansas lawyer Clinton appointed to a judgeship; the wife of a prominent judge; a local reporter; an employee at Arkansas Power and Light, a state-regulated public utility; and a cosmetics sales clerk at a Little Rock department store. Their ages ranged from the early thirties to the early forties. Patterson and Perry said Clinton's extramarital encounters took place at least two or three times a week. Any one of them would come to the residence to see him and be given a "personal tour of the mansion" if Hillary was out. He wouldn't hesitate to seize the opportunity to entertain women at all hours of the day and night and the troopers were instructed to buzz on the intercom if Hillary's car approached.

Or he would visit them in the early morning, perhaps while he was out jogging.

"He would jog out of the mansion grounds very early most mornings and then we would go pick him up at a McDonald's at 7th Street and Broadway," Patterson said. "When we picked him up, half the time he would be covered in sweat and the other half of the time there wouldn't be a drop of sweat on him, even in the middle of July in Little Rock. Sometimes I'd ask him, 'How far did you run today, governor?' And he would say, 'Five miles.' I'd tell him there must be something wrong with his sweat glands because he didn't have a drop of sweat on him. He'd say, 'I can't fool you guys, can I?'"

He may have been cool on the way back, but Gennifer Flowers told *Penthouse* magazine that he always arrived "sweaty but eager".

According to the state troopers, Clinton would also go out on the prowl late at night several times a month. A few minutes after the lights clicked off in the first couple's bedroom, he would get out of bed. He would tell the troopers he was "going out for a drive" and borrow one of their cars as the governor's Lincoln was easily recognizable on the streets of Little Rock. He would leave instructions at the guardhouse that, if Hillary woke up, they should call him on his cell phone. On more than a dozen occasions since 1987, Patterson said he saw one of the troopers' cars parked outside one particular girlfriend's condominium. The woman in question lived just a few doors from Patterson on Shadow Oaks in Sherwood, on the outskirts of Little Rock.

Hillary was a heavy sleeper, but one night she woke to find him gone, flicked on the bedroom light and called down to the guardhouse looking for "the sorry damn son of a bitch" – as she called him when told the governor had gone out for a drive. Perry called Clinton on the cell phone and told him to get back fast.

"He started saying 'Oh God, God, God,'" said Perry. "'What did you tell her?'"

When Clinton arrived home there was a screaming match in the kitchen. Examining the battlefield later, Perry found that the kitchen was a wreck – one of the cabinet doors had been kicked off its hinges.

On other occasions, work would keep him late at the Capitol. Then a trooper would have to drive him direct to a woman's house, where he would have to park unobtrusively and wait for Clinton to emerge. One night, Patterson waited from midnight to 4.30 a.m. But then, as Clinton explained, it was Patterson's responsibility "to cover his ass so he wouldn't get in trouble". After these encounters, Clinton always stopped to wash in the bathroom in the troopers' guardhouse before going back to the residence.

On top of that, there were the brief encounters with women he met at social functions in Little Rock or on the road. The troopers were sometimes used as intermediaries. He would send them off with a message or straightforward propositions, asking the woman in question to retire to a back room, hotel room or empty offices with him.

One day, Clinton eyed a woman at a reception at the Excelsior Hotel in downtown Little Rock. Clinton asked one of the troopers to approach the woman, who he remembered only as Paula, and tell her that the governor found her attractive. He was then to take her to a room in the hotel where Clinton would be waiting. The standard procedure was for one of the troopers to tell the hotel that the governor needed a room for a short time because he was expecting an important call from the White House. While this was not a terribly plausible story during the Reagan and Bush eras, it worked like a charm with hotel clerks in Arkansas. The trooper then stood by in the hall. On this particular evening, the encounter with Paula lasted no more than an hour. As she left, she told the trooper that she would be available to be Clinton's regular girlfriend if he wanted.

Usually, Clinton was discreet. But on more than one occasion Patterson saw the department store clerk fellating Clinton – in a car in the grounds of the governor's mansion or in a parking lot, including the one at Chelsea's elementary school. On that occasion, Patterson was driving Clinton to an annual reception for the Harrison County Chamber of Commerce at the Camelot Hotel in Little Rock. On the way, Clinton suggested they go via Chelsea's school, Booker Elementary. There was only one other car parked there. The sales clerk was in it. Patterson parked across the entrance about 120 feet away. The parking lot was well lit and Patterson stood outside the car, keeping guard.

"I could see Clinton get into the front seat and then the lady's head go into his lap," said Patterson. "They stayed in the car for thirty or forty minutes."

On another occasion she drove up to the governor's mansion. He came out and got into her vehicle. They parked off the rear drive. The troopers then zoomed in the security cameras and the image of Bill Clinton being given a blow job was projected on the twenty-seven-inch screen in the troopers' guardhouse. While they were enjoying this, Chelsea's babysitter turned up. Normally, she would have driven right by where the action was taking place. Patterson stopped her and, explaining that there was a security alert, directed her another way.

When Clinton was finished he came running over to the guardhouse. "Did she see us? Did she see us?" he asked.

Patterson told him what he had done and Clinton said, "Atta boy."

Then there was the time when Patterson met the governor at the airport. He told his bodyguards that he wanted to be driven back to the mansion by an Arkansas lawyer he had met on the plane so that she could show him her new Jaguar. As it was, Clinton drove.

"And she was nowhere to be seen," said Patterson. "Later he told me that he had researched the subject in the Bible and oral sex wasn't considered adultery."

Indeed, it is not even mentioned. This was a defence that would set him in good stead later.

It seems that, when Clinton was not having sex, he was talking about it. "I bet she could give head," he said of a woman reporter, not one he was involved with. Later he complained to Patterson: "If you were a buddy you would fuck her and get her off my ass."

Patterson asked him to sign an autograph for a woman friend. "Does she have big titties?" he enquired.

Another of his aphorisms was: "There are two kinds of fucking redheads. Beautiful fucking redheads and ugly fucking redheads."

Patterson said that, when Clinton was down, all you had to do was talk about sex and he came alive.

During the Flowers eruption, they noted that several calls had been made to the woman living in Sherwood on Clinton's cell phone. As they could not destroy the records of these calls, Betsey Wright asked that, if the records were made public, Patterson would say he made the calls as he lived nearby. Wright then asked Young to write him a cheque. Patterson said he refused to go along with this. Both Wright and Young denied Patterson's account.

Despite this apparent disloyalty, Clinton turned to his trusted state troopers after Flowers went public and asked for their advice. One of them said: "Lie your ass off." It was good advice. He took it and won.

After Clinton was elected president, the Secret Service moved in. The troopers then had to smuggle women through an outer security cordon by saying they were staff or relatives. Before the Clintons left for Washington, one state trooper had to arrange for an employee of Arkansas Power and Light to visit the governor's residence, dressed in a trench coat and baseball cap at 5.15 in the morning. He had to explain to the Secret Service that she was a staff member coming in very early. She was then to be brought in through the basement door to a games room, where Clinton was waiting. The trooper was then instructed to stand at the top of the stairs leading from the basement to the ground floor to alert Clinton if Hillary woke.

By then each mistress had been assigned a trooper whose job it was to call her and find out when Clinton could see her at her home. He would also have to drive her to various events where Clinton was appearing and deliver gifts to her.

"Three times after the [presidential] election I called [the judge's wife] to see if she was at home for the governor," Patterson said.

Clinton also slipped them cash to pay for gifts for the women, which they had to pick up from Victoria's Secret or other shops around town.

"He told us to make sure they were kept in the trunk of the cars and never bring them into the house where Hillary might see them," Perry said.

The trooper whose request for autographed photos for his family Clinton had turned down flat, eventually got his autographs only by insisting on a signature each time Clinton sent him to pick up a gift for a woman.

The troopers agreed that he treated his women well. Clinton even once said that he was in love with one of them, but they could not make out which one it was.

On the day the Clintons headed off to Washington, Clinton asked Patterson to bring one of his women friends to the send-off at Little Rock airport.

"When I got there with [the judge's wife]," said Patterson, "Hillary turned to me and said, 'What the fuck do you think you're doing? I know who that whore is. I know what she's doing here. Get her out of here.'"

Clinton was standing right there and just shrugged, so Patterson dropped her off at a nearby Holiday Inn.

The publication of Brock's Troopergate article prompted Arkansas state employee Paula Jones to file suit against Clinton for sexual harassment. She said she was the Paula that the state trooper had picked up in the Excelsior Hotel. The alleged event took place on 8 May 1991 and she filed suit on 6 May 1994, three days before the three-year statute of limitations ran out. She sought $700,000 in damages for "wilful, outrageous and malicious conduct" at the Excelsior Hotel. Her court papers accused Clinton of "sexually harassing and assaulting" her, then defaming her with denials. She named Arkansas State Trooper Danny Ferguson, the man she said conducted her up to Clinton's room, as co-defendant. Paula also claimed that when she got to the room, Clinton whipped out his cock and, after one look, she politely declined, saying, "I'm not that kind of girl."

Clinton was now in the White House and promptly claimed presidential immunity. When the question reached the Supreme Court in 1997, the justices disagreed and the lawsuit went ahead. Jones's lawyer, conservative-activist Susan

Carpenter-McMillan, then went on the offensive, calling Clinton on national television a "liar", a "philanderer' and even "un-American". I guess that makes George Washington un-American too – though come to think of it he was a Brit until that unfortunate incident in 1776.

"I do not respect a man who cheats on his wife, and exposes his penis to a stranger," she said. I don't think the Puritans who landed on Plymouth Rock spoke like that. No matter.

Trial judge Susan Webber Wright threw the net wider, ruling that Jones was "entitled to information regarding any individuals with whom President Clinton had sexual relations or proposed to or sought to have sexual relations and who were, during the relevant time frame, state or federal employees". But then in a summary judgment she said she found the case without merit. Jones's appeal was dismissed when Clinton settled out of court for $850,000, though poor old Paula only saw $201,000.

By then there had been another bimbo eruption – though not by a state or federal employee, though she claimed to have worked under the governor. A black prostitute called Bobbie Ann Williams claimed that she bore a child by him after one of thirteen sex sessions starting in February 1984. According to Bobbie, she was patrolling her regular patch with two other prostitutes in Little Rock when Clinton, who was jogging, stopped for a chat. She said he returned three days later and told her to walk a hundred yards down the street and wait behind a row of hedges, just yards from the governor's mansion. There she performed a sex act and he paid her $250 instead of her usual $80.

After that, she said they either had sex behind hedges, or his aides would drive her out to a forest cabin around Hot Springs – no, not the one that Vince and Hillary were using. She even said that he took part in an orgy there with her and two other prostitutes.

Clinton was certainly an equal opportunity lover. He had several African-American mistresses, allegedly including

Lencola Sullivan, who had been Miss Arkansas in 1980. At the time of the affair, she was then a reporter on a TV station in Little Rock. When the relationship became too hot, she was shipped off to New York, where the governor, ostensibly on state business, would fly to see her. Later she dated Stevie Wonder.

Then there was Deborah Mathis, a reporter on the *Arkansas Gazette* who, conveniently, went on to become a White House correspondent. Both women deny any involvement. But then, a gentleman never asks and a lady never tells.

When Bobbie Ann was four months pregnant, she said she told Clinton. He rubbed her swollen belly and said: "Girl, that can't be my baby."

That November she gave birth to a ten-pound boy. Although she had an impressive list of customers, she claims Clinton was the only white man she had sex with the month she conceived. Her son grew up tall and fair skinned. In 1991, she went to a lawyer. She underwent two lie-detector tests and gave graphic accounts of the sex sessions she had with Clinton. She also described the aides that drove her out to the cabin itself. Reporters tracked down the cabin and it was exactly as she described.

On 3 January 1999, the *New York Post* ran with the front-page headline: CLINTON PATERNITY BOMBSHELL. It claimed that a DNA test conducted by *The Star* had shown that a sample from Bobbie Ann Williams's thirteen-year-old son Danny matched Clinton's – though the *Post* admitted: "It was unclear how the magazine obtained Clinton's DNA and whether it was a fresh specimen."

However, the following week *Time* magazine said that there was no match and *The Star* did not publish the story. Clinton had ducked under another one.

Then Monica Lewinsky hit the fan. In July 1995, the twenty-two-year-old graduate took a position as an unpaid intern in the office of the White House Chief of Staff Leon Panetta.

According to Lewinsky, she caught the president's eye on 15 November when she flashed her thong at him. It was, she said, "a small, subtle, flirtatious gesture".

Later, the romantic moment was recorded in loving detail in the Starr Report: "At one point, Ms Lewinsky and the president talked alone in the chief of staff's office. In the course of flirting with him, she raised her jacket in the back and showed him the straps of her thong underwear, which extended above her pants."

Things moved fast. On her way to the restroom at about 8 p.m., she passed George Stephanopoulos's office. The president was inside alone, and he beckoned her to enter. She told him that she had a crush on him. He laughed, then asked if she would like to see his private office. Was this a euphemism?

Through a connecting door in Stephanopoulos's office, they went through the president's private dining room towards a small study off the Oval Office.

"We talked briefly and sort of acknowledged that there had been a chemistry that was there before," she said. "We were both attracted to each other and then he asked me if he could kiss me."

Lewinsky said yes. In the windowless hallway adjacent to the study, they kissed. Before returning to her desk, Lewinsky wrote down her name and telephone number for the president.

Two hours later, she was alone in the chief of staff's office and the president approached. He invited her to rendezvous in Stephanopoulos's office in a few minutes, and she agreed. When Monica was asked if she knew why the president wanted to meet her, she said, "I had an idea."

They met in Stephanopoulos's office and again went to the president's private study. This time the lights in the study were off. According to Lewinsky, she and the president kissed. She unbuttoned her jacket and either she unhooked her bra or he lifted her bra up to expose her breasts. She said he touched her breasts with his hands and mouth.

Then the ungallant beast took a phone call, so they moved from the hallway into the back office. Then, "He put his hand down my pants and stimulated me manually in the genital area," Monica said. But for the president it was business as usual and he continued talking on the phone. As he was talking to a senator or a member of congress, she performed oral sex on him.

When he finished his call, after a moment's thought, he told her to stop. She said that she wanted to finish what she was doing, but he said he wanted to wait until he trusted her more. Then he said he had not had "that" for a long time. She took this as a joke. According to the phone records, he talked to two congressmen while she was going down on him. Didn't they notice him moaning? Hold on, they were both southern Democrats. They'd have understood.

Two days later, Monica was working late when some of the staff sent out for a pizza. A piece of it landed on her jacket and she went to the restroom to wash it off. On the way back, the president waylaid her and they kissed. When she said she had to go back to her desk, he told her to come back with a slice of pizza. His secretary Betty Curie ushered her in. Again he got her tits out and gave them a good going over, she said. The door was ajar and Ms Curie came to tell him that there was a phone call for him. It seems they were having a Whitehall farce in the White House.

While the president was on the phone, he deftly unzipped his pants and exposed himself and she went down on him. Again he stopped her before he came. It is not recorded whether the phone call was from a Republican or a Democrat.

Ever the gent, he said he liked her smile – or was it that he liked her mouth? – and told her: "I'm usually around on weekends, no one else is around, and you can come and see me."

And he was serious. In December, she moved to a paid position in the White House Office of Legislative Affairs. Plainly, he needed her on hand.

On 31 December 1995, Clinton had decided how he wanted to see the old year out – or was that the New Year in. Monica told him that he had promised her one of his cigars, so he gave her one. She had thought that he had forgotten what had gone on between them six weeks earlier as he called her "kiddo" rather than using her name. He apologized, saying that he had lost her phone number, though he had tried to find her in the phonebook. Yeah. So he demonstrated beyond doubt that he did remember. He took her into his study.

"And then . . . we were kissing and he lifted my sweater and exposed my breasts and was fondling them with his hands and with his mouth," she said.

She went down on him again and, once more, he stopped her before he came. You have to admire his self-control.

On 7 January 1996, he must have found that illusive phone number because he called her at home.

"I asked him what he was doing and he said he was going to be going into the office soon," said Lewinsky. "I said, oh, do you want some company? And he said, oh, that would be great."

So she went to her office, then they made plans over the phone for a clandestine rendezvous. He would have the door to his office open, and she would pass by with some papers.

"Then . . . he would sort of stop me and invite me in," she said.

Unfortunately, this little drama went awry. There was a uniformed Secret Service officer named Lew Fox outside the Oval Office. But plainly the president was in play-acting mood. He popped out of the office and said: "Have you seen any young congressional staff members here today?"

Officer Fox said, "No, sir."

So Clinton said, "Well, I'm expecting one. Would you please let me know when they show up?"

It worked like a dream. A few minutes later, Monica stopped by and told Fox: "I have some papers for the president."

Fox informed the president she was there and he said, "Oh, hey, Monica, come on in." Then he said to Fox: "You can close the door. She'll be here for a while." He must have thought he was talking to a state trooper.

Monica and Bill talked for about ten minutes in the Oval Office.

"Then we went into the back study and we were intimate in the bathroom," she said.

He gave her the titty treatment again, she said, and he talked about going down on her. But as she was having her period they decided that this might not be a good idea. So Monica did what she was good at and went down on him again.

Back in the Oval Office, they had another little chat.

"He was chewing on a cigar," she said. "And then he had the cigar in his hand and he was kind of looking at the cigar in . . . sort of a naughty way. And so . . . I looked at the cigar and I looked at him and I said, we can do that, too, some time."

The following week they had "phone sex". This made her feel a little bit insecure. She did not know whether he had liked it or not. Nor did she know whether their affair was developing into some kind of a longer-term relationship, or did he have some regular girlfriend who was furloughed? At the time, following a dispute with the Republican-dominated Congress, Clinton had vetoed a spending bill and all non-essential government workers had been furloughed. Monica, of course, was on hand as she was vital to the smooth running of the administration.

On 21 January, the president saw Monica by the elevator and he invited her into the Oval Office. She was quite shirty.

"I asked him why he doesn't ask me any questions about myself," she said. "Is this just about sex? Or do you have some interest in trying to get to know me as a person?"

No, the president laughed and said that "he cherishes the time that he had with [her]". Even Monica thought this was a bit odd, as they had never spent more than a few minutes together.

Then you'll never guess what happened.

He took her into the hallway by the study. With Monica in mid-sentence, "he just started kissing me". Oh, no. Just when she thought he wanted to talk. He got her tits out, then "unzipped his pants and sort of exposed himself", and she went down on him once more. Conversation ceased. As we all know, nice girls don't talk with their mouths full.

Just then someone came into the Oval Office. Bill quickly zippered up.

"I just remember laughing because he had walked out there . . . visibly aroused," she said. "I just thought it was funny."

After dealing with the intrusion, he remembered that an old friend from Arkansas was going to drop by. He gave her a kiss and bundled her out.

Nevertheless on 4 February, he was up for more play-acting. He called her at her desk and she suggested that they bump into each other in the hall. That would be convincing. Then they scurried through into his private study.

"He unbuttoned my dress and unhooked my bra," she said. "He was looking at me and touching me and telling me how beautiful I was."

After working his magic on her breasts, he went for the pussy, first stroking it through her panties, then directly, she said. And, just when they were getting somewhere, she performed oral sex on him. The girl just can't get off her knees.

Afterwards, they talked for about forty-five minutes, like he was "trying to get to know me". Then he kissed her arm and said he would call.

"Yeah, well, what's my phone number?" she said petulantly. The girl's got some spunk. Oh, well, no, she hasn't. Not yet. According to her testimony, he is still holding back.

But then a miracle happened – "He recited both my home number and my office number off the top of his head."

However, the course of true lust never runs smooth. On 19 February, President's Day, he called her at her apartment in the Watergate building – good choice, Monica. She knew from the tone of his voice that something was wrong. She said she wanted to come and see him, but he said he did not know how long he was going to be there. Nevertheless, Monica headed for the White House and stormed into the Oval Office, despite the "tall, slender, Hispanic plain-clothes agent on duty near the door". He was pretty useful at protecting the president then, but who wants to stand in the way of a woman that is about to get the brush-off? Not me.

In his defence, agent Nelson U. Garabito said Ms Lewinsky was carrying a folder and said: "I have these papers for the president." Oh, that old trick.

The president said that he no longer felt right about their intimate relationship and was going to put an end to it. They could go on seeing each other, but just as friends. We've all heard that one. It usually means: "I'm shagging your sister."

After the break-up Monica said that they kept on flirting. Come on, he did that with the American people. After passing in a hallway one night in late February or March, the president telephoned her at home and said he was disappointed that, as she had already left the White House for the evening, they could not get together. Monica thought that the call "sort of implied to me that he was interested in starting up again".

So some added inducement was needed. When a friend named Natalie Ungvari came to town, Monica took her to the White House. They bumped into Bill who seemed to know all about Natalie.

There were more signals that things may rekindle. On 29 March, she spotted that he was wearing a necktie that she had given him.

"Where did you get that tie?" she asked brazenly.

"Some girl with style gave it to me," he replied.

Hillary was away, so Bill phoned Monica at her desk and asked her to come to watch a movie with him. What she had to do was hang about outside the White House movie theatre, he would then bump into her accidentally and invite her in. Even Monica thought this was none too subtle. Instead, she asked to meet him over the weekend. He said he would try.

Again she used the old "I've got some papers for the president" ploy to get into the Oval Office. This time she had a new Hugo Boss necktie in the folder for the chief executive. Then in the hallway by the study "he focused on me pretty exclusively", kissing her bare breasts and fondling her genitals, she said.

At one point, she said, the president stuck a cigar in her vagina, then put the cigar in his mouth and said: "It tastes good."

After that, she needed a walk in the Rose Garden to cool off.

By this time, both White House staffers and the Secret Service had noticed that Ms Lewinsky was spending a lot of time hanging around the West Wing. On one occasion, she had brushed past one member of presidential protection detail, saying breathlessly, "The president needs me." No doubt he did.

Evelyn Lieberman, deputy chief of staff, said she was "always someplace she shouldn't be" and had Monica transferred from the White House to the Pentagon. On Easter Sunday, 7 April, she told the president tearfully that she had been sacked.

"Why do they have to take you away from me?" he said.

They had a "sexual encounter" and he promised to bring her back after the election.

According to Ms Lewinsky: "I think he unzipped . . . because it was sort of this running joke that I could never unbutton his pants, that I just had trouble with it."

She went down on him and, again, he did not come. The girl must be doing something wrong.

Again she did it to him while he was on the phone – this time to Dick Morris, Clinton's aide who resigned after being caught with a prostitute. Then, they were interrupted by deputy chief of staff Harold Ickes who stormed into the Oval Office and hollered: "Mr President."

They always left the door ajar during their sexual encounters.

Clinton "jetted" back into the Oval Office, while Monica slunk off. The Secret Service officer noticed that Monica, still clutching her manila folder, was "a little upset".

Later Bill called her and asked why she had run off.

"I told him that I didn't know if he was going to be coming back," she said. "He was a little upset with me that I left."

Though they did not meet again privately for the rest of the year, he did call to ask how her new job was going, though the telephone conversations regularly ended up with "phone sex". She said that she wanted to make love to him; he asked whether he should stop calling.

They did see each other at public functions. On one occasion when he reached past to shake the hand of another guest, she reached forward and grabbed the commander-in-chief's crotch in a "playful" fashion. Another time, she yelled out: "Hey, handsome – I like your tie."

That night he called. The following day she was going to be in the White House on Pentagon business. He told her to drop by the Oval Office while she was there. But Ms Lieberman was nearby so she did not dare. Then came the famous photograph of Monica shaking hands with the president. She was standing up this time.

Though he was re-elected, she did not hear from him. Nor was she recalled to the White House.

"I kept a calendar with a countdown until election day," she wrote in an unsent letter. "I was so sure that the weekend after the election you would call me to come visit and you would kiss me passionately and tell me you couldn't wait to have me back. You'd ask me where I wanted to work and say something akin to 'Consider it done' and it would be. Instead I didn't hear from you for weeks and subsequently your phone calls became less frequent."

However, Bill Clinton put her encounters on a more formal basis, having his secretary Betty Currie arrange them. Betty would even come to the White House at weekends to make sure that everything went smoothly. She said they were usually alone together in the Oval Office for fifteen to twenty minutes, though once she had to wait thirty or forty minutes because he had another visitor. Monica also sent letters and packages via Ms Currie, who suspected that something was going on.

"He was spending a lot of time with a twenty-four-year-old young lady," she said. "I know he has said that young people keep him involved in what's happening in the world, so I knew that was one reason, but there was a concern of mine that she was spending more time than most."

Clinton was a hands-on sort of guy but Ms Currie knew that "the majority" of the president's meetings with Ms Lewinsky were "more personal in nature as opposed to business".

They even discussed the matter. Monica said: "As long as no one saw us – and no one did – then nothing happened."

"Don't want to hear it," said Ms Currie, flustered. "Don't say any more. I don't want to hear any more."

She did not log Monica's calls, asked the Secret Service officers to admit her without logging her in, and steered her past other staffers who might not approve of her presence. But most of her visits were arranged at night or weekends, so "there would be no need to sneak," said Ms Currie.

On 14 February 1996, Monica Lewinsky posted a small ad in the *Washington Post* that read:

HANDSOME
With love's light wings did
I o'er perch these walls
For stony limits cannot hold love out,
And what love can do that dares love attempt.
– *Romeo and Juliet* 2:2
Happy Valentine's Day.
M

On 24 February, Monica dropped around to the White
House on Pentagon business. She sent a note to the president
but did not see him. However, four days later, she struck
pay dirt. On 28 February, she turned up at the White House
in a navy-blue dress from Gap. They had their photograph
taken together. Then the president told her to go and see Ms
Currie "because he wanted to give her something". She then
accompanied him past the Oval Office to the private study,
then he said discreetly: "I'll be right back." Naturally, she
waited fifteen to twenty minutes before she popped her head
around the door.

Meanwhile the president "started to say something to me
and I was pestering him to kiss me, because . . . it had been a
long time since we had been alone". It's a good way to shut a
politician up too. Why couldn't the Republicans have learnt
that?

Once he had disentangled his mouth, the president said that
he wanted to give her a belated Christmas gift – a hatpin and a
special edition of Walt Whitman's *Leaves of Grass*. Containing
such poems as "To a Common Prostitute" and "I Sing the
Body Electric", it was dismissed as "a mass of stupid filth"
when it was first published. Monica said the book was "the
most sentimental gift he had given me . . . it's beautiful and it
meant a lot to me". It obviously put her in the mood.

"We went back over by the bathroom in the hallway, and
we kissed," she said. "We were kissing and he unbuttoned my

dress and fondled my breasts with my bra on, and then took them out of my bra and was kissing them and touching them with his hands and with his mouth.

"And then I think I was touching him in his genital area through his pants, and I think I unbuttoned his shirt and was kissing his chest. And then . . . I wanted to perform oral sex on him . . . and so I did. And then . . . I think he heard something, or he heard someone in the office. So, we moved into the bathroom . . ."

He liked to lean against the door frame, saying it eased his sore back – a touch of the Kennedys here.

". . . And I continued to perform oral sex and then he pushed me away, kind of as he always did before he came, and then I stood up and I said . . . I care about you so much; . . . I don't understand why you won't let me . . . make you come; it's important to me; I mean, it just doesn't feel complete, it doesn't seem right."

They hugged and, according to Monica, Clinton said "he didn't want to get addicted to me, and he didn't want me to get addicted to him".

They looked at each other for a moment. Then the Starr Report rushed to the climax: "Then, saying that 'I don't want to disappoint you,' the president consented. For the first time, she performed oral sex through to completion."

It seems she was a spitter, not a swallower. Or, at least, a dribbler, not a swallower. Next time she took the dress out of the closet, she noticed stains on the chest and the hip. Well, after holding back so long, there was going to be a lot of the stuff. Rather than sending it out to the dry cleaner, Monica put the dress away safely – as a treasured memento of that first perfect act of love, of course. Later, the FBI found that the stains were the presidential semen, his seal of office, as it were. Ah, the thrills and spills.

It was not quite such a treasured moment for the president. "I was sick after it was over and I . . . I was pleased at that time that it had been nearly a year since any inappropriate contact had occurred with Ms Lewinsky," he said. "I promised myself it wasn't going to happen again."

A month later she was back on her knees again. Ms Currie had set up a meeting in the Oval Office "because he had something important to tell her", according to Monica. He came limping in on crutches, having injured his knee two weeks earlier in Florida.

She started running at the mouth, if you will excuse the expression. He stifled her talk with his lips.

"This was another one of those occasions when I was babbling on about something," she said, "and he just kissed me, kind of to shut me up, I think."

He undid her blouse and fondled her fun bags.

"He went to go put his hand down my pants, and then I unzipped them because it was easier," she said. "And I didn't have any panties on . . ."

Who did she think she was? Marilyn Monroe? Going commando for the commander in chief. How appropriate.

". . . And so he manually stimulated me . . ."

But this was not enough for the poor girl.

". . . I wanted him to touch my genitals with his genitals, and he did so, lightly and without penetration."

Then it is back to standard operating procedure. She performed oral sex on him and, once again, he came.

Afterwards, he told her that he suspected that a foreign embassy was tapping his telephone. In fact, it was someone closer to home.

When no job back at the White House was forthcoming, Monica began to think the president was stringing her along. Then rumours began to circulate about Clinton's late-night phone calls to Monica, which seemed to emanate from Monica's mother and aunt.

Bill got Ms Currie to invite Monica to the White House where he told her that he must end the relationship. He admitted that, early in his marriage, he had had hundreds of affairs, but since turning forty, he had made a concerted effort to be faithful. Well, not very concerted. The year before, he had turned fifty. They kissed and hugged, but there was no more sex, she said. This was three days before the Supreme Court ruled that the Constitution did not give the president immunity against civil lawsuits, allowing the Jones case to resume.

Clinton was still trying to get Monica a job back at the White House, but he was obstructed by Ms Currie and other women staffers. Then things got nasty. Monica said she felt "used" and reminded him in a letter that she had "left the White House like a good girl in April of 1996," when other people might have threatened disclosure to hold on to their job. Ouch.

The response was swift. At a very emotional meeting the next day, he said, "It's illegal to threaten the president of the United States."

She wept. He tried to comfort her with a hug, but she spotted a gardener outside the window. So he took her to the hallway outside the bathroom. She must have been puckering already, thinking her luck was in.

The president was, she said, "the most affectionate with me he'd ever been". He stroked her arm, toyed with her hair, kissed her on the neck, praised her intellect and beauty – though not her naivety, plainly.

"He remarked . . . that he wished he had more time for me." The old charmer. "And so I said, well, maybe you will have more time in three years." Oh, Monica. "And I was . . . thinking just when he wasn't president, he was going to have more time on his hands. And he said, well, I don't know, I might be alone in three years. And then I said something about . . . us sort of being together. I think I kind of said, oh, I think we'd be a good team, or something like that. And he . . . jokingly said, well, what are we going to do when I'm seventy-five and I have to pee twenty-five times a day? And . . . I told him that we'd deal with that."

Come on, she was only twenty-four.

"I left that day sort of emotionally stunned," she said. "I just knew he was in love with me."

But there was already another woman in the frame. Monica told Bill that *Newsweek* were working on an article about Kathleen Willey, a volunteer at the White House who claimed that Clinton had sexually harassed her in the Oval Office. Monica had been told this by Linda Tripp, a colleague in the Pentagon's public affairs office. Tripp, who had formerly worked at the White House, said that she saw Willey emerge from the Oval Office "dishevelled – her face red and her lipstick was off". Tripp later told a grand jury that Willey had pursued Clinton, rather than the other way around. Bill told Monica that the harassment allegation was ludicrous, because he would never approach a small-breasted woman like Ms Willey.

Nevertheless, the president got Monica to talk to Linda Tripp, who was also speaking with *Newsweek*, and try to shut her up. *Newsweek* went ahead with the Willey story, saying that she emerged from the Oval Office not just "dishevelled", but also "flustered, happy, and joyful". Bill must have been on good form that day and was possibly giving her more than Monica was getting. Monica assured Bill that Tripp had been misquoted.

"Well, that's good because it sure seemed like she screwed me from that article," he said.

By then Monica had told Linda Tripp about her relationship with Bill Clinton and Tripp began to record their phone calls. After speaking to literary agent Lucianne Golberg, she also advised Monica not to clean the infamous navy-blue dress.

But Monica was still eager to revive the affair. On 16 August, three days before his birthday, she visited the White House again, where she managed to get into the president's back office. She stuck a candle in an apple square. When he came in, she sang "Happy Birthday" and gave him his presents. (Security was tight that day too then.) Then she asked for a birthday kiss. He said "we could kind of bend the rules that day. And so . . . we kissed."

It was not going to end there. Monica grabbed his penis through his pants and went to go down on him, but he stopped her.

"He said, 'I'm trying not to do this and I'm trying to be good.'"

Still no job in the White House was forthcoming and Monica became miffed that other women who had laid down their panties for the president were enjoying "golden positions". Linda Tripp had heard from a friend at the National Security Council that rumours were spreading about Monica and she would never get another job in the White House. Her advice was to "get out of town". Clinton arranged for Monica to be offered a job at the United Nations in New York, but she turned it down.

Meanwhile, Clinton was being questioned over the Paula Jones case and was asked to list any woman other than his wife with whom he had "had", "proposed having" or "sought to have" sexual relations during the time that he was attorney general of Arkansas, governor of Arkansas and president of the United States. He objected to the scope and relevance of the questions and refused to answer. Those years at Yale Law School were not entirely wasted then.

Lewinsky then became a pain, throwing a hysterical scene when the president of Mexico Ernesto Zedillo was in the White House. On the other hand, she gave Bill an antique paperweight in the shape of the White House – nice – and showed him an email describing the effect of chewing Altoid mints before performing oral sex. She was chewing Altoids at the time, but the president replied that he did not have enough time for oral sex. They kissed, and the president rushed off for a state dinner with President Zedillo.

On 5 December 1997, Paula Jones's attorneys faxed the list of potential witnesses they proposed to call. It included Monica Lewinsky. She attended a Christmas party at the White House with a colleague from the Defense Department. The next day, she turned up at the White House with some Christmas presents and was told that she would have to wait for forty minutes. The Secret Service officer let it slip that Clinton was in a meeting with thirty-seven-year-old actress and TV personality Eleanor Mondale. Lewinsky flew into a rage. The *Washington Post* reported: "Lewinsky 'stormed away, called and berated Mrs Currie from a pay phone.' Currie, in turn, 'hands shaking and almost crying,' told the officers that Clinton was 'irate' that they had told Lewinsky about Mondale and warned a Secret Service supervisor that 'someone could be fired.'"

The *Washington Post* and others implied that he was having a fling with Eleanor Mondale. She denied it.

On 15 December Paula Jones's attorneys asked Clinton to "produce documents that related to communications between the president and Monica Lewisky [*sic*]". Four days later Monica was subpoenaed. She burst into tears. But it was OK. They had already got their cover story sorted out. Clinton's friend and legal adviser Vernon Jordan said he would find her an attorney. But first he asked Clinton one question: "Mr President, have you had sexual relations with Monica Lewinsky?"

Clinton answered: "No, never."

It was best to get in some early practice.

When Judge Wright ruled that the president had to name every state and federal employee with whom he had sexual relations or he had proposed to have sexual relations with since 1986, Clinton answered: "None."

Soon after Christmas, Monica made one last visit to the Oval Office where she finally delivered her presents, which included such tasteful items as a marble bear's head, a Rockettes blanket, a Black Dog stuffed animal, a small box of chocolates, a pair of joke sunglasses and a pin with the New York skyline on it. You have to admit it: the girl's got class.

Bill was overwhelmed. She said that the president rewarded her with a "passionate" and "physically intimate" kiss. "Physically intimate" kiss? We've not gone back to the bathroom scene, have we?

That day Betty Currie drove to Monica's apartment and collected all the gifts that Clinton had given her, though a subpoena required Monica to produce all the gifts he had given her. Vernon Jordan advised her to throw away any correspondence she had had with the president. But Monica remained a class act. She went around to Betty Currie's home to deliver another present for Bill – a book called *The Presidents of the United States*, in case he needed any further inspiration, and a love note inspired by the movie *Titanic*. It said that she wanted to have sexual intercourse with him at least once. The president cautioned her about writing such notes.

"I remember telling her she should be careful what she wrote," he said, "because a lot of it was clearly inappropriate and would be embarrassing if somebody else read it."

Lewinsky's lawyer drafted an affidavit. It said: "I have never had a sexual relationship with the president . . . The occasions that I saw the president, with crowds of other people, after I left my employment at the White House in April 1996 related to official receptions, formal functions or events related to the US Department of Defense, where I was working at the time."

Vernon Jordan and President Clinton reviewed the draft affidavit. "Crowds of people" was deemed implausible and inappropriate – were they having an orgy? That sentence was deleted and "There were other people present on all of these occasions" was added.

Then, with the help of Vernon Jordan, Monica got a job at Revlon. This was unfortunate as Paula Jones's attorneys wanted to call women who had been rewarded for having had sex with Bill Clinton and the Revlon job could be considered a reward.

Meanwhile, Clinton was questioned about his relationship with Monica Lewinsky. He denied having a sexual affair or sexual relations with her. Judge Wright specified, for the purposes of his deposition, that a person engages in "sexual relations" when the person knowingly engages in or causes . . . contact with the genitalia, anus, groin, breast, inner thigh, or buttocks of any person with an intent to arouse or gratify the sexual desire of any person . . . "Contact" means intentional touching, either directly or through clothing.

Later, before a grand jury empanelled by special prosecutor Ken Starr, Clinton argued that this definition "covers contact by the person being deposed with the enumerated areas, if the contact is done with an intent to arouse or gratify", but it does not cover oral sex performed on the person being deposed. According to Slick Willie: "If the deponent is the person who has oral sex performed on him, then the contact is with – not with anything on that list, but with the lips of another person."

He maintained that "any person, reasonable person" would recognize that oral sex performed on the deponent falls outside the definition. So if Monica performed oral sex on the president then, under this interpretation, she was engaged in sexual relations but he was not. He refused to answer whether Ms Lewinsky in fact had performed oral sex on him. He admitted that direct contact with Monica's breasts or genitalia would fall within the definition, but he denied touching them. So here we have Monica half naked on her knees gobbling away, while he stands coolly erect, gripping the edge of the desk. Look, Ma, no hands.

That could even explain the semen on Monica's dress without inviting a charge of perjury. He could come all over her and still not have sexual relations. You need that level of logic to run the world's only superpower.

Still, when he said, "I did not have sexual relations with that woman, Miss Lewinsky", peopled laughed, whatever the definition.

The president then had a word with Betty Currie. He said: "You were always there when she was there, right? . . . We were never really alone . . . Monica came on to me, and I never touched her, right? . . . You could see and hear everything, right?"

Ms Currie said that she got the impression that the president wanted her to agree with him. After all, he was the president.

Sensing they had another Watergate, on 21 January 1998, the *Washington Post* unleashed Zippergate with a story headlined: CLINTON ACCUSED OF URGING AIDE TO LIE; STARR PROBES WHETHER PRESIDENT TOLD WOMAN TO DENY ALLEGED AFFAIR TO JONES'S LAWYERS.

The White House had got wind of the story the night before. Clinton's personal attorney Robert Bennett got in touch with the paper and was quoted in the story, saying: "The president adamantly denies he ever had a relationship with Ms Lewinsky and she has confirmed the truth of that." This time the *Post* had printed the name of Deep Throat.

The following day the *Post* ran a White House statement, approved by the president, saying he was "outraged by these allegations" and that he had "never had an improper relationship with this woman". Again, he proved himself the master of the imprecise phrase.

Meanwhile, he consoled his staff with the repeated assertion: "I want you to know I did not have sexual relations with this woman, Monica Lewinsky. I did not ask anybody to lie. And when the facts come out, you'll understand."

At least, when his definition of "sexual relations" came out they would understand. But this was vitally important. Adultery is a misdemeanour in the District of Columbia with a maximum penalty of $500 or 180 days in jail. But it is a felony in Idaho, Massachusetts, Oklahoma, Wisconsin and Michigan, where the maximum sentence is life. As recently as 1980, a

Massachusetts couple were spotted having sex in a van and, when they admitted they were married but not to each other, they were arrested for adultery and fined $50. If it were proved that Clinton had an affair with Lewinsky or anyone else while he was president, it would constitute one of the "high crimes and misdemeanours" identified in the Constitution as criteria for impeachment.

This is where the oral sex comes in. As Bill Clinton's studies had already shown, there is no mention of oral sex in the Bible. So it is not, technically, adultery. Some states specifically define adultery as sexual intercourse outside marriage. The District of Columbia leaves adultery undefined, so the biblical definition would apply. That meant that Bill Clinton could enjoy oral sex in the White House with as many women as he fancied, though he would have to avoid Kansas and a few other states where oral sex has been written into the criminal code. And it would be best to stay out of Maryland, where Montgomery County Circuit Court Administrative Judge Paul Weinstein ruled that adultery should be understood to include other sexual acts as it was essentially a breach in the trust between a married couple, regardless of the precise nature of the sexual act involved. But otherwise, Monica, suck away.

To others, Clinton played victim. He told his senior aide Sidney Blumenthal: "I haven't done anything wrong. Monica Lewinsky came on to me and made sexual demands on me." She was a maneater, in more than one way. Manfully, he had "rebuffed her", but she had "threatened him. She said that she would tell people they'd had an affair," he said. Apparently "she was known as the stalker among her peers, and that she hated it and if she had an affair or said she had an affair then she wouldn't be the stalker any more."

But generally he was very careful about his denials, so that they fell within the definition he had made for himself. He averred that he spoke the truth: "I said, there's nothing going on between us. That was true. I said I did not have sex with her as I defined it. That was true . . . They may have been misleading, and if they were I have to take responsibility for it, and I'm sorry."

National Public Radio was also on his case. On the programme *All Things Considered*, he was asked whether he had "encouraged a young woman to lie to lawyers in the Paula Jones civil suit. Is there any truth to that allegation?"

"No, sir, there's not. It's just not true," he said.

Then he was asked: "Is there any truth to the allegation of an affair between you and the young woman?"

"No. That's not true either . . . The charges are not true. And I haven't asked anybody to lie," he replied.

Again asking someone to lie in a court case would constitute promoting perjury and be one of those "high crimes and misdemeanors" he could be impeached for.

That evening on *The News Hour with Jim Lehrer*, he said: "There is no improper relationship" with Monica Lewinsky. Asked what he meant by the term "improper relationship", he said, "Well, I think you know what it means. It means that there is not a sexual relationship, an improper sexual relationship, or any other kind of improper relationship."

You are not going to pin Slick Willie down that easily.

The following morning, standing alongside Yasser Arafat, he said, "The allegations are false, and I would never ask anybody to do anything other than tell the truth. That is false."

And he continued the refrain of "no improper relations", "no sexual relations" and "this is untrue".

But by this time there was another lawyer on the case. In 1994, Ken Starr had been appointed by Attorney General Janet Reno as an independent counsel to investigate criminal accusations made against Bill and Hillary Clinton over a failed real-estate venture, known as Whitewater. Before Vince Foster died, he looked into that too. Then he expanded his investigation to the firing of White House Travel Office personnel, potential political abuse of confidential FBI files, Madison Guaranty,

Rose Law Firm, the Paula Jones lawsuit and, most notoriously, possible perjury and obstruction of justice in the cover-up of President Clinton's sexual relationship with Monica Lewinsky.

The polls showed that the American people would forgive the president for adultery – Hillary was never that popular – but they would not forgive perjury or obstruction of justice. So Clinton urged his aides to go easy on Monica Lewinsky in the hope that she would not cooperate with the Starr investigation.

"We don't want to alienate her by anything we put out," he said.

But alienate her he did. On 26 January 1998, he tried to draw a line under the affair, once and for all. At a televised news conference, he said defiantly: "I want to say one thing to the American people. I want you to listen to me. I'm going to say this again: I did not have sexual relations with that woman, Miss Lewinsky. I never told anybody to lie, not a single time. Never. These allegations are false." {Titters off.}

Soon Starr had Tripp's tapes of intimate conversations between Monica and Bill, and he began to request testimony from the Secret Service agents who had guarded the president. He empanelled a grand jury that took testimony from Bill Clinton where, with his legal mind on overdrive, he asserted that he was telling the truth when he told his top aides that "there is nothing going on" between him and Monica Lewinsky.

He said: "It depends on what the meaning of the word 'is' is. If 'is' means is and never has been, that is not – that is one thing. If it means there is none, that was a completely true statement . . . Now, if someone had asked me on that day, are you having any kind of sexual relations with Ms Lewinsky, that is, asked me a question in the present tense, I would have said no. And it would have been completely true."

Looking back, Jim Lehrer and others realized that Clinton had always used the present tense. So he was right. He was not having a relationship with Monica Lewinsky at the time he was talking to them. He had put an end to it.

It was here that he trotted out his definition of "sexual relations", claiming that he had not had sex with Monica Lewinsky because he had not touched her "genitalia, anus, groin, breast, inner thigh, or buttocks".

But this is where it all came apart.

While Monica Lewinsky testified that she had performed oral sex on him and that they had not had sexual intercourse, she maintained that on nine occasions the president fondled and kissed her bare breasts. He touched her genitals, both through her underwear and directly, bringing her to orgasm on two occasions. On one occasion, the president inserted a cigar into her vagina. On another occasion, she and the president had brief genital-to-genital contact. Now that might not be a full-blown shag, but it constituted "sexual relations" under the definition Judge Wright had laid down in the Paula Jones case.

The Starr Report was published on 11 September 1998. The House Judiciary Committee sat on its hands and conducted no investigations of its own into Clinton's alleged wrongdoing, holding no serious impeachment-related hearings before the 1998 mid-term elections, where the Democrats gained a number of seats, though the Republicans still had a majority in both houses.

On 19 December 1998, the House of Representatives impeached Clinton for perjury before a grand jury and obstruction of justice. After a twenty-one-day trial before the Senate, he was acquitted. A two-thirds majority was required to find him guilty. No Democrats voted guilty and a handful of Republicans voted to acquit.

Monica Lewinsky went on to write a bestselling book about the affair with Andrew Morton, the biographer of Princess Diana. It had been the biggest sex scandal in presidential history. Clinton had been a lifelong fan of John F. Kennedy and wanted to follow in his footsteps. He managed that then.

## Earl Long

When the governor of Louisiana Earl Long fell out with his wife, the matronly Miz Blanche, he sought solace in a striptease club in New Orleans called the Sho-Bar. It was there that the sixty-five-year-old politician set eyes on Blaze Starr, the club's headline stripper who had been voted "Queen of the Burlesque" the year before. He fell instantly in love with her. He told her that Miz Blanche had denied him sex for two years. Blaze was prepared to lend a hand at the very least and, in gratitude, Earl set her up in the Flamingo Hotel, just outside town.

When they were caught together there, the scandal hit the headlines. Miz Blanche was fuming, but Earl was not about to come to heel. In front of the astonished audience at the Sho-Bar, Governor Long asked the betassled stripper to marry him.

Miz Blanche and US Senator Russell Long, the governor's nephew, then drew up papers to have Earl committed to a mental hospital. He was dragged from the governor's mansion, flown to Texas and locked up in a clinic. A judge ruled that he could return to Louisiana, provided he checked into another clinic there.

When Earl arrived back in New Orleans, he walked into the front door of a clinic, then straight out the back. He headed for Baton Rouge, but was intercepted on the orders of Miz Blanche and returned to hospital. Finally, he got a judge to release him and, when he got out, he fired the director of the Louisiana Department of Hospitals.

From then on his behaviour became increasingly bizarre. Once, when eating out with Blaze, he put a paper bag over his head and put his false teeth beside him in a jar. When his term of office was over, he invited all the strippers from the Sho-Bar to his farewell party at the governor's mansion. Miz Blanche fled and Blaze did a strip. Then they stuffed all the goodies they could carry in the car and went back to Blaze's apartment.

Earl then ran for Congress and was nominated, but died the following day.

## John Edwards

Former Senator John Edwards was running for the Democratic Party nomination in the 2008 presidential campaign, after having been vice presidential nominee on the ticket with John Kerry in 2004. Two years earlier film-maker Rielle Hunter had pitched the idea of producing a series of webisodes – short TV episodes posted on the web – showing behind-the-scenes life on the campaign trail when she met him in a New York bar. It would cost a mere $100,000. However, what was happening off camera was much more revealing.

On 27 August 2007, the *New York Post* asked: "Which political candidate enjoys visiting New York because he has a girlfriend who lives downtown? The pol tells her he'll marry her when his current wife is out of the picture."

Edwards's wife Elizabeth had been diagnosed with breast cancer in 2004. Treated with chemotherapy and radiotherapy, she continued to work within the Democratic Party and on her husband's One America Committee. Then in March 2007, it was announced that her cancer had returned and had spread to the bone and possibly to her lungs. The cancer was no longer curable.

Following up on the *Post*'s story led reporters to Edwards and Hunter. The webisodes were pulled. On 10 October 2007, the *National Enquirer* ran a story saying that Edwards was having an affair with a campaign worker – it is the traditional thing to do, it seems. The following day, *New York* magazine ran a piece, tying Hunter to the *Enquirer* story.

Naturally, Edwards denied the allegations in the strongest possible terms. The *Enquirer* story was "made-up", he told Associated Press.

"I've been in love with the same woman for thirty-plus years," he said, "and as anybody who's been around us knows, she's an extraordinary human being, warm, loving, beautiful, sexy and as good a person as I have ever known. So the story's just false . . . It's completely untrue, ridiculous."

He was a politician so he must be, er, telling the truth.

Hunter also issued a denial via the political blog MyDD (*My Due Diligence*, later renamed *My Direct Democracy*): "The innuendoes and lies that have appeared on the internet and in the *National Enquirer* concerning John Edwards are not true, completely unfounded and ridiculous . . . When working for the Edwards camp, my conduct as well as the conduct of my entire team was completely professional. This concocted story is just dirty politics and I want no part of it."

So there you have it from both sides.

However, the *Enquirer* stuck by its story – and went further. On 17 December, they published a photograph of Hunter who was visibly pregnant. They even had an unnamed source who said Hunter was claiming that Edwards was the father of the child. However, the story conceded that Hunter had moved into a gated community in Chapel Hill, North Carolina, to be closer to Andrew Young, a member of Edwards's campaign team.

Young, a married man, claimed paternity, but the *Enquirer* continued to claim that Hunter was privately telling friends that Edwards was the father. However, the mainstream media continued to ignore the story.

CBS News journalist Bob Schieffer, asked about the allegations on *Imus in the Morning*, said: "I believe that's a story that we will be avoiding, because it appears to me that there's absolutely nothing to it . . . This seems to be just sort of a staple of modern campaigns, that you got through at least one love child which turns out not to be a love child. And I think we can all do better than this one."

It seems the press did not want to be seen causing any distress to Elizabeth Edwards. Besides the campaign still had a long way to run, so they might as well wait until after the Iowa caucuses. Coming a poor third behind Barack Obama and Hillary Clinton, Edwards dropped out of the race.

That should have been the end of it. But for Edwards's vehement denials it would have been. Then what had been a run-of-the-mill sex scandal now turned into high farce. The *Enquirer* learned that Edwards was going to visit Hunter and her child at the Beverly Hilton in Los Angeles on the evening of 21 July 2008. They sent a team of reporters who cornered Edwards in the hotel at around two in the morning. He was not registered there and locked himself in the men's room until he was escorted from the premises by hotel security.

The guard said the ashen-faced Edwards asked him: "What are they saying about me?" Unfortunately, the security guard did not recognize him and had no idea what he was talking about.

The following day, Edwards was asked about the allegations in New Orleans and said: "I have no idea what you're asking about. I've responded, consistently, to these tabloid allegations by saying I don't respond to these lies and you know that . . . and I stand by that."

Of course, the *Enquirer* had a field day with the story, even claiming they had video footage of Hunter entering a room and Edwards leaving sometime later. Then on 7 August 2008, they published a grainy photograph of what they said was Edwards cradling the baby. By then the story was all over the blogosphere and had been picked up by a number of foreign newspapers.

The following day, Edwards was forced to admit that he had had an affair with Rielle Hunter. He issued a statement saying: "In 2006, I made a serious error in judgement and conducted myself in a way that was disloyal to my family and to my core beliefs. I recognized my mistake and I told my wife that I had a liaison with another woman, and I asked for her forgiveness. Although I was honest in every painful detail with my family,

I did not tell the public. When a supermarket tabloid told a version of the story, I used the fact that the story contained many falsities to deny it. But being ninety-nine per cent honest is no longer enough."

Ninety-nine per cent would have been good. As it was he continued to deny that the child was his and was immediately asked to take a DNA test by Hunter's family.

"I would welcome participating in a paternity test," said Edwards. "I'm only one side of the test, but I'm happy to participate in one."

But maybe he was not so willing. Andrew Young claimed that Edwards asked him to "get a doctor to fake the DNA results. And he asked me . . . to steal a diaper from the baby so he could secretly do a DNA test to find out if this [was] indeed his child."

It was only in 2010, that Edwards admitted that Hunter's two-year-old daughter Quin was his child, which had been conceived several months after she had stopped working on the campaign.

Young went on to write a book about the scandal called *The Politician*. In it he revealed that Elizabeth Edwards had discovered the affair in 2006, shortly after John Edwards and Hunter returned from a trip to Uganda. It seems that his wife answered a mobile phone call to hear Hunter launch into a "romantic monologue". Elizabeth confronted her husband who "confessed to having had a one-night stand but didn't say with whom". He called Hunter in front of his wife to end the affair, but later called her back to say he did not mean it.

While Elizabeth was on a tour for her own book *Saving Graces: Finding Solace and Strength from Friends and Strangers*, Hunter spent time at the Edwardses' home. Young said that Hunter slept in their bed and entertained the children.

Young also said that Edwards would confide in him that he had thought about leaving "crazy" Elizabeth, but she played better with the American voter than he did. He also said that he listened as Edwards told Hunter that one day they would have their own family and have a wedding where her favourite band would play.

Edwards had begged Young to help cover up the affair – even to the point of claiming paternity – to make Mrs Edwards's dying days a bit easier.

"I can't let her die knowing this," said Edwards.

Elizabeth left John in January 2010. The matchmaking *National Enquirer* then reported that Edwards had proposed to Hunter and they planned to move into a $3.5-million beachfront home with their love child. Well, everyone likes a happy ending.

However, this was vigorously denied by Edwards's spokeswoman. There would be no happy ending. Elizabeth Edwards died of breast cancer on 7 December 2010. And on 3 June 2011, Edwards was indicted on felony charges over the alleged use of $925,000 of campaign funds to hide his mistress and baby from the public. He pleaded not guilty and was said to be suicidal at the thought of going to jail for the misuse of campaign funds.

During the hearing it came out that Hunter had made a sex video with Edwards while they had been on the campaign. He exploded, screaming that she was an idiot for not destroying the tape.

"His worst nightmare is that the tape will get on the internet, and destroy what little reputation he has left," said the *National Enquirer*. The video ended up in the possession of Andrew Young, who said he found the tape discarded in a guest room once occupied by Ms Hunter. She hit Young with a lawsuit in a North Carolina court, calling for the tape to be returned to her plus monetary damages.

Speaking about the videotape, Mr Young's wife, Cheri, said on Oprah Winfrey's show last year: 'I won't give any fine details, but I'll tell you yes, he is naked. He is performing sexual acts. The woman is holding the camera. He is aware he is being taped.'

According to the *Wall Street Journal*, Mr Young has described the tape as like "watching a traffic pile-up occur in slow motion – repelling but also transfixing".

# 7

## Musical Bent

### George Michael

One half of the boy band Wham!, George Michael set young girls' hearts athrob the world over. He was, of course, gay – but he kept quiet about it because, he said, he did not want his mother to worry about the possibility of him catching Aids. Luckily, she was dead before it came out in the worst possible way.

Michael had had serious relationships in his life. But his lover, Anselmo Feleppa, a Brazilian designer (no, he did not design Brazilians) whom he met at Rock in Rio in 1991, died of an Aids-related brain haemorrhage in 1993. Michael made the solo album *Older* as a tribute to his "close pal". But still, in interviews, he did not say those three little words those who knew him longed to hear: "I am gay."

In April 1998, he was blasted out of the closet with a rocket up his arse, metaphorically speaking, when he was arrested in a public lavatory in Beverly Hills "engaging in a lewd act".

According to Michael: "I got followed into the restroom and then this cop – I didn't know it was a cop, obviously – he started playing this game, which I think is called, 'I'll show you mine, you show me yours, and then when you show me yours, I'm going to nick you.'

"Actually, what happened was once he got an eyeful, he walked past me, straight past me and out, and I thought, that's kind of odd. I thought, maybe he's just not impressed. And then I went to walk back to my car and, as I got back to the car, I was arrested on the street . . . If someone's waving their genitalia at you, you don't automatically assume that they're an officer of the law . . . I've never been able to turn down a free meal."

Michael pleaded no contest and took his punishment like a man – a fine of $810 and eighty hours of community service. However, he claimed that his arrest involved a conspiracy between the Beverly Hills cops and the British tabloids – who went to town on the story. Michael claimed that he was out already but "it wouldn't seem that way in America because in America there hasn't been that much publicity about me". There was now.

Michael's cottaging activities might also have come as a surprise to his boyfriend of two years, Dallas native Kenny Goss, former cheerleader coach and flight attendant.

"I'm not saying that I have an open relationship with my boyfriend but he knows who I am," Michael told MTV. "He knows that I'm generally oversexed, so he's been very, very good . . . We love each other and he understands that it was a stupid mistake and he's forgiven me, I hope."

He was going to have to be very understanding as Michael was about to take the scandal to a whole new level. In the lyrics to his new single "Outside", he said he was bored with having sex on the sofa, in the hall and on the kitchen table – he wanted to do it outside. Nor was he afraid of prosecution. According to the lyrics: "I'd service the community, but I already have, you see."

The accompanying video starts off like a seventies porno film. Then there is a scene of an arrest. Michael dances in a police uniform in a public lavatory that turns into a disco and it ends with cops kissing. I am sure the LAPD were the first to rush out and buy it.

## Michael Jackson

He was the King of Pop, one of the world's greatest entertainers, but he found himself mired in a sex scandal and a half. After all, he was, well, strange.

In the earlier eighties, when Jackson was already a huge star, he began to change. The good-looking young African-American began to grow pale, eventually turning deathly white. His broad nose became progressively pointy, until you could practically play a record on it and he developed a cleft – or butt – chin. His lips thinned. His forehead broadened, and his cheekbones seemed to migrate northwards.

In January 1984, he carried twelve-year-old Emmanuel Lewis, the diminutive star of the sitcom *Webster* on stage at the American Music Awards as if the boy was a live statuette. The following month, they appeared at the Grammys together. Despite their twelve-year age difference, they were good friends.

"Michael is the best friend you could ever have," said Lewis. "He's gentle, not rough like other guys. I can count on him any time, and he can count on me."

Things got a little more spooky two years later, when it was reported that Jackson slept in a hyperbaric oxygen chamber to slow his ageing process. He was pictured lying down in a glass box. Although the claim was untrue, Jackson had spread the story himself to promote his upcoming film, *Captain EO*. Apparently he wanted to project a more science-fiction image of himself, in keeping with the theme of the film.

Then he adopted a chimpanzee named Bubbles who went to live with him. They shared a life – and a lavatory – and were often seen wearing matching outfits. The story circulated that he had bought the remains of John Merrick, the nineteenth-century "Elephant Man" who had returned to the public attention after a movie of the same name in 1980. Jackson did not rush to deny the story. Again it was thought he had planted it himself. There was little doubt that the boy was weird and the British tabloids began calling him "Wacko Jacko", an epithet he came to hate.

In an interview with Oprah Winfrey in 1993, he claimed that he felt he had missed out on a childhood. So he made himself one. In Santa Barbara Valley, California, he built himself Neverland, former home of Peter Pan, Tinkerbell, the Lost Boys and, apparently, David Beckham. It had a floral clock, numerous statues of children, a petting zoo, two railroads and an amusement park, containing a Ferris wheel, Carousel, Zipper, Octopus, Pirate Ship, Wave Swinger, Super Slide, Dragon Wagon kiddie roller coaster and bumper cars – everything you could need, apart from friends.

But he did have friends. He invited children to stay. And that's where the trouble started.

One of the children who came to stay was thirteen-year-old Jordan Chandler. While Jordan's mother June was sanguine about the relationship, her ex-husband, Jordan's father Evan, was not. He claimed that Jackson was sexually abusing the boy. Eventually, Jordan was persuaded to give a description of Jackson's penis. He even got to draw a picture of the penis in question. Not many thirteen-year-old boys are *asked* to do that. They are usually told not to, repeatedly.

To defend himself, poor old Michael had to drop his kecks and have his private parts photographed. Then there was a heated debate about whether his knob matched the one in Jordan's picture. Surprisingly, one cock can look much like another one.

The Santa Barbara DA Tom Sneddon was convinced, but grand juries in Santa Barbara and Los Angeles could not see the similarity. What's more, opinion polls showed that most people believed that Jackson was innocent. Nevertheless it was a great story that the tabloids were not about to drop. The *New York Post* summed up their attitude with the headline: PETER PAN OR PERVERT. The tabloid TV show *Hard Copy* tried to rope in child actor Macaulay Culkin, star of *Home Alone*. He denied everything. Meanwhile those saying they could confirm the allegations asked for large amounts of money for their stories – rather than going to the police, of course. Geraldo Rivera even set up a TV trial, with a jury made up of audience members, though Jackson had not been charged with any crime.

While no criminal charges had been brought, Jordan Chandler filed a civil suit against Jackson for "repeatedly committing sexual battery" on him. The complaint alleged that Michael Jackson performed oral sex with the boy and masturbated him, and had the boy fondle his breasts and nipples while Jackson masturbated himself. This was more fodder for the tabloids

"This child is getting crucified," said the Chandler's attorney Larry Feldman. "Everyone is batting this kid around in the newspaper."

Clearly, their only concern was to keep Jordan out of the limelight.

In response, Jackson's attorneys filed extortion charges against Evan Chandler and his attorney. These were disallowed as the whole issue disappeared into a legal quagmire. Somehow the authorities had to establish the facts of the case. Hundreds of witnesses were interviewed and detectives flew around the world checking out allegations that had surfaced in the newspapers.

Over Michael's protests, his insurance company settled out of court for around $23 million. Some $15 million would be held in trust for Jordan. His parents would get $1.5 million each and their lawyers would get between $3 million and $5 million. It appears that the insurance company were fully entitled to do this. Jackson explained that he was forced to go along with it because he wanted to get on with his musical career, rather than spend the rest of his life in a courtroom.

As part of the settlement, he admitted no wrongdoing or liability. But that is not the way the press saw it, even though

Jordan Chandler was interviewed by the police and no charges were forthcoming.

A book came out said to be based on Jordan's diary and detailing alleged sexual encounters with Michael. Jackson sued and won $2.7 million. Evan Chandler sued Jackson for $60 million, claiming that Jackson had breached their agreement never to discuss the case. The suit was thrown out of court.

Jackson then went out of his way to prove that he was not a kiddie-fiddler – and that he was all man. He married Elvis Presley's daughter Lisa Marie. Their marriage, she said, was "sexually active". Nevertheless, they broke up. Then he married dermatology nurse Deborah Rowe and had two children before they divorced. Somehow he obtained a third child, which he dangled over a hotel balcony in Berlin.

Then, in 2002, he made the biggest mistake of his life. He agreed to make the programme *Living With Michael* for Granada TV with British TV journalist Martin Bashir, who had come to fame after wringing the details of her failed marriage out of Princess Diana.

Michael took Bashir into his confidence, though he denied having his appearance altered artificially and became quite agitated when Bashir questioned him about it. Bashir got to meet two of Jackson's children, though they were wearing masks. We were back in "Wacko Jacko" territory.

At Neverland, Jackson introduced Bashir to Gavin Arvizo. The thirteen-year-old sometimes stayed with him, Jackson said, but Gavin slept in the bed while he slept on the floor. Jackson explained that he frequently invited young children – Macaulay Culkin and his brother Kieran, then aged twelve and ten, as well as his sisters – to sleepovers in his bedroom and looked injured when Bashir suggested that could seem inappropriate.

He had, he said, "slept in a bed with many children", then added, "It's not sexual, we're going to sleep. I tuck them in . . . it's very charming, it's very sweet."

There was also footage of him holding hands with Gavin and cuddling him, and, at one point, Jackson was filmed seated before a portrait of himself as a Botticelli-esque male Venus surrounded by winged putti. Nevertheless, the *New York Times* said: "As a public relations move, Mr Jackson has done himself more good than harm with this latest interview."

Jackson did not take that view. He issued a statement that said: "Michael feels deeply angry that the programme could have led viewers to conclude that he abuses children in any way. Michael Jackson has never, and would never, treat a child inappropriately or expose them to any harm and totally refutes any suggestions to the contrary."

If that was not bad enough, he went and made things even worse. He issued a rebuttal video where his ex-wife Debbie Rowe claimed that the concept of "sharing a bed" can be misunderstood. For example, she herself likes watching television in bed and, when she has a visitor, they often watch television together in bed. Did she think this made things better?

Gavin Arvizo, his brother Star and mother Janet also appeared, saying that nothing inappropriate happened. They called him a "father figure" – well, hardly pipe and slippers.

The Los Angeles Department of Children and Family Services were also on the case after a school official, who had seen Bashir's documentary, complained. Again the family insisted that nothing untoward happened.

However, Gavin and the Arvizo family were now the subject of intense media interest. Jackson would help them to move while he took them on a family vacation to Brazil. While he was arranging this, they could stay at Neverland, though Janet Arvizo took the opportunity to go and stay with her fiancé, leaving Gavin with Michael.

Janet Arvizo then approached Larry Feldman, Jordan Chandler's attorney. Soon Santa Barbara County Sheriff's Department were back on the case. They interviewed the Arvizo family. Initially, seventy investigators were assigned to the case. Then, when they raided Neverland, it was said that there were more law enforcement officers on hand than on any manhunt for a serial killer in American history. Meanwhile, the district attorney's website was described as an "open casting call" for anyone claiming to have been molested by Michael Jackson.

Jackson was arrested and charged with seven counts of sexual molestation and two counts of administering an intoxicating agent in order to commit that felony. It was alleged that Jackson had given Gavin alcohol – or "Jesus juice" in Jackson-speak – to have his evil way with him. Curiously though, offences were said to have taken place between 20 February and 12 March – starting two weeks after Martin Bashir's documentary had aired in the US.

The Jackson camp claimed that the new allegations of sexual molestation had only come after the Arvizo family had realized that he was not going to go on supporting them indefinitely. Then there was a flurry of allegations against the Arvizo family, claiming that they were crooks and had tried to extort money out of others over sexual molestations charges.

The court case began in January 2005 and went on for five months. It attracted more reporters than the O. J. Simpson trial, though no one was dead. Both Gavin Arvizo and his brother Star gave detailed descriptions of the sexual shenanigans they said Jackson got up to. Much of it revolved around Michael's underpants. However, their stories did not agree. It also came out that the boys had taken acting lessons before an earlier lawsuit their mother had taken against J. C. Penney. In 1998, the Arvizo family was detained after being suspected of shoplifting in the company's store in West Covina, California. Shoplifting charges were dropped after Janet Arvizo claimed she had been beaten by the security guards. Two years later, she claimed that one of the male officers "sexually fondled" her for up to seven minutes. The store settled out of court for $75,000.

When Janet Arvizo took the stand in the Jackson case, she answered questions with a strange series of phrases and non sequiturs. The defence let her ramble, forcing the prosecution to object to the testimony of their own witness. She snapped her fingers at the jurors and provoked them to laughter when she claimed that Jackson aimed to kidnap the boys in a hot-air balloon. She took the Fifth Amendment when asked about welfare fraud and was accused of spending $7,000 shopping and dining out when she said she and her family were being kept captive by Mr Jackson. Then there was an argument over whether she had just had her legs waxed or a full body wax. She later pleaded no contest to felony welfare fraud.

Macaulay Culkin and two other minors Jackson had been accused of molesting denied that any such thing had happened. Then Chris Tucker and Jay Leno were brought in to leaven proceedings. The jury found Michael Jackson not guilty on all counts. When released to speak to the media, the jurors said they were surprised at how insubstantial the case against him had been.

All this might have been dismissed as a comedy of errors where a bunch of stupid people tried to milk a man who had lost touch with reality. However, the allegations continued to circulate on the internet even after he was dead.

## Michael Hutchence

When the lead singer of the Australian rock band INXS Michael Hutchence was found naked and dead in Room 524 of the Ritz-Carlton Hotel in Sydney, the New South Wales coroner ruled it was suicide in November 1997. But his lover Paula Yates was determined to have the verdict overturned. She insisted that his death was due to auto-erotic asphyxiation – a far more dignified way to go.

"He had lots of dignity, no matter what was happening," she told the TV documentary *Excess: The Death of Michael*

*Hutchence* two years later. If it had been suicide, he would have got dressed and written a note, she said.

Hutchence had lived the rock-star life, bedding numerous actresses, models and singers. He was credited with the sexual awakening of actress-turned-singer Kylie Minogue and had a long affair with supermodel Helena Christensen. He once told an interviewer: "The good, sensible thing to do is to be completely drunk, take drugs and have sex all day."

Then he had met Paula Yates, the daughter of Elaine Smith, a former showgirl, actress and writer of erotic novels. She thought her father was Jess Yates, who was known as "the Bishop". He presented the ITV religious programme *Stars on Sunday*, but was fired when it was revealed that he was having an affair with a young actress, Anita Kay. After his death in 1993, DNA testing showed that Paula Yates had actually been fathered by TV presenter Hughie Green.

Posing naked for *Penthouse* brought her into journalism, then TV presenting. In 1986, she married Bob Geldof, lead singer of The Boomtown Rats and organizer of Live Aid. They got married in Las Vegas, with Simon Le Bon of Duran Duran as best man, though there had been rumours that Yates was having a lesbian affair with Annie Lennox, lead singer of the Eurythmics, at the time. She and Geldof had three daughters, though she continued to be sexually omnivorous, maintaining a six-year relationship with actor Rupert Everett even though he was gay.

In 1985 she was an interviewer for Channel 4's rock magazine programme *The Tube* when Hutchence came on as a guest. He invited her back to his hotel room. She said coyly, "Michael, I have a baby."

His road manager warned her off, but she said: "I am going to have that boy."

According to the band's official "autobiography" *INXS: Story to Story*: "Paula was unmoved and began to show up at INXS gigs everywhere for the next few years ... she even brought her daughter."

Ten years later, Yates was a presenter on Channel 4's *Big Breakfast Show*, where she interviewed celebrities on a bed. Michael Hutchence was one of them. The first time they spent the night together, Paula Yates said Michael Hutchence did "six things I was firmly convinced were illegal". Some of them involving oysters. Friends overheard telephone messages from Hutchence, in which he promised to tie her up and torture her with pleasure.

When she left Geldof, there was a huge scandal as, thanks to Live Aid, he was considered a living saint. The following year, she had a child with Hutchence. That autumn the police searched the London home Yates and Hutchence shared, looking for drugs. Along with opium, they found Polaroids, apparently left where the children could find them, of Yates and Hutchence in latex suits and in a variety of sexual situations, using various extreme S&M sex toys. This was hardly going to help in the custody battle Yates was having with Geldof over their three children.

A week later, Hutchence was in Australia, celebrating the twentieth anniversary of the formation of INXS. Those who saw him said he was drinking heavily and taking drugs. There were, as always, other women. After spending a few hours with an ex-girlfriend and her boyfriend, he was found naked with a leather belt around his neck, his hands in his crotch and semen on his thighs.

At first Yates went along with the idea that Hutchence had committed suicide. However this reflected badly on her as they were planning to marry. By choosing to leave life, he was leaving her. So then she began to boast about auto-erotic asphyxiation as if it stemmed from the unfettered sex life they had had together.

On TV she bragged about their sex life. Nothing was out of bounds in the bedroom: "Threesomes, foursomes – whatever."

And she claimed that the Australian police had never asked about Hutchence's sexual tastes, which included orgies.

Hutchence had screwed a ring bolt into an air-conditioning duct and suspended himself from it. Depriving the brain of oxygen provides a more intense orgasm. In fact, Paula, he was just wanking.

Three years later she died of an overdose.

## Jerry Lee Lewis

Rockabilly pioneer Jerry Lee Lewis was at the height of his career in May 1958 when he went on tour in the UK. The British tabloids learnt that his new wife, Myra Gale Brown, was his cousin and was just thirteen years old – Jerry Lee insisted that she was fifteen, not that it made it any better. He was twenty-three at the time. The tour was cancelled after just three shows. There was talk of deporting him before he scuttled back to America, only to find his concerts there had been cancelled too and his single "High School Confidential" stalled at number twenty-one.

As a result of the scandal, he had gone from an artist who could command £10,000 a night to earning $250 in small clubs or beer joints. He slowly rebuilt his career via country music and the spiritual guidance of his cousin Jimmy Swaggart (see page 382).

Lewis could have saved himself a lot of trouble. It seems he and Myra were not even legally married at the time. The young rocker had omitted to complete his divorce from his second wife Jane Mitcham when they tied the knot. That marriage too was of dubious validity, because he had not completed his divorce from his first wife Dorothy Barton.

Explaining the situation to *People* magazine, Lewis said: "I was fourteen when I first got married. My wife was too old for me; she was seventeen. Then I met Jane Mitcham. One day she told me she was going to have my child. Her brothers were hunting me with whips. I was real worried so I married her, but never properly. She divorced me, though she didn't need to. She was never my wife." These things happen in the South.

Nevertheless, Myra was delighted that her beau was free. For the wedding she kept on the shirtwaist dress she wore to her eighth-grade class that morning.

"I was a typical thirteen-year-old – bubble gum, poodle skirt, ponytail," she recalled. "I adored him. He drove me to school if I missed the bus."

They married a second time to make it legal and stayed together for thirteen years. Looking back at his British tour, Lewis said: "It hurt me bad. It's very stupid for a person to flush $50 billion down the commode, which is probably what I did."

His fourth marriage lasted for twelve years, ending when his wife, Jaren Elizabeth Gunn Pate, drowned in their swimming pool. His fifth marriage to Shawn Stephens lasted three months and ended when his wife died of a methadone overdose. He clocked up twenty years on his sixth marriage to Kerrie McCarver. It ended in divorce.

## Gary Glitter

UK glam rocker Gary Glitter never broke through in the US, though cover versions of "I'm the Leader of the Gang" and "I Didn't Know I Loved You ('Til I Saw You Rock 'n' Roll)" charted there. Nevertheless, he was a one-man hit factory in the UK from the early seventies until the late nineties, when the wheels began to come off.

In 1997, he had just shot a cameo role in the Spice Girls' film *Spiceworld the Movie* when he took his laptop in for repair and pornographic images of children were found on the hard drive. His appearance was cut from the film, though the song "I'm the Leader of the Gang" was left in.

Glitter – real name Paul Gadd – pleaded guilty to having over four thousand hardcore photographs of children, mostly young girls, being abused, downloaded from the internet on his computer. He was sentenced to four months in jail. This came only hours after he had been acquitted of having sex with an underage girl some twenty years earlier.

Thirty-four-year-old mother-of-three Alison Brown told the *Sun* that she had been sexually abused by thirty-five-year-old Glitter when she was fourteen.

"He is more than a voyeur," she said. "He is capable of doing all kind of things to children. Hopefully, people who say they have been sexually abused by him will stand up and talk about it. After his acquittal I lost all faith in humanity. But when I had heard he got four months for computer porn, I felt relieved that people would believe me … They should have thrown away the key."

Glitter's ex-tour manager Alan Gee said the star told him of his child-sex fantasies in the eighties. "I wish I had come forward earlier," he said.

A jury had dismissed the charges of sexual assault as Ms Brown had accepted a fee of £10,000 from the *Sun*'s sister paper the *News of the World* and would get another £25,000 if he was convicted. The pay-out was "… highly reprehensible," said the judge. "It is not illegal but it is to be greatly deprecated."

Their relationship had continued for some years and he had threatened suicide if she ended it, Alison Brown said. She had gone to the *News of the World* in 1993 to "get him to leave me alone". She also took the opportunity to reveal that Glitter, known for his extravagant bouffant hair, was now bald and wore a wig.

Released after two months, Glitter fled Britain on his yacht. When he was discovered in Spain, he moved on to Cuba, Mexico, South Africa, Zimbabwe, Colombia, Portugal, Brazil, Venezuela and South-east Asia where he was arrested. After serving time in jail in Cambodia, he was deported to Vietnam, where he was jailed for sexually assaulting two underage girls. He was ordered to pay the girls' families $320 in compensation and jailed for three years, the minimum sentence as he had earlier paid the girls' families $2,000 each in compensation. He claimed to be innocent, the victim of a conspiracy by the British tabloids. A charge of child rape had been dropped due to lack of evidence. It carried a maximum sentence of death before a firing squad.

When Glitter was released, he was denied entry into the Philippines, Thailand and Hong Kong. He returned to the UK when he had to sign the Sex Offenders Register. Then Glitter sought refuge with Gordon Buchanan, a friend of twenty years. Despite threats from vigilantes, Buchanan let Glitter stay in his two-million-pound home in Hampshire. However, after four days, Glitter's bolthole was discovered after he went shopping in Warsash, near Southampton. He was recognized even though he had shaved off the distinctive beard he had grown in the Far East and donned a ginger wig. Glitter was whisked off to a new hideaway, paid for by the authorities.

"It must be costing millions," Buchanan said. "After he was discovered at my house, six police cars escorted us out of Hampshire. We needed petrol and they closed a whole petrol station just for the two of us. It was a massive police operation. I can't begin to think how much it must have cost. And the cost will keep going up because it's only a matter of time before Gary's new hideout is discovered and the whole thing will be repeated again at vast expense to the taxpayer."

Despite everything, Buchanan remained true to his old friend. He believed that Glitter was a schizophrenic and arranged for psychiatrist and child abuse specialist Dr Valerie Sinason to fly from South Africa to treat his pal.

"He needs psychiatric help," said Buchanan. "He needs to be in hospital."

But while Glitter was protected by the full might of the law, Buchanan was left vulnerable to attack by those who wanted to take the law into their own hands.

He said, "My decision to offer him sanctuary has ruined my life."

Gary Glitter may be guilty of paedophilia, but Buchanan was guilty of nothing but loyalty.

## Franz Liszt

Mick Jagger was not the first musician to attract groupies. The lovers of Franz Liszt included Marie Duplessis, the high-class courtesan immortalized by Alexandre Dumas in *La Dame aux Camélias*; the outrageous Lola Montez, who danced naked at the unveiling of the Beethoven Memorial; Princess Cristina Belgiojoso; the poet Bettina von Arnim; the singer Karoline Unger; Princess Caroline Sayn-Wittgenstein; the actress Charlotte Hagn, who Liszt boasted was also the mistress of two kings; the pianist and nymphomaniac Marie Pleyel; Countess Marie d'Agoult, his long-term and long-suffering *maîtresse en titre*, and many many more.

"That so many women want his love and threw themselves at him so passionately does little credit to our sex," wrote Adelheid von Schorn, one of his most dedicated groupies. "Men, naturally, complained about him terribly. This was envy pure and simple."

Born in Hungary in 1811, Liszt planned to become a priest – until he met the blue-eyed Caroline Saint-Cricq, the daughter of the Comte de Saint-Cricq. They were both sixteen, but he was a child prodigy and had taken her on as a pupil. However, when the comte found Liszt creeping out of his house at night, he married his daughter off to a nobleman.

Liszt now realized that he would not reconcile the urges of the flesh with clerical celibacy and fell dangerously ill. The only cure for a broken heart, he found, was "exercises in the lofty French style" – that is, bonking married women. Soon he had a string of lovers.

The elderly Comte Laprunarède made the mistake of having the hot-blooded Hungarian as a houseguest. They were snowed in and Liszt passed the time with the comte's "sparkling, witty, young, beautiful" wife Adèle. When he fled to Paris, he continued writing to her, something he would live to regret.

There he took on more pupils, largely the daughters of the aristocracy who wore him out. Swiss composer Caroline Boissier came to Paris and sought out Liszt to teach her eighteen-year-old daughter Valérie. Both mother and daughter were captivated by him. Madame Boissier paid him over the odds and insisted that he cut down on his other teaching commitments. However, he maintained a select coterie of students, including Charlotte Talleyrand, whose elderly aunt, the Marquise Le Vayer, ran a salon for writers, artists and "women of the world" – one of whom was the Comtesse Marie d'Agoult.

The comtesse was born Marie Flavigy in Frankfurt-am-Main, daughter of a family known for its scandalous affairs. Seething with emotions, the young Marie was described as "six inches of snow covering twenty feet of lava". After completing her education at the Convent of the Sacré-Coeur in Paris, she plunged directly into a torrid affair with the poet Alfred de Vigny. Then she married the Comte Charles d'Agoult, a lame war veteran, fifteen years her senior. It was largely an "open" marriage and Marie amused herself doing the rounds of the fashionable salons.

She was twenty-eight when she met Liszt; he was just twenty-one.

"Franz spoke with vivacity and with an originality that awoke a whole world slumbering in me," she said.

The next day, Marie wrote to Liszt. Soon they were having secret assignations at his mother's apartment, which he called "*Ratzloch*" – the "rat hole". He bombarded her with passionate love letters, which left little to the imagination.

"There is heaven and hell, and everything else, inside you," he wrote, "yes, inside you."

However, some of the letters he wrote to Adèle Laprunarède came into her hands. There was a jealous row. Liszt confessed everything, swearing that he now belonged to her alone.

Then her eldest daughter fell ill and died. Excluded from her life by her grief, Liszt wrote to Marie, saying he was leaving Paris and wanted to see her one last time. It was a passionate reunion. Nine months later their first child was born.

While she was pregnant, Marie and Franz eloped to Switzerland. She wrote to her husband, telling him that their marriage was over and begging his forgiveness.

"As for me," she wrote, "I ask only for your silence in the face of the world which is going to overwhelm me with insults."

They settled in Geneva. They could not marry, but Liszt gave her the ring from his finger. When the baby was born, Liszt registered the birth under his own name at the registry office. But for the sake of Marie's reputation, a false name was used to conceal the mother's identity.

Then the writer George Sand turned up and made a play for him. It was also rumoured that Sand and Maria had a friendship "*à la Dorval*". Sand said they were the "galley-slaves of love who don't know the value of any chain". Nevertheless, Marie conceived a second child with Liszt. They went to Italy. Maria stayed at Como to have the child while Liszt visited Rossini in Milan. Then he went on tour where she suspected he was being unfaithful.

In Frankfurt, he met the young Clara Wieck, who later became Clara Schumann. She told him of a terrible flood in his native Hungary. The ladies of Vienna held a fund-raiser. Liszt sent a letter to Marie. The envelope bore the coat of arms of a well-known Austrian lady. As the arms were also on the notepaper inside, it was clear to Marie that it had been written in the lady's boudoir.

When he returned to her, Marie upbraided him, but he said he would hardly give the brush-off to women who were raising money for the flood victims. Marie rebuked him as a "Don

Juan *parvenu*". He said he was deeply hurt by this, but soon got over it as Marie was pregnant once more.

Now with a growing family to support, Liszt had no choice but to go out on the road again.

Marie was worried. "I fear that trouble will come from the way you can no longer willingly submit to any restraint," she said. "I cannot believe that a man ought to surrender himself so completely to his instincts." In pique, she gave him his ring back.

"I don't know why, but in putting this ring back on my finger I felt as if I were recovering from a long illness," he wrote. Soon he left the ring off altogether. "I felt a curious pleasure in abandoning this symbol of our union to chance," he wrote.

In October 1839, they parted in tears in Florence. They both knew it was all over between them.

"I am willing to be your mistress, but not one of your mistresses," she wrote.

Liszt travelled to Trieste where he spent a great deal of time in the company of the singer Karoline Unger, explaining to Marie that he and "*La* Unger" were just good friends. Then he headed back to Vienna to do more charity work for flood victims, ostensibly.

Returning to Paris, Marie met the British diplomat Henry Bulwer-Lytton, who proposed to her. She wrote to Liszt and asked for "*une petite permission d'infidélité*". He knew all about Bulwer-Lytton and told her to go ahead. Marie was naturally upset that he betrayed no hint of jealousy. She wrote back saying, "your way of looking at things will always be incomprehensible to me".

She insisted that she was too ill to have an affair with Bulwer-Lytton. But she still tried to provoke Liszt to jealousy, saying that the Polish expatriate Bernard Potocki had also asked to marry her. Then she spelt out in detail her relationship with George Sand. After all, it was driving Sand's new lover

Frédéric Chopin mad with jealousy. Once again, Liszt was unmoved.

Marie's friend Delphine de Girardin introduced her to her husband Émile, editor of *La Presse*. Émile persuaded Marie to write for him under the name Daniel Stern and began an affair with her.

Liszt wrote, admitting a trifling affair – "a passion of forty-eight hours". But she no longer minded. Indeed, she was even pleased that he had told her about it, rather than lying about his infidelity as he had done so often in the past. When he returned to Paris, Liszt took up with Princess Cristina Belgiojoso. Marie simply dismissed her rival as "*La Comedienne*".

When he took off on tour again, she kept him posted with the latest development of her affair with Émile de Girardin. He hit back by reminding her cruelly: "In the loveliest days of my youth, I had similar feelings for Piff [George Sand] and I spoke of an eternal bond between us."

But in the public's eye, his affair with Marie was forgotten. The whole of Europe was now engulfed in "Lisztomania", decried at the time as a scandalous manifestation of "women's idolatrous worship of men of genius".

Female fans flocked to see him, trembling in his presence and fainting when he played. A glove he left on a piano was torn to shreds. Princesses in St Petersburg fought over the rind of an orange he had sucked and discarded. Women stole his cigar butts and hid them down their cleavages. Plainly, the phallic symbolism was not lost on them. Years later, when a youthful fan had grown smelly with age and finally died, a rotting cigar butt was found lodged in her corset.

Four noted beauties carrying his bust in the Prussian court represented themselves as caryatids, the bare-breasted maidens that act as pillars in Greek temples. One Polish countess received him in her boudoir ankle-deep in rose petals. One young fan spoke for them all when she said: "If Liszt would only love me for a single hour – that would be joy enough for life."

Twenty-one-year-old actress Charlotte von Hagn seduced him with a love poem. After she married, she wrote to him, saying, "You have spoiled all others for me. No one can stand the comparison." It did not matter to her that, at the time, she was sharing him with Bettina von Arnim, an intimate of both Beethoven and Goethe.

After a brief and fruitless reconciliation with Marie, he met the most scandalous love of his life, Lola Montez.

Born plain Eliza Gilbert in Limerick, she eloped to India with Captain James, an officer in the British Army, at the age of eighteen, when her mother tried to marry her off to a sixty-year-old judge. But her husband ran off with the wife of an adjutant. On the ship home she met a Captain Lennox. Arriving in London, they checked into the Imperial Hotel together. The result was the scandalous court case *James* v. *Lennox* as reported in *The Times* of 7 December 1842.

Eliza then decided to become an actress, but had no talent for it. So she took to the stage of the Haymarket Theatre in London as Doña Lola Montez. Never having visited Spain, as a flamenco dancer she was a flop. But her bust wasn't. It piqued the interest of a number of European impresarios. Doña Lola toured the Continent, taking a series of theatre managers as her lovers to help keep her career on the road.

Lola then planned to use her natural assets to ensnare a great man. She met Liszt in Dresden in 1844. He was more than willing to accommodate her with a one-night stand. But then he could not shake her. She pursued him around Germany. While he was giving a concert, she would persuade the manager of the hotel where Liszt was staying to let her into his room and slip naked into his bed. Once he left her locked in the room with instructions that she was not to be let out for twelve hours while he fled town. She caught up with him at the dinner after a memorial concert in honour of Beethoven in Bonn. Liszt was the guest of honour, though Berlioz and Hallé were there, along with King Friedrich Wilhelm IV and his queen. Lola blagged her way in, saying she was a guest of Liszt's. She then leapt on a table, stripped off and gave an uninhibited exhibition of her talent as a dancer. The other guests fled, only to be drenched in a thunderstorm outside.

Liszt was unimpressed, but when she flashed her boobs at King Ludwig I of Bavaria, he bought her a house in Munich. She became his favourite "sultana" and it was rumoured that he enjoyed spanking her naked bottom – at least, that's how cartoonists depicted it at the time.

Lola dropped her stage name, became Countess von Starhemberg and ruled Bavaria alongside her lover. As a result, there was a revolution. King Ludwig was deposed and Lola banished. She headed to America where she quickly ran through the huge fortune she had amassed and died in penury at the age of forty-three.

Despite the turmoil, Liszt continued his correspondence with Marie d'Agoult and Lola's antics were a source of amusement to both of them. He also detailed his encounters with Charlotte von Hagn, Balzac's Polish mistress Eva Hanska and the insatiable pianist Marie Pleyel.

In November 1845, Liszt met the beautiful courtesan Marie Duplessis, "*La dame aux camélias*". It seems that he was her last great love. When she died just eighteen months later, aged twenty-three, a portrait of Liszt was found among the meagre possessions left in her squalid room at 15 Boulevard de la Madeleine. Liszt settled her doctor's bills after she died.

Liszt was away in Poland at the time. He wrote to Marie saying that Marie Duplessis was "the first woman I fell in love with ... Fifteen months ago she said to me: 'Take me, take me with you wherever you want. I will not be a burden to you. During the day I will sleep. In the evening I will go to the theatre. At night you can do anything you want with me.'"

Next Liszt fell for Princess Carolyne zu Sayn-Wittgenstein, the estranged wife of Prince Nicolas zu Sayn-Wittgenstein, who had huge estates in the Ukraine. Though she was no beauty, she was rich and titled, and Liszt was a snob. They also shared a religious mania. Her bedroom was modelled on a monk's cell and positively groaned with crucifixes. When people remarked that she was ugly, he said: "I, who can claim to be a connoisseur in such matters, maintain that she is beautiful, because her soul lends her face the transfiguration of the highest beauty."

Marie wrote saying:

> If this woman is of noble character, she will certainly not want to share you with anyone else. She will not want to be just *one of your mistresses*. During these past four years, you must have reached satiation and have become disgusted with loveless pleasure. You must grasp this thread, so that it can pull yourself out of the labyrinth . . . for the greatest joy of my heart would be to see you straighten out.

But he was not about to straighten out. A string of new lovers awaited him in Russia, including one he called the Snow Queen. When he headed westwards again Princess Carolyne was still waiting on her knees, with her Bible. They settled in Weimar, where Liszt had been appointed music director by Grand Duke Karl Alexander. Princess Carolyne tried to regularize the situation by divorcing her husband. This was a complex business as she was a Catholic, made more difficult as she managed to alienate the Grand Duchess by smoking cigars at court.

Eventually, they went to Rome to appeal directly to the authorities. They planned to marry there on Liszt's fiftieth birthday, but her husband feared the scandal would affect the marriage prospects of their daughter. He and the tsar put pressure on the Vatican to prevent the divorce. The Russian government also impounded her estates, considerably diminishing her attractions in Liszt's eyes. He took holy orders. But even when he was an abbé women were still attracted to him.

"Does the cassock make no difference?" asked a fellow cleric.

"On the contrary, it excites them all the more," he was told. "He now has the added attraction of being forbidden fruit."

Another cigar-smoking proto-feminist, the so-called "Cossack Countess" Olga Janina fell for him in 1869. In fact, she was the daughter of a boot-polish manufacturer in Lemburg. When he dropped her, she achieved notoriety by publishing three highly fictionalized accounts of the affair, including *Souvenirs d'une Cosaque*.

When he refused a Russian countess, she burst into his study with a loaded pistol. Unfazed, Liszt simply said, "Fire." The woman dropped the gun and fled in tears.

But this was a rarity. Despite his reacquaintance with the Ten Commandments, he said, "I shall never abjure love, for all its profanations and false pretences."

## Ludwig van Beethoven

After the composer Beethoven died, a long, passionate, three-part letter, dated 6–7 July 1812, written to an anonymous woman was found in his desk. It was addressed to "My angel, my everything, my very self" and, more famously, "Immortal Beloved". In the second part of the letter, he writes "I must go to bed . . ." then the words "oh go with, go with me" are crossed out.

The son of a penniless, alcoholic musician, Beethoven never married. As a romantic, he liked to fall in love with unattainable women. And as a music teacher, this was a cinch. He was regularly thrust into the company of aristocratic young women, far above his station. Any liaison with them would, of course, have been scandalous.

He was shy around women of his own class, so relieved himself furtively with prostitutes. This filled him with shame. His diary is full of entries promising never to go to the brothel again. It was a promise he failed to keep. Once, when caught red-handed in a red-light district, he said simply, "Blame it on my dick."

His use of prostitutes may have resulted in his deafness, a condition that can be caused by syphilis. He kept a copy of *How to Guard Against and Cure Sexual Diseases* on his bookshelves, alongside works on how to treat diseases of the ear.

In May 1799, Countess Anna von Brunsvik brought her daughters, twenty-four-year-old Thérèse and twenty-year-old Josephine, to Vienna to take piano lessons with the twenty-nine-year-old Beethoven who was already a rising star. He was immediately attracted to Josephine, but any relationship with her was impossible. He tried to suppress any feelings he had for her. But in 1805 he wrote: "Oh beloved J., . . . when I met you for the first time – I was determined not to let a spark of love germinate in me . . ." Clearly, he had failed.

What's more, his feelings were reciprocated. In the winter of 1806/7 she wrote: "My soul was already enthusiastic for you even before I knew you personally – this was increased through your affection. A feeling deep in my soul, incapable of expression, made me love you. Even before I knew you, your Music made me enthusiastic for you. The goodness of your character, your affection increased it."

However, in 1800, Josephine was married off to the wealthy fifty-year-old Count Joseph von Deym. Beethoven turned elsewhere – to another unattainable aristocrat, the sixteen-year-old Countess Julie "Giuletta" Guiciadi. He dedicated the "Moonlight Sonata" to her.

"I am now leading a slightly more pleasant life, for I am mixing more with my fellow creatures," he wrote. "This change was brought about by a dear fascinating girl, who loves me and who I love. After two years I am again enjoying a few blissful moments."

Again, he knew he could not marry her. They were not of the same class. In 1803, she married the aristocratic young composer Count Wenzel Robert Gallenberg and moved to Italy, then abruptly returned to Vienna.

"She sought me out, crying, but I scorned her," he told his secretary Anton Schindler.

Eventually a triangular relationship developed.

"She loved me very much," he told Schindler, "far more than she ever loved her husband. Meanwhile, he was more of a lover to her than I was. Heaven forgive her. She did not know what she was doing."

He went on to help out her husband when he fell on hard times, finding him a rich sponsor, and she remains a candidate for the "Immortal Beloved".

Even though Josephine was married, Beethoven continued as her piano teacher. After some initial difficulties, her marriage seems to have been a happy one, with the couple knocking out a baby every year. Josephine was pregnant with her fourth child when, in January 1804, Count von Deym died suddenly of pneumonia.

Beethoven continued to see the young widow. This alarmed her younger sister Charlotte, who called her "Pepi". "Beethoven is very often here, he gives Pepi lessons – this is a bit dangerous, I must confess," Charlotte wrote.

Her older sister Thérèse agreed. "It's just a little dangerous," she wrote. "May she be on her guard . . . her heart must have the strength to say no."

It seems it did not. According to Thérèse's diaries, Josephine gave herself "freely without concern", then was mortified by guilt afterwards. Just twenty-four, Josephine had sworn an oath of chastity after her husband's death. Nevertheless Beethoven and Josephine maintained a passionate correspondence.

"That I cannot satisfy this sensuous love, does this cause you anger?" she wrote. "I would have to break holy vows were I to listen to your desires."

Beethoven gave her a gentlemanly reassurance. "Oh beloved J., it is no desire for the other sex that draws me to you," he wrote, "it is your whole self with all your individual qualities."

Yeah. Tell me lies, tell me sweet little lies.

"You have conquered me," he wrote.

"I love you inexpressibly," she responded.

If she was not giving herself to him, he reasoned in a fit of jealousy, she must be giving it to someone else.

"Do not doubt me," she wrote. "I cannot express how deeply wounding it is to be equated with low creatures."

However, her family put pressure on her and she was out when he came to call. She travelled to Switzerland where she met Baron Christoph von Stackelberg, who travelled back to Austria with her. Heedless of her vow of chastity, Josephine fell pregnant. But as Baron von Stackelberg, an Estonian, was not a Catholic, her family opposed the marriage. Their daughter, Maria Laura, was born in secret in December 1809. Three months later, in a remote town in Hungary, with no guests, they married.

Although a second daughter Theophile was born nine months after the wedding, the marriage was soon in difficulties. There were financial problems, rows, lawsuits. In June 1812, von Stackelberg left her.

On 3 July 1812, Beethoven travelled via Prague to Teplitz where he wrote the letter to his "Immortal Beloved" and seems to have met her there. Nine months later, Josephine gave birth to her seventh child, Minona.

In 1814, von Stackelberg turned up to demand custody of the children. When Josephine refused to give them up, he called the police who removed them forcibly. According to Beethoven's biographer Rita Steblin, Josephine then "hired the dubious mathematics teacher Andrian [Karl Eduard von Andrehan-Werburg] ... she gradually fell under his charismatic spell, becoming pregnant and giving birth to Emilie, hiding in a hut".

While she was pregnant, von Stackelberg returned. He then

slandered her to the police, concerning an incident of incest among her children.

"The morality of the Countess does not appear to enjoy a good reputation," read a police report of 1815. "It is stated that she cannot be absolved from having given grounds for conjugal quarrels."

She seems to have met Beethoven again in Baden in the summer of 1816, where they seem to have spent some time together. When she died on 31 March 1821, Beethoven composed his last piano sonatas, which musicologists see as requiems and contain elements of what they call "Josephine's theme".

Sister Thérèse is also a candidate for the "Immortal Beloved". Miriam Tenger, a friend in later life, claimed that Thérèse had been secretly engaged to her piano teacher. Beethoven always included a sprig of *immortelle* in his love letters to Thérèse, Tenger said. When they broke it off, Beethoven returned her love letters in a bundle and tucked a note under the ribbon which read: "*L'Immortelle à son Immortelle – Luigi.*"

When Thérèse died, thirty years after Beethoven, it is said that she was laid to rest with her head cushioned on the sprigs of *immortelle* taken from the letters.

There was another Thérèse in the frame – Thérèse von Malfatti, the niece of Beethoven's doctor. He dedicated some piano pieces to her. He complained of the "volatile Thérèse who takes life so lightly" – but she was nineteen, when he was forty. Nevertheless, he drew up marriage plans with her in 1810. But the volatile Thérèse, who took life so lightly, promptly married someone else.

Other scholars think that the "Immortal Beloved" was Antonie Brentano – wife of his close friend Franz Brentano – or Bettina von Arnim, née Brentano, an intimate of Goethe who also knew Liszt. He wrote passionate love letters to her, but slightly less passionate than the one to the "Immortal Beloved". Then there is the Countess Anna-Marie Erdödy and the singer Amalie Sebald, whom he called "a nut brown maid of Berlin". She was with him in Teplitz. He was working on his Eighth Symphony at the time, but he recorded that it did not "prevent him making love with much ardour". When he decided to leave Teplitz, she was so upset she did not even say goodbye. He was angry with himself over the incident, writing to a friend at Teplitz: "It is a frightful thing to make the acquaintance of such a sweet creature, and to lose her immediately. Nothing is worse than to have to confess one's own foolishness like this." And he urged a friend to give Amalie "an ardent kiss – if there is nobody there to see". She married someone else.

There were plenty of other women in his life as he became more famous and he was always on the lookout for a casual conquest. He openly admired the "magnificent arse" of the young wife of his friend, the conductor Counsellor Peters. When Peters went off on a trip to Italy, he suggested that Beethoven sleep with his wife "because it is cold".

"When I am away my place is taken by amenable friends," he said. It was better than her sleeping with an obdurate stranger, I guess.

Beethoven also received a note from the wife of the singer Franz Janitschek, another friend, saying, "Why don't you come and visit me? My husband is away." Janitschek and his wife split up soon after.

There were other flirtations and more prostitutes. The latter were procured for him by his friend Baron Nikolaus Zmeskall. Beethoven liked the girls to come around between half past three or four o'clock, so he could have his evenings free. But there were no more "Immortal Beloveds".

However, there was another potential scandal in his life. At one time he was close to Johanna Reiss, the daughter of a prosperous Viennese upholsterer. When she was four months pregnant, she married Beethoven's younger brother Kaspar. The child, Karl, was nine when Kaspar died. Beethoven became the child's guardian, accusing Johanna of being a whore and forbidding the child to see his mother.

Beethoven and Karl lived together with a couple of loose-living chambermaids. One, Karl complained, "sat up in bed with her breasts exposed and looked at me in a brazen way".

There is a theory that Beethoven was the father of Karl, and Kaspar, who was already terminally ill, married Johanna to save his brother from scandal.

Despite the cruel insults Beethoven threw at her, Johanna never responded in kind. He even had sexual fantasies about her, imagining her turning up naked to the Artists' Ball and offering herself to him for twenty guilders. And it may not all have been fanstasy. As a widow, Johanna had an illegitimate daughter that she called Ludovica – the feminine form of Ludwig.

Later in life, after Karl tried to kill himself, Beethoven and Johanna were reconciled. She may have even been the mysterious, heavily veiled woman who visited Beethoven on his deathbed. She may even have been his "Immortal Beloved", but he did not know it.

# 8

## Religious Vices

### Eamon Casey and Michael Cleary

Most sex scandals in the Catholic Church involve child abuse and there is nothing at all funny about that. But Eamon Casey, Bishop of Galway, was not that way inclined. While he and the prominent Irish priest, TV personality and host of a late-night phone-in Father Michael Cleary were on the liberal wing of the Church, they continued to speak out for clerical celibacy and against extramarital sex.

In 1992, a newspaper discovered that Casey had had an affair with American divorcee Annie Murphy. She gave birth to his son in 1974, when he was Bishop of Kerry. She said that he tried to persuade her to give up the boy for adoption at birth, but she raised him with the help of her parents. Father Cleary had demanded to know who the father was, but she refused to tell him. He also upbraided her for not giving up the child.

Casey paid her £7,000 from diocesan funds to keep quiet, though he paid the money back when the scandal broke. When Casey discovered that the *Irish Times* were going to publish the story, he resigned and left the country to become a missionary in Ecuador, even though he did not speak Spanish. Annie Murphy later published a blow-by-blow account of the affair in a memoir deliciously entitled *Forbidden Fruit*.

She said when she first met Bishop Casey at Shannon airport in 1973, she instantly saw him as a delightful person who was larger than life. She felt he was terribly lonely and she was wounded by her divorce at the time. So they decided to throw the rules out the window.

"Here was a perfect opportunity to say 'to hell with it, let's go' and we did," she said.

While Bishop Casey had to face the scandal, Father Cleary managed to take his secret to the grave with him. Three weeks after he died in 1993, the Irish news magazine *The Phoenix* revealed that he had been living with his common-law wife for twenty-six years. In 1967, Phyllis Hamilton had moved in as his housekeeper. She was seventeen when they first made love. He was some ten years older. According to her memoir, *Secret Love: My Life with Father Michael Cleary*, they had taken marriage vows, though no third party was present.

They had two children together. The first was given up for adoption; the second, Ross, they brought up themselves. DNA tests later proved that he was Cleary's son.

Phyllis was terrified when Annie Murphy went public. When the story broke she had sat looking at the newspaper for three hours before she could bring herself to read it.

"I didn't like Annie at all," she said. "I felt this is the end for all of us."

Father Cleary had been out of the country with a group of golfing friends in Spain and had learned about it on Sky News. He was furious. When he came home a few days later, he was still "whiter than white". He was afraid and he was shaking, she said. Casey knew about his relationship with Phyllis, though he did not know if Annie did. A close personal friend, Dr Ivor Browne, warned Cleary to end the relationship with Phyllis, but he refused.

Phyllis described Father Cleary as "terribly hypocritical" but in his role as priest he was "delivering what he was told to deliver". She said there were three parts to him – the priest, the performer and the man at home. But she loved him and, when he spoke off the cuff, he was "the best person on the planet".

The Church was good to her, up to a point. After Father Cleary died, she was allowed to stay on in the house they had shared. But when she died in 2001, they told her son to leave. When he refused, they started legal proceedings against him. Eventually, though, they paid him £40,000 to move out – then went on to sell the property for £700,000.

But that did not put anyone off. In 2006, seventy-three-year-old Reverend Maurice Dillane from Woodford, County Galway, admitted fathering a child by a thirty-year-old local schoolmistress. The local bishop said that it was a "private matter". Father Dillane, it was said, was recovering from back surgery – understandably.

## Pope Alexander VI

Fathers Casey, Cleary and Dillane were following in a long line of sex scandals that emanated from the pontificate itself. There have been many bishops of Rome who have failed to live up to their vow of celibacy. The most scandalous was the Borgia pope, Alexander VI.

Born in Spain in 1431, Rodrigo Borgia was probably the illegitimate son of the Archbishop of Valencia, Alfons de Borja – Borgia is the Italian spelling of Borja. He had at least six illegitimate children in Spain before he moved to Italy at the age of twenty-two after "Uncle" Alfons was elected pope.

Rodrigo studied law in Bologna and was ordained as a deacon, though this did not diminish his appetites. According to his tutor, Gaspare de Verona: "Beautiful women are attracted to love him and are excited by him in a quite remarkable way, more powerfully than an iron is attracted by a magnet."

As Callistus III, Alfons made two of his "nephews" cardinals. One of them was Rodrigo who also took over as Archbishop of Valencia. Back in his native Spain, he began fathering more illegitimate children. He seduced a ravishing Spanish widow, then ravished her two daughters, "initiating them into the most hideous voluptuousness". When the mother died, he sent the older daughter to a convent and gave the younger one three children. Her great-great-great-grandson went on to become Pope Innocent X who, before his election at the age of seventy in 1644, devoted himself chiefly to "knightly exercises and the pleasures of love," according to the Venetian ambassador. He was also said to have come under "the influence of a bad and reckless woman". This was his sister-in-law and, probably, mistress Donna Olimpia Maidalchini. Her presence in the Vatican was so conspicuous that his papacy was known as "the Pontificate of Donna Olimpia".

Thanks to "Uncle" Callistus, Rodrigo picked up a number of lucrative offices, including the vice-chancellorship of the Holy See in 1457, and became extremely wealthy. When Callistus died, Rodrigo expected to succeed him. Instead, Pius II was elected. Born Enea Silvio Piccolomimi, he had written pornography to amuse the court of the anti-Pope Felix V. As a youth, he had visited Scotland, where "the women are fair, charming and easily won". Indeed, he fathered a son there. In England, he travelled with two servants, a guide and a hundred women. Two of them took him to a chamber strewn with straw, "planning to sleep with him if they were asked, as was the custom of the country", according to his *Secret Memoirs*. Back in Italy, he fathered a child by the widow of King Alfonso of Naples. He had another child by the wife of a tradesman in Strasbourg and wrote to his father about it. When the old man chided him, he responded: "Certainly you, who are flesh, did not beget a son of stone or iron. You know what a cock you were and I am no eunuch . . ."

His pornographic novel *Lucretia and Euryalus* was widely read and the erotic comedy *Chrysis* brought him fame. Quiting the service of Felix V, he joined the court of the Holy Roman Emperor Frederick III where he both preached and practised sexual freedom, fathering at least two more bastards.

The historian Ferdinand Gregorovius claimed he fathered at least twelve illegitimate children in all. As pope he seemed to have behaved himself, though in his *Secret Memoirs* he raved about Queen Charlotte of Cyprus who kissed his feet. She got everything she asked for. He considered allowing priests to marry – as they were more likely to be saved that way. He also dissolved the nunneries of St Clara and St Bridget, "lest the nuns should harbour under religious habits lascivious hearts". But there was little he could do to curb Cardinal Rodrigo.

Meeting at Mantua, Pius II remarked: "The vice-chancellor is twenty-five and looks capable of every wickedness."

Rodrigo was staying with the Marchesa of Mantua, who shared his passion for sport. He also entertained himself with the wife of a dim-witted nobleman. The Pope withdrew to Siena. From there he wrote to Rodrigo, saying:

> Judging from the manner of your life, you seem not to have chosen to govern the state of the Church, but to enjoy pleasure. You do not abstain from hunting or games, or from intercourse with women; you give dinners of unseemly magnificence; you wear costly clothes; you have an abundance of gold and silver plate, and you keep more horses and servants than any man can need.

Rodrigo took no notice. After a christening on 7 June 1460, he and Cardinal Estouteville held a private party in a walled garden to which only their servants and the ladies were admitted. Their menfolk were specifically excluded. Soon Italy was abuzz with scandal.

When this came to Pius's ears on 11 June, he wrote to Rodrigo, saying:

> Beloved Son: We have learned that your worthiness, forgetful of the high office with which you are invested, was present from the seventeenth to the twenty-second

hour, four days ago, in the gardens of Giovanni de Bichi, where there were several women of Siena, women wholly given over to worldly vanities. Your companion was one of your colleagues, whose years, if not the dignity of his office, ought to have reminded him of his duty. We have heard that the dance was indulged in, in all wantonness; none of the allurements to love were spared, and you behaved yourself as if you were one of a group of young laymen. In order that your lust might be all the more unrestrained, the husbands, fathers, brothers and kinsmen of the young girls were not invited; you and a few servants were the leaders and inspirers of this orgy. It is said that nothing is now talked of in Siena but your vanity, which is the subject of universal ridicule. Certainly, here at the baths, your name is on everyone's tongue. Our displeasure is beyond words.

Pius had regular cause to ask Rodrigo if it was right for a man in his position "to court you women, to give those you love presents of fruit and wine, and to give no thought to anything but sensual pleasure" and he asked Rodrigo not to appear again at an orgy dressed in his cardinal's vestments.

Bartomeo Bonatti, the Mantuan envoy to Siena, remarked: "If all the children born within the year arrive dressed like their fathers, many will appear as priest and cardinals."

He reported back to his mistress, the Marchesa of Mantua, that Rodrigo had been seen "in the company of the most beautiful woman that ever was". This was Nachine, a high-class courtesan, whose liaison with the Cardinal was well known.

At Mantua in 1461, Rodrigo met the eighteen-year-old Roman beauty Vannozza Catanei. He had already slept with her mother and, probably, her sister. But, no matter, he took "Rosa" as his long-term lover. However, to avoid any further scandal, instead of taking her back to Rome, he installed her in a palazzo in Venice where she had four children by him – Cesare, Juan, Lucrezia and Jofré. He wrote to her, begging for her to be patient until "I shall have what he whom they called my uncle has left me for an inheritance, the See of St Peter. Meanwhile take particular care of the education of our children, because they are destined to govern nations and kings."

In anticipation of becoming pope and moving his family to Rome, he built a splendid palazzo, which Pius II compared to the house of the famously debauched Roman emperor Nero.

When Pius II died in 1464, Rodrigo did not succeed him. Paul II did. He was known by his cardinals as "Our Lady of Pity" and liked to see naked men racked and tortured. He wore a papal tiara that "outweighed a palace in its worth" and, it was said, died of a heart attack, in 1471, while being sodomized by one of his favourite boys.

At forty, Rodrigo was still considered too young to become pope. Next up was Sixtus IV. To fund a war against the Turks, he built a new brothel that opened its doors to both sexes and taxed every prostitute in Rome. He found a new stream of income by taxing priests who kept mistresses and sold indulgences to rich men who wanted to "solace certain matrons in the absence of their husbands".

Sixtus swung both ways. Six of his "nephews" – either his illegitimate sons or his catamites, or both – became cardinals. Two of them, Pietro Riario – said to be his own son by his sister – and Giuliano della Rovere were rumoured to be "the instruments of his infamous pleasure". Riario became rich courtesy of the papal treasury but "succumbed to his dissipations" in 1474. Della Rovere went on to become Pope Julius II, who was called the "great sodomite" and was accused of wearing himself out "among prostitutes and boys". He was also the patron of Michelangelo, who shared his tastes.

According to a chronicler of the age: "The following most execrable act was alone sufficient to render the memory of Sixtus IV forever infamous: the family of the Cardinal of St Lucia, having presented to him a request to be permitted to commit sodomy during the three hot months – June, July and

August – the pope wrote on the bottom of the petition: 'Let it be done.'" They couldn't just do it in the cold months then?

He also sanctified the erotic and blasphemous vision of a monk named Alano de Rupe. According to a version published in Germany at the time: "Upon a time the ever-blessed Virgin Mary entering the cell of Alano de Rupe, being locked, she took a hair of his head and made a ring, with which she espoused the father, and made him kiss her and handle her breasts, and, in a word, grew in a short time as familiar with him as women used to be with their husbands."

He was responsible for the building of the Sistine Chapel, which bears his name, and he began the Spanish Inquisition.

When Sixtus died in 1484, it was still not Rodrigo's turn. Instead it was Innocent VIII. Innocent? It was said that "his private life was darkened by the most scandalous proceedings". He had an impressive CV: "Having been educated among the people of King Alfonso of Sicily, he had contracted the frightful vice of sodomy. His uncommon beauty had introduced him, in Rome, into the family of Philip, Cardinal of Bologna, to serve his pleasures; and after the death of his protector, he became the favourite of Paul II and Sixtus IV, who created him a cardinal."

Despite this, he fathered eight sons and eight daughters – "Rome might with good reason call him father," it was said. He did not even pretend they were his nephews and nieces, but acknowledged them openly. He found them jobs and officiated at their weddings. His reign was called the "Golden Age of Bastards".

Though Catholic historians said he gave up his mistress when he became pope, it was widely rumoured that he had other concubines. "His Holiness rises from the bed of harlots," it was said, "to open the gates of purgatory and heaven."

When it was suggested that priests should give up their mistresses, Innocent dismissed the idea. "Even among the Curia, you will hardly find one without a concubine," he said.

Innocent was more concerned with the outbreak of witchcraft and his papal bull condemning those who had sex with the devil forms the foreword to the book *Malleus Maleficarum* – *The Witches' Hammer* – a handbook on discovery and torture.

On his deathbed, Innocent craved mother's milk and a wet nurse was found for him to suck on. Perhaps, like Casanova, he wanted the comfort of a woman's breast while he was dying.

Under Sixtus IV, Rodrigo saw no reason to exercise discretion and brought Vannozza and the children to Rome. He passed her off as the Countess Ferdinand of Castile and Rodrigo's agent passed himself off as her husband. On the pretext of meeting his compatriot, he visited her every night. Such pretence was hardly worthwhile when Innocent VIII came to the throne. By then there were fifty thousand prostitutes on the streets of Rome.

When Innocent VIII died, Cardinal della Rovere was tipped to take over. But Rodrigo had been vice-chancellor under four popes and bought himself votes. Only two were outstanding. One belonged to Cardinal Gherardo of Venice. He was ninety-five, probably senile, and neither asked for nor accepted a bribe. But he voted for Rodrigo anyway.

The casting vote was held by a Venetian monk. All he wanted was five thousand crowns and a night with Rodrigo's daughter, twelve-year-old Lucrezia. The deal was done and Rodrigo became Pope Alexander VI.

The cardinals who had elected him had no illusions. Giovanni de'Medici said to Cardinal Cibò: "We are now in the clutches of perhaps the most savage wolf the world has ever seen. Either we flee or he will, without a doubt, devour us."

Giovanni de'Medici went on to become Leo X. While he had a number of illegitimate children, he had been practising sodomy vigorously for so many years that he had to be carried into the conclave on a mattress. He liked putting on masked balls for his cardinals and their mistresses, though he himself preferred banquets where naked boys appeared from the puddings. He also put on a play involving eight hermits and a "virgin". When they see her naked, praying to the goddess

Venus, they take it in turns to become her lover, then kill each other over the love of her.

Leo X was the patron of the writer Pietro Aretino whose *Dialogue of Whores* was the scandal sheet of the day, lampooning the proclivities of the great and the good in Rome, until he was run out of town in 1527.

Like other popes, Leo X made his catamites cardinals. One of them, Aflonso Petrucci, was ambitious and thought he had the makings of a pope himself. He bribed the doctor who was treating Leo X's ulcerated backside to stick poison up the Pope's backside. But Leo's secret police intercepted a note outlining the plot. Under torture, the doctor confessed and was hanged, drawn and quartered. Petrucci fled. But Leo sent word via the Spanish ambassador offering his safe passage if he returned to Rome. Petrucci accepted, returned and was arrested.

"No faith need be kept with a poisoner," he said.

Petrucci was tortured. When he confessed, he was sentenced to death. But Leo would let no Christian lay hands on a prince of the Church, so had him strangled by a Moor instead. Afterwards, Leo comforted himself with the choirboy Solimando, grandson of Sultan Mehmet, the Turk who had taken Constantinople in 1453.

When Alexander VI became pope, Giovanni della Rovere went into hiding in France.

The historian Edward Gibbon described Alexander VI as the "Tiberius of Christian Rome", after another famously scandalous emperor. He loved entertainments that featured naked women. During festivals, he had an average of twenty-five courtesans a night laid on for his amusement. Wherever he went, he was accompanied by a troupe of scantily clad dancing girls to the outrage of the rest of Christendom. On one occasion, he interrupted Mass with a giggling young woman and, it was said, the Host was trampled underfoot.

Naturally Alexander advanced his own children. Following family tradition, his villainous son Cesare was made Archbishop of Valencia. To take the post, Cesare, theoretically, had to be legitimate, so Alexander issued a papal bull saying that Cesare was the son of Vannozza Catanei and her "husband". In a second, secret bull, he acknowledged Cesare as his own. That did not stop Cesare packing his house in the Trastevere with girlfriends, while Rodrigo regularized his domestic arrangements by moving Vannozza and his daughter into the Vatican.

To recoup the money he had expended in bribes to become pope, Alexander let murderers off – for a fee. To increase the money he earned from simony, bribes taken for office, he took to poisoning cardinals. The dead cardinal's property reverted to the Church – that is, Alexander – and he received an exorbitant fee from the new appointee. He also sold indulgences, pardoning sins yet to be committed. One nobleman paid 24,000 gold pieces to be allowed to commit incest with his sister. Peter Mendoza, Cardinal of Valencia, bought permission to call his catamite his natural son. After all, Alexander needed to keep his mistress in the opulent style to which she had become accustomed.

Or, rather, his mistresses. At the age of fifty-eight, he took the fifteen-year-old Giulia Farnese – "Giulia Bell" or "Julia the Beautiful" – as his mistress. As part of the arrangement, he officiated over her marriage to the compliant Orsino Orsini and made her nineteen-year-old brother, Alessandro, a cardinal. He was known as "Cardinal Petticoat" and went on to become Pope Paul III, who indulged in incest and murder. He commissioned Michelangelo to paint the Last Judgement in the Sistine Chapel and excommunicated Henry VIII for divorcing Catherine of Aragon and marrying Anne Boleyn, while ordering the spilling of so much Lutheran blood that "their hordes should be able to swim in it". After Giulia moved into the Vatican, she became known as the "Bride of Christ" and they had two children together.

From a young age, Alexander's daughter Lucrezia was used sexually by both Rodrigo and Cesare, among others. It is still a matter of debate whether the father of her first child was her father or her brother. Cesare and Juan used to compete for their father's favour by supplying beautiful women for his private harem. At one point, Juan outshone Cesare by supplying a Spanish beauty who moved Rodrigo to ecstasy. In jealousy, Cesare stabbed his brother and threw his body in the Tiber. Rodrigo was so upset that he mended his ways, but not for long.

It is said that Alexander and Cesare imprisoned and raped the most beautiful young man in Italy. His body was later found in the Tiber with a stone tied around his neck. But normally Rodrigo preferred women.

Giulia and Lucrezia became so tight that Alexander decided to have his daughter married off. For the ceremony, he wore a gold Turkish robe whose train was carried by an African slave girl. He amused himself by throwing confetti down the low-cut bodices of the ladies' dresses. Then, when the moment came for the marriage to be consummated, Alexander accompanied the couple to the bridal chamber.

"There such shocking and hideous scenes took place as no language can convey or describe," wrote one chronicler. "The Pope played the part of matron for his daughter; Lucrezia, that Messalina who, even while a child, had been by her father and brothers initiated into the most hideous debauchery, played, in this instance, the part of an innocent in order to prolong the obscenities of the comedy; and the 'marriage' took place in the presence of the pontifical family."

Even after she married, Lucrezia remained in the papal apartments. When Giulia Farnese took her to visit her husband, Alexander was beside himself with jealousy. He wrote letters that threatened them with eternal damnation if they did not return. When they did, he was soon back to his normal self, sleeping with three other women – "one of them a nun from Valencia, another a Castilian, a third a very beautiful girl from Venice, fifteen or sixteen years of age," Ludovico Sforza told the Milan Senate.

Ludovico was the uncle of Lucrezia's first husband, but the marriage was annulled by Alexander on the grounds of non-consummation. As part of the procedure, a papal commission had to declare that Lucrezia was a virgin – "a conclusion that set all of Italy laughing," said a chronicler. "It was common knowledge that she was the biggest whore there ever was in Rome." To cap it all, when the divorce was finally granted, she was pregnant with the miraculous papal child known as the "*Infans Romanus*" – "the child of Rome".

Visiting the Isle of Elba, Alexander invited the prettiest girls on the island to dance for him. "A party with a Borgia could not end otherwise than with orgies," wrote the historian Edward Gibbon.

But there was a dark side. Cesare, particularly, revelled in the cruelty of the times.

"It was so agreeable to him to see blood shed that, like the Emperor Commodus, he practised butchery in order to keep alive his thirst for blood," wrote Johann Burchard, Bishop of Ostia. "One day he went so far as to have the square of St Peter enclosed by a palisade, into which he ordered some prisoners – men, women and children – to be brought. He then had them bound, hand and foot, and being armed and mounted on a fiery charger, commenced a horrible attack upon them. Some he shot, and others he cut down with his sword, trampling them under his horse's feet. In less than half an hour, he wheeled around alone in a puddle of blood, among the dead bodies of his victims, while his Holiness and Madam Lucrezia, from a balcony enjoyed the sight of that horrid scene."

But usually, the entertainment was much more wholesome. Cesare organized a hunting party for his father that involved a horde of prostitutes and dancing girls, protected by 500 knights and 600 infantrymen. According to the historian Thomas Tomasi: "They passed for entire days in the woods of Ostia, amusing themselves in surpassing all that imagination could invent in lewdness and debauchery." He added despairingly: "It would be impossible to enumerate all the murders, the rapes and the incests which were everyday committed at the court of the Pope. Scarcely the life of a man could be long enough to register the names of the victims murdered, poisoned or thrown alive into the Tiber."

These excesses reached a pinnacle with what became known as "The Joust of Whores" put on in the papal apartments to celebrate Lucrezia's third wedding – Cesare had murdered her second husband. Buchard wrote:

> This marriage has been celebrated with such unexampled orgies as were never before seen. His Holiness gave a supper to the cardinals and grandees of his court, placing at the side of each guest two courtesans, whose only dress consisted of a loose garment of gauze and garlands of flowers; and when the meal was over, those women, more than fifty in number, performed lascivious dances – at first alone, afterwards with the guest. At last, at a signal given by Madam Lucrezia, the garments of the women fell down, and the dance went on to the applause of His Holiness.
>
> They afterwards proceeded to other sports. By order of the Pope, there were symmetrically placed in the ballroom, twelve rows of branched candelabras covered with lighted candles; Madam Lucrezia threw upon the floor some handfuls of chestnuts, after which the naked courtesans on hands and knees gathered them up, wriggling in and out among the candelabra . . . The swifter and more successful obtained from His Holiness presents of jewels and silk dresses. At last, as their prizes for the sports, there were premiums for lust, and the women were carnally attacked at the pleasure of the guests; and this time Madam Lucrezia, who presided with the Pope on the platform, distributed the premiums to the victors.

The men who had copulated the most times with the prostitutes got prizes.

When Alexander died in 1503, the corpse swelled up and turned black. Cesare suffered so badly from syphilis that his face was eaten away. He had to wear a mask and only went out at night. He was killed in an ambush in Spain in 1507, just thirty-one years old. Lucrezia's third marriage to Alfonso d'Este, Duke of Ferrara, was a success, though she had an affair with Francesco Gonzaga, who had taken Cesare's place as military commander of the church. She particularly relished this affair as Gonzaga was married to Alfonso's sister whom she hated. But Gonzago got a little overenthusiastic and tried to invade Ferrara and carry her off. While Alfonso was away fighting him, Lucrezia acted as regent and turned Ferrara into one of the centres of letters during the Renaissance. She died in childbirth at the age of thirty-nine.

## Jim Bakker

But not all scandalous priests were Catholics as TV evangelist Jim Bakker helped to demonstrate. He and his wife Tammy Faye were the stars of *The PTL Club*, a popular evangelical Christian television programme. PTL stood for "Praise the Lord" or "People That Love" – which was certainly true in Jim's case.

Bakker was proud of his virtue, telling anyone who would listen: "I have never been involved with wife-swapping. I am not a homosexual. And I've never been to a prostitute." While Tammy Faye would regularly harangue Satan.

"I've been telling the devil, you stay away from Jim Bakker," she told viewers. But it seems that the devil, Bakker and, for that matter, Tammy Faye could not resist. Twenty-year-old church secretary Jessica Hahn told Larry King: "Tammy Faye was having an affair with the choir director or something like that. Jim Bakker came along. He said, 'Jessica Hahn, listen. You're a virgin.'"

She was, of course.

Then she was told to go down to Clearwater Beach, Florida to "make Jim Bakker feel better". She was to look after the kids while Jim and Tammy Faye did a telethon. After all, you can never have too much money.

Hahn said that another minister named Jim Fletcher put some thing in the water or the wine she was drinking. Then the televangelist she idolized came to her motel room. There were bodyguards outside the door.

"Jim Bakker walks in with his little itty-bitty shorts. He rips up the bedspread. He takes off my dress. And he lays me down on the bed," she recalled. "He said, you know, my wife doesn't make me feel like a man anymore. And, you know, when you help the shepherd, you help the sheep. And so . . . your mind is like, oh my God, I know this is wrong, but your body just gives in."

She was terrified of getting pregnant. But King could not help probing deeper.

"It hurt like hell," she said. "And then, after that, John Fletcher comes in, who was the middle man, and said, you know, you can't just be with Jim Bakker. You've got to be with me. He threw me on the floor, head back. I had blood coming out of my back. And, you know, he just went nuts on me."

Jessica Hahn decided to keep quiet "because I love God . . . I don't want to hurt God's people."

For eight years she said nothing and Jim Bakker gave her $20,000 to get counselling, along with $400,000 to buy her silence, though she later returned it. The money came from funds that Bakker later went to jail for obtaining fraudulently. But then the story broke when the *Charlotte Observer* found out about the pay-off.

At first Bakker denied everything, then said, "I was set up by that female."

Later, in a book, he would say, "Most of all, I did not rape Jessica Hahn. The sexual encounter, for which we both are now famous, was completely consensual."

"Consensual, my ass," Hahn responded.

But it could not have been his fault and he called her a professional who knew every trick of the trade – not very Christian. Jessica Hahn said that she was told that she should go after Billy Graham.

When the whole thing came out, Tammy Faye said that she lay on the floor for three days and cried. But she stood by her man. He was not a womanizer and she could not divorce him "because he was hurting too bad".

Rival preacher Jerry Falwell said, "Jessica, come over to my place. I'm going to hide you out."

Instead Hahn moved into the Playboy Mansion. She slept with Hugh Hefner, but provided "no sexual favours," she said. Then she posed nude for his magazine. Hefner protected her, she said, " . . . that was my church. Those guys, they never took advantage of me. They took care of me. They fed me. They protected me and I'd love to do it again."

She went on to have a career as an actress.

Bakker was forced to resign. Jerry Falwell took over and accused him of homosexuality and called him "the greatest scab and cancer on the face of Christianity in 2,000 years of Church history", which is a bit harsh after Alexander VI.

When Jim Bakker went to jail, Tammy Faye, now penniless, divorced him and married his friend and business partner Roe Messner, who went to jail for fraud soon after. When Bakker came out of jail, he began a new evangelical show with his new wife Lori. The Lord moves in mysterious ways.

## Jimmy Swaggart

Jim Bakker and his ilk were condemned as "pompadoured pretty-boys with their hair done and their nails done who call themselves preachers" by another televangelist, namely, Jimmy Swaggart. But Swaggart also found it hard to kick the sins of the flesh. And it all began because he had had a fellow minister Marvin Gorman in the Assemblies of God defrocked for having an extramarital affair with a bereaved parishioner. It was part of his grief counselling, apparently. And Gorman, a good Christian, was determined to get his own back.

He got his son Randy and son-in-law Garland Bilbo to stake out the Travel Inn on Airline Highway in New Orleans. They photographed Swaggart with prostitute Debra Murphree going into room seven. They then let Swaggart's tyres down and called Gorman. The deal was simple. All Swaggart had to do was to say publicly that he had lied about Gorman's affair and Gorman would stay silent about room seven.

When, after a year, Swaggart still had not fulfilled his side of the bargain, Gorman went to the leaders of the Assemblies of God and showed them the photos, along with further pictures of men going in and out of room seven, showing that it was a place used for prostitution. Swaggart was suspended from broadcasting for three months.

But first a tearful Swaggart went on TV, confessed to unspecified sins and begged for forgiveness. Four days later, his playmate in room seven, Debra Murphree, went on the morning news in New Orleans and said that while she stripped off for Swaggart, a regular customer, they did not have sexual intercourse. Did he just like to look, or was this the Clinton defence? According to the *Sunday Times*: "First, he picked a prostitute who looked like his mother, told her his name was 'Billy', and regularly claimed he couldn't afford more than ten bucks per servicing. He insisted on wearing condoms during oral sex, and not simply because he feared Aids. Presumably, it made him feel as if he wasn't entirely cheating on his wife. Usually, though, Jimmy just wanted to snap photos of the soon-to-be-notorious Debra Arlene Murphree posed on the cheap mattress. And, of course, these wouldn't be the last such pictures taken of Jimmy Swaggart's 'dream date'. Many would be featured in the very magazines Swaggart had been boycotting at Seven-Elevens across the country."

Swaggart soon tried to blag his way back on to television. "If

I do not return to the pulpit this weekend, millions of people will go to hell," he said. The Assemblies of God immediately defrocked him. Nevertheless, he staggered on regardless – both in Bible-bashing and conducting an unsavoury private life

On 11 October 1991, he was caught with another prostitute, Rosemary Garcia, driving in a white Jaguar that belonged to a board member of his ministry in a red-light district of Indio, California. Swaggart had propositioned Garcia on the side of the road, asking whether there were any motels around that showed pornographic movies.

They were pulled over by the Highway Patrol after driving down the wrong side of the street. When Garcia was asked why she was with Swaggart, she replied: "He asked me for sex. I mean, that's why he stopped me. That's what I do. I'm a prostitute" – thereby giving Swaggart an eloquent object lesson in professional integrity.

While Swaggart was clearly up for some "laying on of hands", Ms Garcia remained in awe of her God-fearing client.

"He's the same guy who cries on TV for all these people to feel sorry for him," she said, "to give him all their money. For what? So he can come give it to us. That's pretty good."

Instead of begging for forgiveness from his congregation, he told them: "The Lord told me it's flat none of your business." His son Donnie quickly stepped in, announcing that his father would be temporarily stepping down as head of Jimmy Swaggart Ministries in order to have "a time of healing and counselling". Donnie would take over the ministry until "Brother Swaggart gets back on his feet".

# 9

## Royal Romps

### Prince Charles and Diana

It began with a fairy-tale wedding. On 29 July 1981 the heir to the British throne and his shy virgin bride tied the knot at St Paul's Cathedral to the cheers of the crowds as over 750 million people around the world looked on. Just eleven years later, with the publication of Andrew Morton's *Diana: Her True Story*, the fairy tale turned into a farce and the greatest royal scandal for more than half a century began to unravel. The couple divorced in 1996 and the scandal saga ended in tragedy the following year.

It is not difficult to see how the scandal came about. In royal families, it is generally accepted that married people fool around, but stay together for the sake of propriety. As Prince of Wales, the heir to the British throne is in a good position to sow a few wild oats. According to the tabloids, Charles lost his virginity to Lucia Santa Cruz, daughter of the Chilean ambassador, when he was a student at Cambridge. She was a post-graduate student, three years older than him. Later, the prince scaled the walls of the all-women Newham College to sample the delights of Sybilla Dorman, daughter of the governor general of Malta. Soon after, he was snapped escorting Audrey Buxton to the May Ball.

He tried out the daughters of dukes and marquesses, entertaining them at Broadlands, the country estate of his

Uncle Dickie – Lord Mountbatten. There was a good deal of fevered press speculation about Prince Charlie's relationship with Lady "Kanga" Tryon, who was married at the time, and some snobbish tut-tutting about his sipping at the lips of Sabrina Guinness, daughter of the famous brewing family.

When he took up with Davina Sheffield, her jilted lover James Beard spilt the beans in the Sunday papers. Prince Charles's dalliance with Lord Manton's daughter Fiona Watson was a gift for the tabloids. The bountiful Fiona had once stripped off for *Penthouse*, so here was a royal scandal complete with juicy pictures.

Then in 1972, Charles met the love of his life, Camilla Shand. He was introduced to her at the upmarket Mayfair disco Annabel's by guards officer Andrew Parker-Bowles, later the husband of Camilla whom Charles would comprehensively cuckold. Camilla connived from the off. She introduced herself as the great-granddaughter of Alice Keppel – the last mistress of Edward VII, the legendary Bertie, Prince of Wales. A married woman, Alice famously remarked that her role as royal mistress was to "curtsy first and then hop into bed".

Camilla and the prince shared a love of riding, the countryside and gardening – and a juvenile sense of humour. But as heir to the throne, Charles had to do his bit in the armed forces. In 1973, he left Camilla on the dockside and shoved off in his ship HMS *Minerva*. It had already been made clear to Camilla that she was not the stuff future queens were made of. That is, she was not a virgin. Four weeks after she had kissed her sailor prince goodbye, she accepted the proposal of Andrew Parker-Bowles. Within months they were married and, the following year, Prince Charles became godfather to the couple's first child.

Prince Charles saw other women. Prince Andrew told a girlfriend that Charles was trying to compete with Warren Beatty, then at the height of his seductive powers. The prince's valet would often find discarded women's underwear left around his apartment in Buckingham Palace. These would be laundered and returned in an Asprey's box, if the owner could be identified. Otherwise they would be handed out to members of the palace staff, many of whom were gay. The *Daily Mail* said that Charles had a slush fund to buy the silence of women whom he had used and cast aside.

During this promiscuous period, Charles was seeing Sarah Spencer, Diana's older sister, but she was deemed unsuitable because she was a heavy smoker. Meanwhile, Andrew was having a brief dalliance with Di herself.

Now thirty, Charles was under pressure to do what heirs to the throne were born to do – produce more heirs. The hunt was on to find a suitable wife. Foreign princesses were vetted. But all those of the right age were Catholics. Under the Act of Settlement of 1701, the heir to the British throne cannot marry a Catholic.

So royal matchmakers looked closer to home and their eyes alighted on Diana. She had all the right qualifications. She was upper class, naive, none too bright – by her own admission – and a virgin. At least this was the assertion of her uncle Lord Fermoy; no one questioned how he was in a position to know. Randy Andy had got nowhere with Diana, apparently. Neither had author and socialite George Plumptree who had been going out with her for more than a year. No one asked and they were not saying. Besides, she looked the part. Her soft complexion and doe eyes were everyone's image of the unsullied maiden who gets to marry Prince Charming.

But Charles was no Prince Charming. His coolness towards his mouth-watering young bride was palpable. When asked whether he was in love with her, he replied, "Yes, whatever that may mean."

The problem was not just that Diana was not Camilla. She had not been brought up privy to the aristocratic game and learnt to overlook her husband's misdemeanours. A modern

young woman, she expected more and she was not going to
put up with her fiancé fooling around.

While they were courting, Charles was still seeing Davina
Sheffield and Anne Wallace. He also maintained his interest
in Camilla Parker-Bowles. Weeks before the wedding, Diana
found a bracelet in Charles's desk drawer. At first, she thought
this expensive gift was for her. But then she spotted the initials
"F" and "G" engraved on it. Camilla shared Charles's love
of the fifties radio comedy programme *The Goon Show* and
they addressed each other by the names of two of the stock
characters "Fred" and "Gladys".

Diana was heartbroken, but Charles could not see what the
fuss was about. He was simply doing what royals do, carrying
on his love life privately, while at the same time discharging his
public duty. After all, his father, the Duke of Edinburgh, had
been doing that during the long years of his marriage to the
queen. There was no turning back now. The wedding plans
were almost complete. The TV networks had cleared their
schedules. Heads of state from around the world were on their
way. The fairy-tale wedding had to go ahead.

The nightmare Diana had innocently blundered into
immediately became apparent. The first night of their married
life would be spent at Broadlands, where he took his conquests
in his bachelor days. In the morning, instead of lingering
lovingly with his bride, he leapt from the marriage bed at first
light to go fishing with Uncle Dickie.

Things improved during their honeymoon on the Royal
Yacht *Britannia*. They rose late and went to bed early. It was
said that they took saucy pictures of each other. Some were
supposed to have fallen into the hands of the press, but no
newspaper dared publish them.

However, instead of having intimate meals alone together,
dinners on-board were formal affairs, attended by numerous
staff. When they were alone things were worse. Charles was a
man fond of his own opinions. Old beyond his years, he would

propound his great thoughts on world affairs, religion and mysticism. A normal twenty-year-old airhead whose interests did not extend beyond clothes, make-up, pop music and babies, she wanted some small talk. She was bored by him – and hurt. During the cruise, she came across pictures of Camilla. She also realized the significance of the entwined CCs on his cufflinks. Fortunately, there were plenty of handsome young sailors to flirt with.

Within a year of his marriage, Charles made it clear to Diana that he had no intention of giving up Mrs Parker-Bowles. She would be *maîtresse en titre*. Soon after giving birth to Prince William in 1982, Diana overheard Charles on the phone saying, "Whatever happens I will go on loving you."

These were the words every young mother would love to hear on the lips of her husband, but not when he was saying them to his mistress.

In 1984, she gave birth to Prince Harry. Having produced an heir and a spare, her duty was done. Publicly, she did her job as a loving mum and turned up at Charles's side at state occasions. The rest of the time her life was her own. Soon the press discovered that, like his mother and father, they slept in separate rooms.

The gossip columns noted that Diana had a number of close male "friends". She took advantage of Charles's absence to attend an all-night party. Then, she spent the weekend with banker Philip Dunne. She was seen at a David Bowie concert with guards officer Major David Waterhouse. There was Mervyn Chaplin, who had called her "Duch", short for Duchess, since they had been teenagers; Roy Scott, a friend of hers from the days before she was married; and Nicky Haslam, hi-fi dealer to the aristocracy. Haslam claimed to have had affairs with Antony Armstrong-Jones, later Lord Snowdon, husband of Princess Margaret and Charles's uncle, and Princess Margaret's lover Roddy Llewellyn.

While teaching Prince William to ride, Captain James Hewitt also eased Diana back into the saddle. When Hewitt was sent to

the Gulf War, they exchanged torrid love letters. He denied being
the father of Prince Harry, despite the striking likeness, saying
that the affair did not begin until after Harry had been born.

Then there was the upper-class car dealer and scion of
the gin family James Gilbey. At 8 p.m. one evening in 1989,
journalists tailing Diana saw her bodyguard drop her off at
Gilbey's flat. They waited. No one left or entered the apartment
for the next five hours. She finally emerged at 1 a.m., looking
slightly dishevelled. When reporters asked Gilbey what the two
of them had been doing for five hours, he said gallantly that
they had been playing bridge. You need four to play bridge.

It was now clear that there was something wrong with the
royal marriage. For a while Buckingham Palace managed to
keep a lid on it. But then Andrew Morton's book *Diana: Her
True Story* let the cat out of the bag. The marriage, the book
said, was a sham from the start. The royal family only wanted
her as a baby machine. As a result, she fell prey to the eating
disorder bulimia nervosa. And Charles's cold and unfeeling
behaviour drove her to attempt suicide.

While Morton stoutly denied that Diana had been the
source for his book, it became clear after her death that she had
colluded. It was quickly followed by *Fall of the House of Windsor*
by Nigel Blundell and Susan Blackhall, which took Charles's
side. Diana's petulant tantrums had alienated the royal family
and Charles had been driven into the arms of another woman
by his young wife's unreasonable behaviour. It also mentioned
the existence of the scandalous "Squidgygate tapes".

On New Year's Eve 1989 retired bank manager Cyril Reenan
and secretarial agency manager Jane Norgrove, who both listened
on non-commercial radio frequencies, independently recorded
mobile phone conversations between two people who were
lovers. They called each other "darling" and the man addressed
the woman repeatedly as "Squidgy" or "Squidge", lending the
tapes their name. For anyone who had ears to hear, the man on
the tapes was James Gilbey, the woman the Princess of Wales.

Although the tapes were touted around Fleet Street for two years, it was not until they surfaced in the US in 1992 that the *Sun* decided to run them. There were attempts to question the veracity of the tapes, but they soon proved to be the real McCoy. Now the royals had a full-scale scandal on their hands.

The tapes begin in mid-conversation, with the man asking: "And so, darling, what other lows today?" The woman replies: "I was very bad at lunch, and I nearly started blubbing. I just felt so sad and empty and thought, Bloody hell, after all I've done for this fucking family ... It's just so desperate. Always being innuendo, the fact that I'm going to do something dramatic because I can't stand the confines of this marriage ... He makes my life real torture, I've decided."

The tapes continued:

Gilbey: You know, all I want to do is to get in my car and drive around the country talking to you.

Diana: Thanks (laughs).

Gilbey: That's all I want to do, darling. I just want to see you and be with you. That's what's going to be such bliss, being back in London.

Diana: I know.

Gilbey: Kiss me, darling. (Blows kisses down the phone.)

Diana: (Blows kisses back and laughs.)

Gilbey: Squidgy, laugh some more. I love it when I hear you laughing. It makes me really happy when you laugh. Do you know I am happy when you are happy?

Diana: I know you are.

Gilbey: And I cry when you cry.

Diana: I know. So sweet. The rate we are going, we won't need any dinner on Tuesday.

Gilbey: No. I won't need any dinner actually. Just seeing you will be all I need ...

(Pause.)

Diana: Did you get my hint about Tuesday night? I think
you missed it. Think what I said.

Gilbey: No.

Diana: I think you have missed it.

Gilbey: No, you said: "At this rate, we won't want anything
to eat."

Diana: Yes.

Gilbey: Yes, I know. I got there, Tuesday night. Don't
worry, I got there. I can tell you the feeling's entirely
mutual . . .

Then they talked about making babies.

Diana: You didn't say anything about babies, did you?

Gilbey: No.

Diana: No.

Gilbey: Why darling?

Diana: (laughs) I thought you did.

Gilbey: Did you?

Diana: Yes.

Gilbey: Did you, darling? You have got them on the brain.

Diana: Well yeah, maybe I . . .

(Pause.)

Diana: I don't want to get pregnant.

Gilbey: Darling, it's not going to happen.

Diana: (Sighs.)

Gilbey: All right?

Diana: Yeah.

Gilbey: Don't worry about that. It's not going to happen,
darling. You won't get pregnant.

The tapes continued in the same vein.

Gilbey: Oh Squidgy, I love you, love you, love you.

Diana: You are the nicest person in the whole wide world.

Gilbey: Pardon?

Diana: You're just the nicest person in the whole wide world.

Gilbey: Well, darling, you are to me too.

Gilbey: You don't mind it, darling, when I want to talk to you so much?

Diana: No. I love it. Never had it before.

Gilbey: Darling, it's so nice being able to help you.

Diana: You do. You'll never know how much.

Gilbey: Oh, I will, darling. I just feel so close to you, so wrapped up in you. I'm wrapping you up, protecting.

Diana: Yes please. Yes please.

Gilbey: Oh, Squidgy.

Diana: Mmm.

Gilbey: Kiss me please. (Blows more kisses.) Do you know what I'm going to be imagining I am doing tonight at about twelve o'clock. Just holding you so close to me. It'll have to be delayed action for forty-eight hours.

Diana: (Titters.)

Gilbey: Fast forward.

Diana: Fast forward.

These were plainly two people who could not wait to get their hands on each other. But they must be careful.

Diana: I shall tell people I'm going for acupuncture and my back being done.

Gilbey: (Giggles) Squidge, cover them footsteps.

Diana: I jolly well do.

Part of the transcript was so explicit that the newspapers decided not to publish it on the grounds of decency. But journalists and other insiders knew what was said and it helped fuel the scandal. The omitted section was an indelicate discourse on masturbation.

Gilbey: Squidgy, kiss me.

(Sounds of kisses being exchanged.)

Gilbey: Oh God, it's wonderful, isn't it? This sort of feeling. Don't you like it?

Diana: I love it.

Gilbey: Umm.

Diana: I love it.

Gilbey: Isn't it absolutely wonderful? I haven't had it for years. I feel about twenty-one again.

Diana: Well, you're not. You're thirty-three.

Gilbey: Darling, mmmm. Tell me some more. It's just like sort of . . . mmmmm.

Diana: Playing with yourself.

Gilbey: What?

Diana: Nothing.

Gilbey: No, I'm not actually.

Diana: I said it's just like, just like . . .

Gilbey: Playing with yourself.

Diana: Yes.

Gilbey: Not quite as nice. Not quite as nice. No, I haven't played with myself, actually. Not for a full forty-eight hours. (They both laugh.) Not for a full forty-eight hours.

While no one could doubt the authenticity of the tapes, there was still a mystery that surrounded them. From the tapes it is plain that Gilbey was talking on the mobile phone in his car. As he drove, the call would automatically be passed from one mast to the next within the cell network. So an amateur radio enthusiast would only catch a snatch of the conversation before it jumped frequency. The recording would have to be made using a bug in the landline at Diana's end, then rebroadcast on a fixed frequency in the hope that someone would pick it up.

Suspicions fell on the security forces. Clearly, orders to tape Diana's phone would have to come from the highest authority.

Diana's supporters accused Charles, saying that he used the security forces to gather evidence he could use in a divorce, but then they had leaked the information to get his own back for Diana's collusion in *Diana: Her True Story*, which he had seen as an act of betrayal.

Gilbey went to earth, while Diana pressed home her advantage. She demanded an immediate divorce with a large financial settlement, unimpeded access to her sons and the retention of her royal titles. The Palace put out the story that Charles and Diana had had a romantic reconciliation at the annual Ghillies' Ball at Balmoral and cooperated with ITN in the production of an hour-long documentary aimed to assure the world that divorce was not on the agenda. Then the unhappy couple were despatched to South Korea. The state visit would be a glittering occasion with plenty of photo opportunities for the world's press. But it was plain from their body language that the royal couple could not stand each other.

The marriage was over and it fell to the luckless prime minister, John Major, to make a statement to the House of Commons. It was later revealed that he had also indulged in an extramarital affair with Edwina Currie when she was a fellow government minister.

"It is announced from Buckingham Palace that, with regret, the Prince and Princess of Wales have decided to separate," he told the packed chamber. "Their Royal Highnesses have no plans to divorce and their constitutional positions are unaffected. Their decision has been reached amicably, and they will both continue to participate fully in the upbringing of their children. Their Royal Highnesses will continue to carry out full and separate programmes of public engagements and will, from time to time, attend family occasions and national events together. The queen and the Duke of Edinburgh, though saddened, understand and sympathize with the difficulties that have led to this decision. Her Majesty and His Royal

Highness particularly hope that the intrusion into the privacy of the prince and princess may now cease. They believe that a degree of privacy and understanding is essential if their Royal Highnesses are to provide a happy and secure upbringing for their children, while continuing to give wholehearted commitment to their public duties."

Major added that the succession was unaffected and that, if he became king, Charles would still become head of the Church of England. Some doubt that. The *Sun* declared that John Major's statement was a "Victory for Di". But she felt that she had been outmanoeuvred by the Palace, who were out to sideline her. The story was about to take a new twist though.

There was another, even more inflammatory tape. On the night of 18 December 1989 – two weeks before the Squidgygate tapes were recorded, another amateur radio enthusiast had recorded a telephone conversation between Prince Charles and Camilla. He sold it to a national newspaper, but they decided that the content was too tawdry to use. However, in January 1993, an Australian magazine called *New Ideas* got hold of a copy of the transcript and broke the story down under. Within minutes, copies were being faxed around the world. Now there was no reason for the British papers to hold back.

It seems that Camilla was at her family home in Wiltshire – she was still married at the time. Charles was a guest at the Cheshire country home of the Duke of Westminster and lying on the bed with a mobile phone. Again the recording began when the conversation was already underway:

Charles: . . . he was a bit anxious actually.

Camilla: Was he?

Charles: He thought he might have gone a bit far.

Camilla: Ah well.

Charles: Anyway you know, that's the sort of thing one has to be aware of and sort of feel one's way along with, if you know what I mean.

Camilla: Mmm. You're awfully good at feeling your way along.

Charles: Oh stop! I want to feel my way along you, all over you and up and down you and in and out . . .

Camilla: Oh.

Charles: Particularly in and out.

Camilla: Oh, that's just what I need at the moment.

Charles: Is it?

Camilla: I know it would revive me. I can't bear a Sunday night without you.

Charles: Oh God.

Camilla: It's like that programme *Start the Week*. I can't start the week without you.

Charles: I fill up your tank.

Camilla: Yes, you do.

Charles: Then you can cope.

Camilla: Then I'm all right.

Charles: What about me? The trouble is I need you several times a week. All the time.

Camilla: Oh God, I'll just live inside your trousers or something. It would be much easier. (She laughs.) What are you going to turn into, a pair of knickers? It would be much easier. (They both laugh.) Oh, you're going to come back as a pair of knickers.

Charles: Or, God forbid, a Tampax. Just my luck. (He laughs.)

Camilla: You're a complete idiot. (She laughs.) Oh, what a wonderful idea.

Charles: My luck to be chucked down a lavatory and go on and on forever swirling around the top, never going down . . .

Camilla: Oh, darling.

Charles: . . .. until the next one comes through.

Camila: Oh, perhaps you could come back as a box.

Charles: What sort of box?

Camilla: A box of Tampax so you could just keep going.

Charles: That's true.

Camilla: Repeating yourself. (She laughs.) Oh, darling. Oh, I just want you now.

Charles: Do you?

Camilla: Mmm.

Charles: So do I.

Camilla: Desperately, desperately, desperately. I thought of you so much at Yearly.

Charles: Did you?

Camilla: Simply mean that we couldn't be there together.

Charles: Desperate. If you could be here – I long to ask Nancy sometimes.

Camilla: Why don't you?

Charles: I daren't.

Camilla: Because I think she's so in love with you.

Charles: Mmm.

And so it goes on. She tells him that she loves him eleven times; he tells her twice. She calls him "darling" eighteen times; he calls her "darling" seven times. Her husband is referred to dismissively as "A" or simply "him". At one stage, she says, "He won't be here Thursday, pray God."

They arrange an assignation. Then she tells him to get some sleep and to call her in the morning. Then they say goodnight to each other no fewer than nineteen times. The final sequence goes like this:

Camilla: . . . night, night.

Charles: Night, darling, God bless.

Camilla: I do love you and I am so proud of you.

Charles: Oh, I am so proud of you.

Camilla: Don't be silly, I've never achieved anything.

Charles: Yes, you have.

Camilla: No, I haven't.

Charles: Your great achievement is to love me.

Camilla: Oh darling. Easier than falling off a chair.

Charles: You suffer all these indignities and tortures and calumnies.

Camilla: Oh darling, don't be so silly. I'd suffer anything for you. That's love. It's the strength of love. Night, night.

Charles: Night, darling. Sounds as though you're dragging an enormous piece of string behind you, with hundreds of tin pots and cans attached to it. I think it must be your telephone. Night, night, before the battery goes. (He blows a kiss.) Night.

Camilla: Love you.

Charles: Don't want to say goodbye.

Camilla: Neither do I, but you must get some sleep. Bye.

Charles: Bye, darling.

Camilla: Love you.

Charles: Bye.

Camilla: Hopefully talk to you in the morning.

Charles: Please.

Camilla: Bye. I do love you.

Charles: Night.

Camilla: Night.

Charles: Night.

Camilla: Love you forever.

Charles: Night.

Camilla: Goodbye. Bye, my darling.

Charles: Night.

Camilla: Night, night.

Charles: Night.

Camilla: Bye, bye.

Charles: Going.

Camilla: Bye.

Charles: Going.

Camilla: Gone.

Charles: Night.

Camilla: Bye. Press the button.

Charles: Going to press the tit.

Camilla: All right, darling. I wish you were pressing mine.

Charles: God, I wish I was. Harder and harder.

Camilla: Oh darling.

Charles: Night.

Charles: Love you.

(Camilla yawns.)

Camilla: Love you. Press the tit.

Charles: Adore you. Night.

Camilla: Night.

Camilla: Night.

(Camilla blows a kiss.)

Charles: Night.

Camilla: Goodnight my darling. Love you . . .

Finally Charles hangs up – no doubt, to the great relief of the reader.

Not only was the Tampax exchange distasteful, no one could figure out why a man who was married to one of the most beautiful women in the world should be besotted by a woman who, not to put too fine a point on it, needed ironing. She was thirteen years older than his radiant young wife and over a year older than him.

Again there were concerns about where the Tampax tape had come from. The author and former MI6 officer James Rushbridger pointed the finger at GCHQ, the government listening centre in Cheltenham. A year later he was found hanged in his West Country home in mysterious circumstances.

The next blow in the "War of the Waleses" came from James Hewitt. In 1994, a "novelized" version of the torrid love affair between Hewitt and Diana called *Princess in Love* was published by Anna Pasternak, a distant relative of the author of *Dr Zhivago* and former girlfriend of Hewitt.

Then the battlefield moved to the TV. Diana appeared on *Panorama*, where she admitted committing adultery and begged to be "Queen of Hearts". However, having admitted to being unfaithful to the heir to the throne, she was technically admitting treason, but no one from the Metropolitan Police Force was sent to arrest her.

Charles responded by filming an extended TV interview with an obsequious Jonathan Dimbleby, giving him the chance to plug his authorized biography of Charlie boy. He too admitted adultery and having three separate affairs with the winsome Mrs Camilla Parker Bowles.

Diana threw herself into a new charm offensive. She seized numerous photo opportunities showing her with sick children and began a one-woman campaign against landmines. She won a £15-million divorce settlement, but was forced to cash in the title "Her Royal Highness". Rumours that she was having an affair with England rugby captain Will Carling lost him his wife, but did little to dent Diana's popularity.

However, she misjudged things when she began an affair with Dodi Fayed, son of Harrods' boss Mohamed Fayed. Fayed senior had been refused a British passport and there had been questions about his business methods. And while Dodi Fayed himself listed his profession as "movie producer", the newspapers referred to him more accurately as "millionaire playboy".

Dodi and Diana's love blossomed on his yacht on the Côte d'Azur in front of the telephoto lenses of the world's paparazzi. Meanwhile, Charles walked out with the freshly divorced Camilla, laying on her fiftieth birthday bash. They could hardly compete.

Milking the publicity his son's royal affair afforded him, Mohamed Fayed bought the house in Paris where Edward and Mrs Simpson, the last British royals to be ousted by scandal, had spent their exile. There were rumours of marriage. Was this to have been the Princess of Wales's home too?

It seems they might have been heading there, on the night of 30 August 1997, after a romantic dinner at the Ritz Hotel in Paris when their car smashed into a pillar in an underpass, killing them both.

Any criticism of Di ended right there. Fears that the mother of the heir to the throne – and hence a future head of the Church of England – might marry a Muslim were quietly forgotten, as was any further mention of the fact that Di's marriage to Dodi would be opposed by the establishment because he was, shall we say, tinted. However, the idea that the powers that be were so against the match that they had the happy couple bumped off has spawned a lively new outlet for conspiracy theorists, encouraged by Mohamed Fayed, who claimed M16 had knocked them off on the orders of the Duke of Edinburgh.

The press, perhaps feeling a little guilty over their own role in the hounding of Di, now went into reverse. The fairy-tale princess had died in the arms of her handsome young sheikh. When the royal family maintained their usual regal decorum, they were pilloried for being cold, old-fashioned and out of touch. The fresh young modernizing Prime Minister Tony Blair had to step in, dubbing Diana "the People's Princess".

Nevertheless the tabloid-reading public blamed the paparazzi for pursuing Di to her death. Echoing public sentiment, the press were vilified from the pulpit at the funeral by Diana's brother, the adulterous Earl Spencer, whose own messy divorce was already attracting the newspapers' disapprobation.

Now Prince Charles had no one to upstage him on the global stage. Soon there were pictures of him in a kilt teaching his sons rural pursuits that they, plainly, had no interest in. Camilla emerged as dowdy stepmother-in-waiting. In 2005, she and Charles married in a civil ceremony, despite doubts about its legality. The Marriage Act of 1836 specifically excludes members of the royal family from contracting civil marriages, not to mention the fact that Camilla's first husband was a Catholic. But, then the royal family hold themselves above the law.

The twenty-first century has now had its fairy-tale wedding with the nuptials of Prince William and Kate Middleton in 2011. Both are young and have the rest of their lives to entertain us with their sex scandals.

## Mike Tindall

Six weeks after marrying Zara Phillips, thirteenth in line to the throne, Mike Tindall was leading the England rugby team at the World Cup in New Zealand where he was caught kissing and groping a girl in a nightclub.

According to the *Sun*:

> One particularly beautiful blonde went straight for Mike. But rather than reject her advances, unfortunately he was extremely responsive. They were flirting with each other and getting very touchy-feely. Then they went into the doorway, where the girl gestured Mike towards her chest.
>
> She pulled his head towards her breasts and she rubbed the back of his head as she did so. The girl was absolutely stunning and all over him. He clearly thought it was a case of 'What happens on tour, stays on tour'. But it's not the behaviour you would expect of a man who is not only England captain but also now a member of the Royal Family.

He was later seen canoodling with his ex, twenty-nine-year-old Jessica Palmer. Spotting the danger signs, Zara flew to New Zealand to see what was going on down under. But after they returned to the Northern Hemisphere for a belated honeymoon in Cyprus, they were seen to kiss and make up.

Zara may not have chastised him, but the Rugby Football Union were not amused. They fined him £15,000 and booted him out of England's elite players squad, but then had him back. Not such a naughty boy then.

## Edward and Mrs Simpson

The Abdication Crisis of 1936 was a sex scandal like no other because, for the British people, it came like a bolt from the blue. As Prince of Wales, Edward VIII, or David as he was then known, had been popular. He had visited the front during World War I and genuinely seemed to sympathize with the plight of the unemployed during the Great Depression. But for several years, he had been having a torrid affair with American divorcee Wallis Simpson. He wanted to marry her and thought he could when he came to the throne in January 1936.

While the foreign press was full of the royal romance, the newspaper barons in Britain were pillars of the establishment and nothing about the relationship was published. But once the new king had come to the throne, the matter was bound to come to a head. The American papers were predicting that they marry before Edward's coronation, scheduled for May 1937, so that Wallis could be crowned queen alongside him. But they had not counted on the redoubtable Prime Minister Stanley Baldwin who was implacably against the match.

Over the years the waters have become muddied. Some say that the government opposed the marriage because Wallis Simpson was an American. Others think it was because she was a divorcee – twice over. Still others say it was because she was a commoner. And there are those who believe that Edward had already exhibited pro-Fascist sympathies and that the scandal surrounding the marriage was simply an excuse to oust him.

Ironically, the crisis was sparked by someone who knew nothing about the affair. The Bishop of Bradford, Dr Alfred Blunt, spoke out against the king's playboy lifestyle in the diocesan conference in December 1936. True, before he met

Mrs Simpson, David had been a bit of a playboy, siring two illegitimate children along the way.

His first sexual experience was in a brothel in Calais on his way to the front during World War I. He said he found the prostitutes "perfectly filthy and revolting", but that did not stop him having a second go in Amiens, or taking up with a courtesan in Paris.

Returning to England, he began seeing Lady Sybil Cadogan, but was soon in love with Mrs Marian Coke, a married woman twelve years older than him. It was convenient to have affairs with married women. One of his long-time lovers was Freda Dudley Ward, the wife of a Liberal MP. She was half-American and they met during a Zeppelin raid when she ran into a house where he was having dinner to take cover. The affair lasted several years though there were many others along the way. They came from a class that would not kiss-and-tell in the newspapers. Besides, the owners of Fleet Street were peers of the realm and it was not in their interests that such things were printed.

The Prince of Wales liked Americans. He visited the US several times and set his cap at Audrey James, the daughter of an American industrialist. She rebuffed his advances while single but, once married, she succumbed.

Next came Lady Thelma Furness, the daughter of an American diplomat. She was both married and a divorcee. At sixteen, she had eloped with a man twice her age. The marriage did not last. Once she had got rid of her first husband, she snared Viscount Furness, who was famous for his consumption of brandy and women.

Lady Furness accompanied Edward on safari in Kenya in 1930. There, she said, she felt "as if we were the only two people in the world". In her diary she recorded: "This was our Eden, and we were alone in it. His arms about me were the only reality; his words of love my only bridge to life. Borne along on the mounting tide of his ardour, I felt myself inexorably swept from the accustomed moorings of caution. Every night I felt more completely possessed by our love."

This is definitely a step up from Squidgygate or the Tampax tapes.

The affair came to an end when she had a fling with Prince Aly Khan, racehorse owner and head of the Ismaili Muslims. At the age of eighteen, he had been trained in the art of delaying ejaculation in the brothels of Cairo. He had so perfected the technique that, in aristocratic circles, it was said, like Father Christmas, he only came once a year.

With competition like this, the Prince of Wales could hardly stand up. Thelma openly complained of Edward's poor sexual performance and that he was not very well endowed, scandalizing society by openly calling him "the little man". This had not gone unnoticed. When he was at Osborne Naval College, the other pupils joked that he should be called "Sardines" rather than "Whales".

Ill equipped to satisfy women, he may well have experimented with men. The gay writer Lytton Strachey tried to pick him up once in the Tate Gallery, only to flee when he realized who his prey was. Later, Strachey wrote ruing what might have been.

When Dr Blunt spoke out, Edward had been faithful to Mrs Simpson for several years. But the Bishop's ill-judged remarks breached the dam.

The press pact was already under strain. Soon after Edward came to the throne, he began to put his marriage plans into action. First he had to arrange a speedy divorce for Mrs Simpson. Her husband Ernest was discovered in the bedroom of a Thames-side hotel with a professional co-respondent named Buttercup Kennedy. When Lord Beaverbrook, the Canadian-born owner of the *Express* newspaper group, heard that the divorce proceedings were to be heard at Ipswich on 27 October 1936, he called Mrs Simpson's solicitor and warned him that he intended to report the proceedings in the London *Evening Standard*. The solicitor assured him that Mrs

Simpson had no intention of marrying the king and that the notoriety that her friendship had brought her was causing her great distress. Beaverbrook bought it and, together with Lord Rothermere, owner of the *Daily Mail*, persuaded the rest of the papers to continue their code of silence on the matter.

However, the pressmen did turn up for the divorce hearings, but they were locked in the courtroom, while Mrs Simpson made her escape. Two enterprising photographers tried to photograph her as she sped away in a car driven by the king's chauffeur, only to have their cameras smashed by the police. Nevertheless, while the divorce proceedings did make the British papers, they were published without comment.

In America, it was a sensation. One newspaper ran the memorable headline KING'S MOLL RENO'ED and they began calling Wallis Simpson "Queen Wally". Even the House of Commons began to suspect something was going on. On 17 November 1936, Labour MP Ellen Wilkinson asked the President of the Board of Trade why two or three pages had been ripped from distinguished American magazines that were coming into the country.

"What is it that the British public are not allowed to know?" she asked.

It was not until 3 December, when Dr Blunt made his remarks that she got an answer. Although Dr Blunt claimed that he knew nothing about Mrs Simpson, the newspapers assumed he did. As a senior churchman, he was an insider. The establishment, the press thought, were breaking ranks. Suddenly, the whole thing was out in the open and a national debate raged.

"Why shouldn't the king marry his cutie?" asked Winston Churchill.

"Because England does not want Queen Cutie," replied Noël Coward.

Stones were thrown through the windows of Mrs Simpson's London home. Letters and telegrams of abuse arrived by the sack full. Terrified, she fled to the South of France.

Edward's mother, Queen Mary, was against the marriage instinctively. But Baldwin's opposition was more reasoned. If the abdication of the king would cause a scandal, his marriage would cause a bigger one. The British secret service had already compiled a weighty dossier on Mrs Simpson's activities. It did not make pretty reading, especially if the papers got their hands on it.

Of Virginian stock, Wallis had been born in Baltimore. Her first husband, navy flier Lieutenant Earl Winfield "Win" Spencer had been an alcoholic and a sadist who liked to tie her to the bed and beat her. He had numerous extramarital affairs with both men and women. Wallis, for her part, launched herself on the diplomatic scene in Washington, bedding the Italian ambassador and a senior Argentine diplomat who was said to be the best tango dancer in DC.

In a belated honeymoon, Win took her on a trip to the Far East where together, and separately, they visited the brothels of Shanghai and Hong Kong. Wallis particularly liked watching girls performing lesbian acts and would sometimes join in threesomes without her husband. In these famous "singing houses", Wallis learnt the ancient erotic arts of Fang Chung. In ancient China, emperors would employ a mature woman as a sexual adviser to pick new wives and concubines for him, and advise him how to satisfy the hundreds of wives and concubines he accumulated. Over the centuries, these women had distilled their knowledge of sex into pillow books.

Fang Chung is a method of relaxing a sexual partner. It involves massaging hot oil into their nipples, stomach and inner thighs. Only when the recipient is totally relaxed are the genitals addressed. Those adept at Fang Chung are said to be able to arouse even the most passionless of men by concentrating on the nerve centres and delicate brushing of the skin.

Despite Wallis's growing abilities in the erotic arts, Win decided that he was gay after all and moved in with a handsome young artist. This left Wallis free to practise her newfound techniques on a string of other men. These included a young American called Robbie, the Italian naval attaché Count Galeazzo Ciano, who would become Italy's foreign minister after he married Mussolini's daughter, and American millionaire Herman Rogers. With Rogers's wife Katherine, they set up a ménage à trois. Around this time, Wallis suffered a botched abortion that left her unable to bear children.

Wallis met her second husband Ernest Simpson, a British subject, in New York. He, too, was married, but they quickly divorced their respective spouses and moved to London. Married life changed nothing. They were members of a fast set that included the Mountbattens and Lady Thelma Furness. Wallis went on a women-only holiday to the South of France with Consuela Thaw and Gloria Vanderbilt, who was having a lesbian love affair with Nada, wife of the Marquess of Milton Haven and lover of Edwina Mountbatten, at the time. Consuela and Wallis shared a bedroom. And they went out together on the pull.

After Wallis was introduced to the Prince of Wales by Lady Furness, the two of them would often make up a foursome with Wallis's husband and Mary Raffray, Ernest Simpson's mistress. In 1934, the prince holidayed with Mrs Simpson in Biarritz. Sadly, Mr Simpson could not join the party, so Wallis was chaperoned by her aunt Bessie.

In February 1935, the prince was photographed with Mrs Simpson leaving a lingerie shop in Kitzbühel where they were enjoying a skiing holiday together. In May, the gossip came home to London when the prince danced with Mrs Simpson at his parents' Silver Jubilee Ball.

In June, he told the British Legion that they should extend the hand of friendship to Germany, where Hitler had come to power two years earlier. Meanwhile, Wallis found a way to express her pro-German sympathies more directly. It was rumoured that she was having a brief fling with the German ambassador to the court of St James, Joachim von Ribbentrop, who later became Hitler's foreign minister. But that did not stop her holidaying with the prince in the South of France and then on Corsica.

On 27 May 1936, the new king invited Mr and Mrs Baldwin to dinner – along with the Mountbattens and the notorious swingers the Duff Coopers – to meet Wallis. Baldwin was impressed by her and with how much the king loved her. But he knew that a woman with her track record could not become queen.

The British press respected the king's privacy when he set off on a cruise in the Adriatic with Mrs Simpson that summer, but the rest of the world's press and the newsreels followed their every move. They noted that her husband was nowhere to be seen. The Foreign Office was outraged when The king paid an unauthorized visit to the Greek dictator Ioannis Metaxas, who drove them through cheering crowds. Mrs Simpson was received like a queen. They also visited Kemal Ataturk, Turkey's dictator, and invited him on a state visit to Britain. All this was done without the knowledge of the British government or parliament. Edward was getting above himself.

Baldwin bided his time and waited for public opinion to turn against the king. Edward cancelled a visit to Aberdeen to open a hospital extension, sending his brother instead, on the grounds that the court was still in mourning. However, Edward had already been on a Mediterranean cruise and been seen at Ascot. It was noted that, at the time of the hospital visit, rather than being in mourning, the king was actually hosting a house party at Balmoral. According to the Court Circular, Mrs Simpson was on the guest list.

While the press barons were still keeping the news out of the British papers, the Canadians knew what was going on and were sending letters of protest to the government and prominent members of the establishment in London.

Baldwin put pressure on the king to halt Mrs Simpson's divorce proceedings. Edward refused on the grounds that it would be wrong to interfere in Mrs Simpson affairs as she was "just a friend". From Edward's point of view, there could be no delay. As Mrs Simpson would have to wait six months after the decree nisi was issued before she got a decree absolute and could marry again, if she was to be by his side at his coronation in May, the divorce had to go ahead as planned.

Friends counselled caution. If he waited until he was crowned, he could introduce Mrs Simpson slowly to the public. Once he got the people on his side, he could marry her. He rejected this, saying that he would be "being crowned with a lie on my lips".

Once the divorce was completed, Baldwin knew nothing could prevent a constitutional crisis. In mid-November, he called a Cabinet meeting to discuss what could be done. The rest of the government were with him, firmly rejecting any marriage to Mrs Simpson. But Edward was not without his supporters. He set out for Wales where thousands of unemployed miners turned out to sing hymns of praise, in Welsh, to the man they still considered to be their champion.

Once Dr Blunt had broken the press pact, Edward withdrew to his country house, Fort Belvedere, near Virginia Water in Surrey, and spent hours on the phone to Wallis who was in Cannes. They had already discussed the possibility of a morganatic marriage, one that denied her and her heirs any position in the succession. Edward put this to Baldwin. Under the 1931 Statute of Westminster, to make any alteration to the succession required not just the approval of the British parliament, but also the parliaments of all the Dominions. Under the king's instructions, Baldwin put it to them. They rejected it.

In Britain, not only the government was against the marriage, but the opposition was against it too. Baldwin told the king that, if he married against the government's advice, he would resign and force an election on the issue.

With the press now free to discuss the matter, the king could get some sense of public opinion. The *Daily Mirror* issued a challenge on its front page.

"God save the King," it said. "Tell us the facts Mr Baldwin . . . The nation insists on knowing the king's full demands and conditions . . . The nation will give you its verdict."

Others were not so equivocal. They mistrusted Mrs Simpson's hold over the king and her Nazi sympathies. It was rumoured that Mrs Simpson was blackmailing him, that Edward had punched his brother the Duke of Gloucester on the nose for criticizing the liaison, that the next in line to the throne, the Duke of York, was an epileptic, that American newspaper tycoon William Randolph Hearst had offered £250,000 for Mrs Simpson to file her divorce petition in America and name the king as co-respondent and that the king was a closet Fascist. This last was not without foundation. He refused to meet the exiled king of Abyssinia, ousted by the Italian invasion, when asked to do so by the Foreign Secretary.

Although there were, on balance, more papers against the marriage than for it, the embattled couple did not think that the situation was irretrievably lost. Mrs Simpson suggested that the king take a leaf out of the American president's book and go on the radio for a cosy "fireside chat". She felt sure that when his people heard the story of their romance from the king himself, they would back him.

Edward agreed, but he showed a draft to Baldwin who pointed out that such an appeal to the people over the heads of the government was unconstitutional. Baldwin insisted that whatever the king did he should not divide the British people. The king offered to abdicate.

Wallis Simpson issued a press release, offering to withdraw from the situation. She even sent a message to the prime minister, offering to drop her divorce petition. But it was too late. The king had been outmanoeuvred by Baldwin. Even his one parliamentary champion Winston Churchill gave up after being shouted down in the House of Commons.

"Our cock won't fight," said Beaverbrook.

On Thursday, 10 December 1936, just seven days after the scandal had broken in the press, Edward signed the Instrument of Abdication, renouncing the crown of Great Britain and Ireland. He also resigned as head of state of the Dominions and as Emperor of India, and all the other titles and positions those posts entailed. He did, however, keep the £1 million settled on him by his grandmother Queen Alexandra.

The following day, Edward was driven to Windsor where he broadcast to the Empire explaining that he could no longer go on being king without the woman he loved. The whole world listened. People wept openly. Even tough New York cab drivers pulled over, amazed that the king of Great Britain would renounce everything for the love of a woman. This, everyone agreed, must be the greatest love story ever told.

Well, not exactly. Cynics have suggested that the tricks that Wallis picked up in the singing houses of China were deployed to such good effect that the thought of living without her was unbearable. She was also adept at fellatio and, it is said, had an operation to have her vagina tightened to help stimulate his undersized genitals.

Prominent socialite Lady Ottoline Morrell claimed he was also taking injections to make him more virile that were driving him quite mad. There was also talk of him being a foot fetishist, which Wallis ruthlessly exploited. She also acted as his dominatrix. One day, in front of friends, she turned to Edward and ordered: "Take off my dirty shoes and bring me another pair." To everyone's amazement, he did.

There was talk of elaborate nanny–child scenes enacted

between them. Freda Dudley Ward also commented on this side of his nature.

"He made himself the slave of whomsoever he loved and became totally dependent on her," she said. "It was his nature; he was like a masochist. He liked being humbled, degraded. He begged for it."

After the broadcast, Edward sailed into exile on-board a Royal Navy destroyer. This was ironic as the current joke was that Edward had resigned as Admiral of the Fleet only to sign on as third mate on a Baltimore tramp.

In June 1937, Edward and Mrs Simpson married in France. No members of the royal family attended the ceremony and most of their friends stayed away. He was created Duke of Windsor. Although he retained his HRH, the Duchess was refused one. "A damnable wedding present," he called it.

But that was not the end of the scandal. In the run up to the war, Edward and Wallis paid a social call on Adolf Hitler. That Edward was sympathetic was beyond doubt. He encouraged friends to contribute to the Nazi cause and liked to speak German in private.

In 1937, he told a cheering crowd in Leipzig: "What I have seen in Germany is a miracle."

At the outbreak of World War II, he joined the British Army, but he was considered a security risk. When France fell he sought refuge in Fascist Spain with friends who were openly pro-German. There was even talk that, should Britain fall, Edward would be restored to the throne as Hitler's vassal.

To get him out of harm's way, the government despatched Edward to Bermuda as governor general. There he became embroiled with illicit currency deals, making money out of the war. This all went disastrously wrong when one of his friends, Sir Harry Oakes, who was also involved, was murdered. A relative of Oakes's was framed but, in court, was acquitted. No one has ever got to the bottom of the Oakes scandal.

Low-level scandal continued to follow the Duke and Duchess of Windsor for the rest of their lives. By the fifties, rumours spread that Wallis had grown tired of his cloying love and was seen everywhere with Woolworth heir Jimmy Donahue.

Donahue was homosexual, but the rumour was that Wallis was trying to convert him. Others said that it was the Duke that was sleeping with Donahue, although it was widely known that he despised all homosexuals.

Noël Coward, who moved in the same circles as the Windsors after the abdication, explained the situation.

"I like Jimmy," he said. "He's an insane camp but he is fun. I like the Duchess; she is the fag hag to end all fag hags, but that's what makes her likeable. The Duke . . . well, although he pretends not to hate me, he does because I'm queer and he's queer. However, unlike him, I don't pretend not to be. Here she's got a royal queen to sleep with and a rich one to hump."

The Duke and Duchess lived out the rest of their lives in Paris. The Duke never set foot in England again. But when he died in 1972, at the age of seventy-seven, his body was flown home. He was laid in state for two days in St George's Chapel, Windsor. Nearly 58,000 people filed past his body.

## Bertie, Prince of Wales

While Edward VIII's one public peccadillo robbed him of the crown, his grandfather Edward VII's life was attended by sexual scandal every step of the way and he got away with it. When he was just fifteen, he was in Königswinter on the Rhine to improve his German, and he groped a serving wench and tried to kiss her. Prime Minister William Ewart Gladstone, that great reformer of fallen women, condemned his behaviour as "this squalid debauch, a paltry affair, an unworthy indulgence".

At Oxford, the Prince of Wales – universally known as "Bertie" – began a life of drunkenness, debauchery and gluttony under the tutelage of the flamboyant aristocrat

Henry Chaplin, known to one and all as "Magnifico". At the sumptuous meals laid on by Magnifico's private chef, Bertie was regaled by stories of London life – the womanizing, the dog fights, the boxing matches, the opium dens and the brothels. Life in Oxford was tame by comparison, but the story is told of Bertie and Magnifico meeting a peasant woman on a country road. They pulled her dress up over her head and stuffed a five-pound note into her drawers.

After Oxford, Bertie was sent to the army and posted to the Curragh, a military camp near Dublin. After a drunken mess party, his fellow officers decided that nineteen-year-old Bertie should lose his virginity. They put a naked young girl, an actress named Nellie Clifden, in his bed. Bertie plainly enjoyed the experience. His diary for 1861 records: "September 6, NC First time; September 9, NC Second time; September 10, NC Third time . . ."

Gossip about Bertie and his "Princess of Wales" soon reached the London clubs, the foreign press and then the ears of the queen. She was appalled, especially as Nellie was also sharing her affections with Charles Wynn-Carrington, later governor of New South Wales. Prince Albert warned that if his son did not stop the affair "the consequences for this country and for the world would be too dreadful".

"I knew that you were thoughtless and weak," wrote Prince Albert, "but I could not think you depraved!"

He travelled to Cambridge to tell his son off in person. But there was an outbreak of typhoid in the city at the time. Prince Albert caught it and died.

To save him from further scandal, Bertie was married off to the Danish Princess Alexandra of Schleswig-Holstein-Sonderburg-Glucksburg. Immediately after their wedding in 1863, Bertie and his bride moved into their own private residence, Marlborough House in Pall Mall. Freed from the constraints of Queen Victoria's court, which was still in mourning, the prince began partying in earnest.

While he loved his wife, Bertie could not resist pretty women. Fortunately, Alexandra was happy to stay home with the children while he gallivanted. Despite his love of gambling, sumptuous food, fine wines, good cigars and amorous adventures, Bertie was surprisingly popular, especially compared to his mother who had swathed herself in black and withdrawn from public life. Bertie turned the London social scene into one long round of banquets, balls and gala nights out. The only person he was not popular with was Queen Victoria, who still blamed him for the death of her beloved Albert. She kept up a constant barrage of letters condemning his debauched lifestyle.

As well as relishing the high life, the Prince of Wales also took his pleasure in the low life, visiting brothels and illegal cockfights. With photography still in its infancy, Bertie could enjoy a discreet tryst with a young woman in Cremorne Pleasure Gardens in Chelsea or sex with a lady of the street in the back of a hansom cab without much fear of appearing on the front page.

Nevertheless, for the sake of discretion, he would often indulge himself abroad. As a young man he had enjoyed himself in Egypt and the Middle East, but it was easier to travel to the debauched spa towns of Germany, particularly Marienbad. One prostitute travelled all the way from Vienna to sleep with him there. When she found that he was otherwise occupied, she insisted that another gentleman from his entourage enjoy her favours so she could cover the train fare.

In Paris, Bertie became something of a legend. One brothel, Le Chabanais, carried his coat of arms over the bed in one of its rooms. It also contained a copper tub with a half-woman half-swan figurehead where he would bathe in champagne with selected prostitutes. The tub was later bought by the surrealist painter Salvador Dalí. Bertie also kept a specially constructed *siege d'amour* there. This was a "love seat", allowing easier access to oral and other types of sex to the overweight prince and two or more women. The chair is now owned by the Soubrier furniture-making family, who originally custom-built it for Bertie.

The Duc de Gramont took him to visit Guilia Beneni, who worked under the name of La Barucci and proudly claimed to be the "greatest whore in the world". On being introduced, she promptly let her dress fall to the ground, without a word of warning. When she was reprimanded for this breach of protocol, she exclaimed: "What, did you not tell me to behave properly to His Royal Highness? I showed him the best I have, and it was free!"

Bertie also asked to see Cora Pearl, a prostitute from Plymouth whom Napoleon III had once paid £10,000 for a single night. She had herself served up to the prince on a silver salver. When the lid was removed, she was naked except for a string of pearls and a sprig of parsley.

These excesses went unreported. However, when Bertie took up with Hortense Schneider, a singer and actress so well known for distributing her favours to European royalty she was known as Le Passage des Princes, *The Times* condemned this scandalous "friendship".

In an attempt to be more discreet, he began passing himself off as the Duke of Lancaster or the Earl of Chester. But his portly figure and his whiskers were so well known that, when he visited the Moulin Rouge one night, a dancer yelled from the stage: "Hello, Wales."

He had a long affair with Princesse de Sagan. But her son grew jealous. One day, when he found the Prince of Wales's discarded clothes outside his mother's bedroom door, he threw them in a fountain. The Prince of Wales had to find his way back to his hotel in a pair of borrowed trousers that were far too small.

Back in England, the prince used the Earl of Rosebery's London home for his afternoon's entertaining, later moving to the ultra-discreet Cavendish Hotel in Jermyn Street. Largely, the public tolerated his shenanigans with chorus girls and prostitutes, but it was a different matter when he was subpoenaed to appear in a divorce case.

The lady concerned was Harriet Moncreiffe, one of the eight beautiful daughters of Sir Thomas Moncreiffe of that Ilk. She had been a close friend of the prince's before her marriage, at eighteen, to Sir Charles Mordaunt, the Conservative MP for South Warwickshire.

The year after their wedding, in 1866, Mordaunt noticed his wife reading a letter from the notorious Bertie.

"I don't approved of your friendship with the prince," he said.

On one occasion it is said that Mordaunt returned home to find his wife with the prince and two white ponies. After expelling Bertie from the premises, he had the two ponies shot in her presence.

In 1869, Harriet gave birth to a daughter, who doctors feared was blind. Harriet became hysterical. When Mordaunt tried to comfort his wife, she said: "Charlie, I have deceived you. The child is not yours. It is Lord Cole's."

The implication was that the child's eyesight problems were caused by syphilis caught from Viscount Cole, the third son of the Earl of Enniskillen. She went on to confess to sleeping with Lord Lucan, the man responsible for the disastrous Charge of the Light Brigade, Sir Frederic Johnstone, the Prince of Wales and others. Apparently, the prince had made a habit of visiting her at home several times a week. When Bertie's interest flagged, Lord Cole and Sir Frederic Johnstone, friends from his Oxford days, took over as her suitors.

Furious, Mordaunt broke into his wife's writing desk to find a Valentine card from the prince along with one of his monogrammed handkerchiefs and a dozen letters. He also found letters from Lucan and hotel bills made out to Johnstone. Immediately, Mordaunt began divorce proceedings, citing Sir Frederic Johnstone and Lord Cole as co-respondents, along with "others" – generally thought to include the Prince of Wales.

Bertie was summonsed. Both his wife and his mother were sympathetic. Queen Victoria wrote to the Lord Chancellor, saying: "The fact of the Prince of Wales's intimate acquaintanceship with a young married woman being publicly proclaimed will show an amount of impudence, which cannot but damage him in the eyes of the middle and lower classes, which is to be deeply lamented, in these days when the higher classes, in their frivolous, selfish and pleasure-seeking lives, do more to increase the spirit of democracy than anything else."

The Lord Chancellor regretfully told the queen that there was no way the Prince of Wales could be excused. The prince's own solicitor, Sir George Lewis told Bertie: "You must go into the witness-box. It is the only way to clear your name."

Meanwhile Harriet fled to her father's home in Perthshire, where an eminent physician found no sign of syphilis on her or the child. However, her emotional state had begun to deteriorate, so her father petitioned the divorce courts, arguing that she could not be sued due to her mental condition. Mordaunt claimed that she was feigning madness to save herself from public disgrace. But the divorce petition was put on hold and, in 1869, a trial was ordered to determine Harriet's sanity.

When the trial opened before Lord Penzance on 23 February 1870, evidence was presented that Harriet had tried to kill her own child, smeared herself with excrement, walked around the house at night naked except for stockings and a cloak and had tried to batter down the butler's door with a hammer. Mordaunt's barrister quickly conceded that Harriet was, indeed, insane.

But that was not the end of the case. Johnstone wanted to clear his name. This was unfortunate for Viscount Cole as extracts from Harriet's diary seemed to indicate that he was indeed the father of her child, conceived while her husband was away on a fishing trip in Norway.

The Prince of Wales was then called to the stand. He admitted a close friendship with Harriet Mordaunt. She had visited him frequently at Marlborough House. Then came the crucial question: "Has there ever been any improper familiarity or criminal act between yourself and Lady Mordaunt?"

The prince was emphatic. "There has not," he said.

The jury took less than ten minutes to find Lady Mordaunt unfit to plead. But the damage had been done. *Reynold's Newspaper* wanted to know why the prince was "so eager to pay weekly visits to a young married woman when her husband was absent, if it was all so innocent?" And it accused him of "bringing dishonour to the homestead of an English gentleman". He was booed when he arrived at Ascot with Princess Alexandra and a meeting in Hyde Park called for the abolition of the monarchy.

The scandal did not cause Bertie to mend his ways. In 1871, the widowed Lady Susan Pelham-Clinton wrote to him telling him that she was six or seven months pregnant. "Without any funds to meet the necessary expenses and to buy the discretion of servants, it is impossible to keep this sad secret," she said.

Bertie gave her £250 and sent her to Ramsgate with his personal physician.

In 1875, Bertie was embroiled in another scandalous divorce. During a royal tour of India, his companion Lord Aylesford received a letter from his wife, saying she was eloping with the Marquess of Blandford.

"Blandford is the greatest blackguard alive," commented the prince, sympathetically, neglecting to mention that he, too, had enjoyed Lady Aylesford's favours.

Lord Aylesford dashed home to begin divorce proceedings. Both the families of Lady Aylesford and the Marquess of Blandford tried to hush up the matter. When Aylesford refused to drop his suit, Blandford's brother Randolph Churchill, Winston's father, asked the Prince of Wales to intercede. He refused, so Churchill went to Princess Alexandra and told her of her husband's involvement with Lady Aylesford. He had copies of their letters that he threatened to make public if the prince would not rally to his support.

Bertie was outraged. He challenged Churchill to a duel in France. This was ridiculous. They both knew it. Duels were illegal and Churchill could hardly look forward to a comfortable future if he shot the heir to the throne. What's more, it would hardly endear him to his wife, the American beauty Jenny Jerome, Winston's mother, who was another of Bertie's mistresses.

The queen again supported her errant son. Princess Alexandra went very publicly to meet her husband when he returned from India. That night, the royal couple made a great show of going to the opera together. Crowds that had booed him before now cheered and clapped.

Ironically, Bertie's greatest popularity came with his very public liaison with Lillie Langtry, "the Jersey Lily". The daughter of a clergyman, Lillie – née Emilie Charlotte Le Breton – had been born on the island of Jersey and longed to get off it.

At the age of twenty, she saw a yacht in the harbour. "To become mistress of that yacht," she said, "I married the owner."

His name was Edward Langtry. A widower, his family owned shipyards in Belfast. But he was a brute. When other men paid compliments to Lillie's stunning good looks, he said, "You should have seen my first wife."

When they arrived in London three years later, the violet-eyed Lillie was the smash of the season. Artists begged her to sit for them and her image became very popular on postcards, which had recently been introduced. She was next to the Prince of Wales at a dinner party given by Arctic explorer Sir Allen Young.

Princess Alexandra was away at the time. When she returned, Bertie and Lillie were the talk of the town. They dined out together openly and rode together in Hyde Park. In Paris, he kissed her in full view of everyone in the middle of the dance floor at Maxim's. He built the Red House, now Langtry Manor Hotel, in Bournemouth to her design as a private retreat.

"I've spent enough on you to build a battleship," he once complained.

"And you've spent enough in me to float one," she replied.

Lillie revelled in the notoriety that being a royal mistress gave her. She had her negligees trimmed with ermine. Society matrons such as Lady Cadogan would stand on chairs just to catch a glimpse of her. And she was so famous that she hardly dared venture out on the streets.

"People ran after me in droves," she complained, "staring me out of countenance and even lifting my shade to satisfy their curiosity."

Although the whole world knew that Lillie was the prince's mistress, they still had to maintain a thin veneer of decorum. Bertie even managed to have Lillie and her husband presented to Queen Victoria. And she even developed a cordial relationship with Princess Alexandra.

After falling out with Lillie at a fancy-dress party where she put an ice cube down his back, Bertie took up with the notorious French actress Sarah Bernhardt. Lillie had other lovers too, including the Earl of Shrewsbury and Prince Louis of Battenberg, the father of Lord Louis Mountbatten.

Her love affair with Bertie went on for four years and Bertie only gave her up after the birth of her daughter Jeanne-Marie in 1881, leading Prince Louis to believe the child was his. This sparked a mucky divorce that the prince decided it best to stay out of. Nevertheless, he gave Lillie the money to go to Paris with another lover, Arthur Clarence Jones, where she had the baby.

Lillie now needed money. She decided that she wanted to become an actress and Bertie persuaded the manager of the Haymarket Theatre to give her the lead in a charity performance of *She Stoops to Conquer*. The prince's presence on the first night assured the success of her debut.

In 1891, the Prince of Wales was summonsed to appear in court again, not in a divorce case this time but in what was known as the Baccarat Scandal, or the Tranby Croft Affair. The previous September, Bertie had been invited to a house party at Tranby Croft, where Lieutenant-Colonel Sir William Gordon-Cumming had been accused of cheating. He sued the other guests – with the exception of the Prince of Wales – for slander. Again Bertie was called as a witness. The jury found the defendants not guilty and Sir William was ruined. But the scandal did not reflect well on the prince and the defendants were booed when they left the court.

Wisely, Bertie gave up baccarat, but he could not give up dangerous liaisons with women – though his next affair did not threaten to break as a scandal until after his death.

The woman in question was Frances Brooke, whom Bertie called Daisy. She was beautiful, intelligent and rich. The Prince of Wales and Princess Alexandra were the guests of honour at her magnificent wedding to Lord Brooke.

An aristocrat, young "Brookie" did not object to Daisy sating her seemingly unquenchable sexual desires elsewhere, especially if her lovers were rich and powerful. But Daisy was a jealous woman. When the wife of her lover Lord Charles Beresford fell pregnant, she wrote him a scalding letter. This fell into his wife's hands and she threatened to make it public.

Hoping to avoid a ruinous scandal, Daisy turned to the prince for help. He was very understanding, she said, and she was a woman who knew how to show her gratitude. From early 1891, he was a regular visitor to her home, Easton Lodge. She had a private railway station built nearby so he could reach her on the royal train. They would meet for assignations in the summer house she had built in the gardens of the estate.

In London, they would be seen dining in his favourite restaurants. They even went to church together. And, when they were apart, they would exchange passionate letters several times a week.

Her wealth was further increased when her father, the Earl of Warwick, died. She became Countess of Warwick, inheriting Warwick Castle and a vast fortune. At around the same time, she became a passionate socialist under the guidance of W. T. Stead, the idealistic editor of the *Pall Mall Gazette*. And she began squandering her fortune on good causes.

She and Bertie, inevitably, broke up as both had numerous new partners. After his death, her debts had mounted to some £100,000. With the help of the infamous journalist Frank Harris, Daisy decided that her only way out was to publish the king's love letters. Their scandalous content would ensure a bestseller.

As soon as the Palace heard about the plan, they hit her with a writ. George V claimed, as his father's heir, he owned copyright. Naturally, the courts were sympathetic to the new king's view and found in his favour. This kept the letters out of the public domain for another fifty years.

When Queen Victoria finally died, Bertie abandoned the name his father had given him – Albert – and decided to reign as Edward VII instead. The public were still in two minds about him. But he got lucky. The coronation was planned for 26 June 1901, but Edward was struck down with peritonitis and almost died. Some 300 legs of mutton, 2,500 quails, snipe, oyster, prawns and sole poached in Chablis had already been prepared. This was distributed among the poor of the East End, giving Edward VII a much needed boost in public esteem.

When he was eventually crowned on 9 August, his mistresses turned out in force. In Westminster Abbey, a block of seats above the chancel was reserved for them. This was known as "the king's loose box". Noting this, the American writer resident in London Henry James dubbed the new king "Edward the Caresser".

In 1898, Bertie had met Alice Keppel, who became his last important mistress. The wife of George Keppel, she was already an accomplished adulterer and her husband seemed flattered that the prince should take an interest in her. When Edward came to the throne, the government used her as an intermediary with the king and even Queen Alexandra praised her good sense. They holidayed each Easter together in Biarritz, but he still made time to visit Paris and Marienbad alone. And there were always a number of society ladies that he would visit.

When Edward was dying, the queen sent for Mrs Keppel so she could visit him on his deathbed. After his death, the Keppels' home was plunged into mourning. Alice's two daughters considered the king their uncle and one of them asked her father: "Why does it matter so much Kingy dying?"

George Keppel replied generously, "Because Kingy was a very, very wonderful man."

Alice Keppel was still alive in 1936. When she heard the news of the abdication, she said, "We did things much better in my day."

## Prince Eddy

In 1889, the police had raided a homosexual brothel called the Hundred Guineas Club at 19 Cleveland Street. When the owners of the brothel were arrested, they dropped the names of their aristocratic clients. These included Lord Arthur Somerset, the Earl of Euston and Prince Eddy, who was known there as "Victoria". He was also the oldest son of Bertie, grandson of Queen Victoria and third in line to the throne. The names of these high-born gentlemen were kept out of the subsequent trial, which earned the low-born brothel keepers nine months' hard labour. However, Ernest Parke, the crusading editor of the *North London Press*, published the names of Somerset and Euston.

Somerset fled to France where he stayed until his death in 1926, but Euston sued Parke for libel. He claimed that he had been given a flier advertising "*poses plastiques*" – where nude girls posed in classical Greek tableaux – at 19 Cleveland Street. Naturally, when he got there and discovered what was going on, he was appalled and fled, he said.

However, a young boy named Saul who worked at the brothel had a different story. He said that Lord Euston had picked him up on the street and he had taken him back to Cleveland Street for sex. But Euston was ". . . not an actual sodomite," Saul said. "He likes to play with you and then 'spend' on your belly." The judge dismissed Saul as a "loathsome object". He later wrote *Recollections of a Mary-Ann*. Parke went down for a year with hard labour, while Lord Euston was fully rehabilitated and was appointed aide-de-camp to Edward VII at his coronation in 1901.

Although Eddy's name was kept out of the proceedings, more scandalous accusations clung to his dissolute reputation. In 1888, it was rumoured that he was Jack the Ripper. It was also said that he murdered a baby he had fathered by a prostitute. Fortunately, Eddy died, probably of syphilis, before he could succeed to the throne.

## Mrs Brown

Queen Victoria is seen as a paragon of virtue, the fulcrum of Victorian values. In fact, scandal was never far from her door.

Her father Edward, Duke of Kent, was so dissolute that his father King George III exiled him to Gibraltar where he took a French mistress named Julie St Laurent. There and in Montreal he sadistically disciplined the regiment put under him, sentencing one man to 999 lashes. His unit rebelled, inviting even more brutal punishment. Returning to London with his long-standing mistress, he ran up such enormous debts that they had to flee to Brussels. To put himself back in the good books of his father and get him to pay off what he owed, he contracted a royal marriage. His Madame St Laurent only found out that he had married Princess Victoria of Leinigen when it was reported in the Continental newspapers. They had been together for twenty-five years.

And the Duke of Kent was by no means the worst of the family. His younger brother Prince Ernest, Duke of Cumberland, was said to have committed incest with his sister Princess Sophia in a mirrored room in St James's Palace. He was accused of attempting to rape the wife of the Lord Chancellor in her own drawing room, and Lord Graves slit his throat when he heard the prince was having an affair with his fifty-year-old wife.

Princess Sophia gave birth to an illegitimate child, sired by an equerry at the palace who was thirty-three years her senior. Her sister Princess Augusta fell in love with the king's equerry, Major-General Sir Brent Spencer. She never dared ask the king whether she could marry him. And when she plucked up the courage to ask the Prince Regent, he forbade it. This did not stop them being lovers and they may have married in secret. Princess Amelia also fell for one of the king's equerries, a middle-aged philanderer named Charles Fitzroy who was descended from one of Charles II's bastards. They never married but she considered herself to be his wife and left everything she had to him when she died. Then there was Princess Elizabeth who was rumoured to be pregnant while unmarried at the age of sixteen. She did not marry until she was forty-seven.

George III's youngest son, Prince Augustus Frederick married Lady Augusta Murray secretly in Rome, in direct contravention of the Royal Marriage Act. When she fell pregnant, they married again publicly in St George's, Hanover Square. He used the name Mr Frederick Augustus. The marriage was ruled invalid and Prince Augustus was exiled. His wife's passport was seized to prevent her following him. However, using forged papers, she escaped and caught up with him in Berlin. For ten years, they lived happily there until the lure of £12,000 and the Duchy of Sussex persuaded him to abandon her and return to England. He then sued for the custody of their children and married again, bigamously, to Lady Cecilia Buggin, the widow of a city grocer. Condoning the match, Queen Victoria created her Duchess of Inverness.

The Duke of Kent had died less than two years after marrying. But in that period, Princess Victoria of Leinigen produced a daughter who would become Queen Victoria. The young Victoria knew of her father's murky past and sometimes referred to his former mistress as "the old French lady" or "the discovery of St Lawrence". The misbehaviour of her uncles and aunts was simply overlooked, though she remained on friendly terms with her cousin King Leopold of the Belgians who was partial to feather boas and high-heeled shoes. However, the scandalous behaviour of her widowed mother brought more shame to the young queen. She took as her lover the Irish upstart Sir John Conroy and made no effort to hide her physical familiarity with him in front of her impressionable young daughter. Together they tried to dominate the princess, but when Victoria became queen she banned Conroy from court.

Victoria became convinced that Conroy was using one of the Ladies of the Bedchamber, Lady Flora Hastings, as a spy. After Lady Hastings travelled back from Scotland with Conroy in 1838, her belly swelled and Victoria was convinced that she was pregnant by "that Monster and Demon incarnate".

Flora consulted the royal physician, Sir James Clark, a poor diagnostician, who quickly concluded that she was indeed pregnant. The other Ladies of the Bedchamber broadcast the fact. But when she was given a thorough examination, she was found still to be a virgin. The scandal had reached such proportions that Flora's uncle Hamilton FitzGerald had to publish an open letter exonerating the girl in *The Examiner*.

Once the public realized that Lady Flora was not pregnant but gravely ill, Queen Victoria's scandalous treatment of her made her very unpopular and she was hissed at by the crowds at Ascot. In 1839, this turned into a full-scale political scandal called the "Bedchamber Crisis".

When Victoria's prime ministerial favourite, Lord Melbourne – a two-time divorcee who once complimented Victoria on her "full and fine bust" – fell from power, he was replaced by Sir Robert Peel, who insisted that she dismiss her gossiping Ladies of the Bedchamber. Victoria refused. In the street, mobs hurled abuse at her. They called her "Mrs Melbourne", suggesting that the former prime minister was more than just an adviser. Eventually she had to give way.

When Lady Hastings died on 5 July 1839, it was found that the cause of the swelling was a tumour on her liver. The *Morning Post* described the queen's behaviour in the affair as "the most revolting virulence and indecency".

Victoria's husband, the strait-laced Prince Albert, was not free from the whiff of scandal either. His mother outraged the good people of Saxe-Coburg-Gotha by having an affair with the court's Jewish chamberlain, who may have been Albert's real father. His parents divorced when he was five. His mother married an army officer and never saw her son again, while his father, in proper Hanoverian style, consoled himself with a series of mistresses.

Albert's brother took after his father and died of syphilis, but the young Albert prided himself on being a pillar of moral rectitude. He went to an all-male university and forswore contact with women.

As soon as she saw him, Victoria was bowled over by his looks. "Albert's beauty is most striking," she remarked.

At their third meeting, she asked him to marry her, while remarking that she was quite unworthy of him. He eventually consented, but warned that he would not be "corrupted" by her.

Albert was good to his word. The time they spent together on the first night of the honeymoon was shockingly brief, the diarist Charles Grenville noted.

"I told Lord Palmerston that this is not the way to provide us with a Prince of Wales," he wrote.

Queen Victoria was a woman of robust sexual appetites though and she knew how to get the best out of Albert. She hung their bedroom at Osborne House with paintings of male nudes, though she hated getting pregnant, as Albert believed that sex was for procreation and not recreation. He would abstain for the nine months of the pregnancy and at least another three months after she had given birth. She would have to go without sex for over a year. Nevertheless, they had nine children in all. When Albert said that there should be no more, Victoria said, "Can we have no more fun in bed?"

When Albert died in 1861, she went into prolonged mourning, ordering that his rooms were to remain as they were on the day of his death. Brooding alone at Osborne, the home on the Isle of Wight they had built together, those around the queen feared that she might become unhinged. To snap her out of it, they sent for her carriage and her favourite ponies from Balmoral. These were brought by her Scottish ghillie John Brown in bonnet and kilt. A giant of a man with a great shock of red hair, when she saw him, it is said, she smiled for the first time since Albert's death.

As her "personal Highland servant", he was told to take orders from no one but herself. This put the nose of her equerry, General Sir Charles Grey, out of joint. When Grey protested, she offered him an obscure posting in a remote part of India. Brown's salary was bumped up to £120 a year, five times what he was earning at Balmoral. Anything but deferential, he addressed the queen merely as "woman" and told her off if she was dressed too lightly for the cold weather.

The queen's own daughters joked that Brown was "Mama's Lover", while Foreign Secretary Edward Stanley, 15th Earl of Derby, wrote in his diary that Brown and Victoria slept in adjoining rooms "contrary to etiquette and even decency".

With Brown's encouragement, she came out of mourning and began to fulfil her public duties again. In 1866, she attended the state opening of parliament for the first time since Albert's death. And Brown accompanied her when she reviewed the troops at Aldershot. This did not go unnoticed. *Punch* magazine began calling her "Mrs Brown" and published a spoof Court Circular detailing their activities. In September 1866, the Swiss newspaper *Gazette de Lausanne* ran a story from the special correspondent in London, saying that Queen Victoria and Brown had married secretly and she was pregnant. Indeed leading Liberal politician Victory Lewis "Loulou" Harcourt recorded that Queen Victoria's Scottish chaplain, the Reverend Norman Macleod, confessed on his deathbed that he had presided over their marriage. He said he had heard of this via Macleod's sisters and concluded that Miss Macleod would be unlikely to have concocted the story and, because of its source, those who heard it would be "almost inclined to believe it, improbable and disgraceful as it sounds".

When this scandalous rumour reached the ears of the republicans, they published a pamphlet alleging that the queen had hatched a morganatic marriage with Brown. He was even blamed for the queen's withdrawal from public life as it was said that she would rather spend time at Balmoral with her ghillie than attend to affairs of state. Cartoons showed him eyeing the empty throne.

Fearing unrest, the government asked the queen not to appear in public with Brown, but she refused to leave him at home. However, in 1867, the execution of Emperor Maximilian of Mexico – a remote relative by marriage – was used as an excuse to plunge the court back into mourning and cancel the queen's public engagements.

She returned to public life in February 1872 for a thanksgiving service for the Prince of Wales's recovery from typhoid. On her way to St Paul's Cathedral, she was confronted by a man, who pointed a pistol in her face. Brown, who was riding on the box of the queen's carriage, jumped down and thrust the man aside. He made a dash for it. Brown pursued and caught him. Instantly, Brown was a national hero, even though the would-be assassin was found to be deranged and the pistol did not work. In gratitude, the queen had a special award – the Devoted Service Medal – struck and Brown was awarded an annuity of £25 a year.

When John Brown died in 1883, at the age of fifty-six, he lay in state in Windsor Castle for six days and his obituary in the Court Circular was longer than Disraeli's. In a recently discovered letter, Victoria wrote of her loss: "Perhaps never in history was there so strong and true an attachment, so warm and loving a friendship between the sovereign and servant . . . Strength of character as well as power of frame – the most fearless uprightness, kindness, sense of justice, honesty, independence and unselfishness combined with a tender, warm heart . . . made him one of the most remarkable men. The Queen feels that life for the second time is become most trying and sad to bear, deprived of all she so needs . . . the blow has fallen too heavily not to be very heavily felt . . ."

Brown's room at Windsor was given the same treatment as Albert's, until Edward VIII came to the throne and turned it into a billiard room. Edward also had the statue of John Brown removed from the hallway at Balmoral.

Queen Victoria had already published a book dedicated to Brown. It was called *More Leaves from the Journal of a Life in the Highlands*. She began on *The Life of John Brown*. The Dean of Windsor read the manuscript and found it so scandalous that he threatened to resign if she published it. Eventually she gave in.

After John Brown's death, Victoria turned to her beturbaned Indian secretary Munshi Hafir Abdul Karim, whom she called Munshi. Although he was still in his twenties, she gave him a cottage at Windsor and a staff of his own. The government became concerned about their relationship and told her that it was inappropriate for her to be on such intimate terms with a black man. She pointed out that, as Empress of India, she could do what she liked with him.

*Royal Romps*

## George IV and Queen Caroline

If the divorce of Prince Charles and Diana caused a scandal, it was as nothing compared to the divorce proceedings of George IV and Queen Caroline, which resulted in fifty-two days of detailed testimony before the House of Lords in 1820. And it was but one incident in the scandalous life of one of the most hated monarchs ever to sit on the British throne. When George was crowned at the age of fifty, the poet Leigh Hunt wrote in *The Examiner* that the new king was "a violator of his word, a libertine head over heels in debt and disgrace, the companion of gamblers and demi-reps . . . and a man who has just closed half a century without one single claim on the gratitude of his country or the respect of posterity". Hunt was fined £500 and jailed for two years for libel. Under English law, speaking the truth is no defence.

George IV began his scandalous sex life with one of his mother's maids of honour when he was sixteen. Queen Charlotte admonished the boy for keeping "improper company" in his rooms after bedtime. Taking his mother's advice to heart, he began an affair with an actress, Mary Robinson, who came to his apartments dressed as a boy. The prince promised her £21,000 on her twenty-first birthday for services rendered. It was one of many debts he did not pay. So when they broke up, she threatened to publish a number of highly charged letters he had sent her. To prevent a scandal, his father, George III, had to recover them. It cost him £5,000, plus a pension of £500 a year.

Soon after, wealthy divorcee Mrs Grace Elliot claimed that the Prince of Wales was the father of her daughter, who she named Georgina in his honour, though she had been entertaining two other men at the time. Besides society ladies, George scythed his way through maids, cooks, prostitutes and actresses. At eighteen, another scandal befell the prince when he fell for the "divinely pretty" Countess von Hardenburg, wife of the ambassador of Hanover. When her husband read about it in the *Morning Herald*, he wrote a curt note to the prince. The countess wrote too, begging him to elope with her. Unsure what to do, the prince confided in his mother, who cried a lot. His father expelled the Hanoverian ambassador and again admonished his son for bringing shame on the family.

A born troublemaker, the prince teamed up with the radical politician Charles James Fox – whose future wife he had already seduced – to oppose his father's policies in parliament. Otherwise, he continued his career as a playboy and got into drunken brawls in the Vauxhall pleasure gardens. The king complained that there was something bad about him in the newspapers every day. Even *The Times*, a pillar of the establishment, described him as a man who "preferred a girl and a bottle to politics and a sermon".

At the age of twenty-three, he fell in love with Mrs Maria Fitzherbert and tried to kill himself when she refused his advances. When that failed, he threatened to abdicate so he could emigrate with her to the newly independent United States of America. But she would only entertain his propositions when he promised to marry her.

Not only was she twice divorced, like Mrs Simpson, any marriage between them was quite illegal. In an effort to curb the excesses of his offspring, George III had passed the Royal Marriages Act in 1772, which prevented members of the royal family under the age of twenty-five marrying without the sovereign's consent. And he was not about to give in. Even if he had consented, Mrs Fitzherbert was a Catholic so marrying her was also illegal under the Act of Settlement of 1701. She was also six years older than George and a commoner. But in 1785 the Prince of Wales went ahead and married her anyway.

Even the way the ceremony was carried out was scandalous. George paid £500 to get an Anglican priest out of debtors' prison. He then married them on the promise of a bishopric. For political reasons, Mrs Fitzherbert was sworn to secrecy.

But George himself failed to be discreet. He set up home with "Princess Fitz" quite openly in Park Street, Mayfair, and she bore him ten children.

If that were not scandalous enough, when drunk, he would attack her. More than once, she had to flee from his unsheathed sword. And he was constantly unfaithful to her.

A fresh scandal erupted when Lucy Howard bore him an illegitimate child. He paid £10,000 and a fine selection of jewellery to bed Anna Crouch, star of John Gay's West End hit *The Beggar's Opera*. Her husband, a naval officer, demanded another £400 not to drag him through the divorce courts. George also left them a sheaf of passionate love letters, which assured them a healthy income for many years to come.

He began a very public affair with Frances Villers, Countess of Jersey, though she was forty and a grandmother nine times over. There was a problem though. He could not afford both Lady Jersey and Mrs Fitzherbert on the £50,000 a year his father gave him. Although it was considered a fortune at the time, his stables alone cost him £31,000 a year and his gambling debts were legendary.

By 1791, his debts topped £630,000. He was now in the embarrassing position of being refused credit and Mrs Fitzherbert, once a wealthy woman, had to pawn her jewellery to stave off the bailiffs.

George III and Prime Minister William Pitt the Younger then cooked up a deal. The government would settle the prince's debts, provided he married and gave the country a much needed heir. The pretty, intelligent, Louise of Mecklenburg-Strelitz was their favoured candidate. But Lady Jersey considered her too formidable a sexual rival, so the prince plumped instead for the short, fat, ugly and smelly Princess Caroline of Brunswick. She was considered "excessively loose" even by German standards and a distinct odour followed in her wake, even though the British envoy sent to Germany to bring her to England persuaded her to wash herself and her underwear before they left.

Whatever charms she might have possessed were hidden beneath the unflattering gowns and heavy make-up that Lady Jersey, who had somehow inveigled herself into the position of the Caroline's Lady of the Bedchamber, persuaded her to wear. When the prince first saw her, he said, "Pray, fetch me a glass of brandy. I am unwell."

For the next three days up to the wedding ceremony, he continued consuming brandy at an alarming rate. On the morning of the wedding, he sent his brother to tell Mrs Fitzherbert that she was the only woman he ever loved. That did not stop him leering drunkenly at Lady Jersey throughout the ceremony.

On the wedding night, he was so drunk that he slept with his head in the fireplace. The following morning, he did his duty though. To everyone's surprise, Caroline gave birth to a daughter, Princess Charlotte, nine months later. The honeymoon was a surprisingly passionate affair, but only because George had the foresight to take Lady Jersey along.

With the birth of Princess Charlotte, George considered that he had fulfilled his side of the bargain he had made with parliament and he told Caroline that he had no intention of sleeping with her ever again. When the news broke, the public were overwhelmingly on the princess's side. When George went out, mobs howled: "Where's your wife?"

The scandal also affected the palace and the king was forced to take a hand.

"You seem to look on your union with the princess as merely of a private nature," he wrote, "and totally put out of sight that as Heir Apparent to the Crown your marriage is a public act, wherein the kingdom is concerned."

The Prince of Wales tried to smooth things over. He wrote to the princess, explaining that "our inclinations are not in our power". He also reminded her of the importance of "being polite". Caroline asked the politician George Canning what George meant by "being polite". Canning said that George was giving her permission to sleep with whomever she wanted, provided she was discreet. Caroline immediately took advantage of this warrant and promptly slept with George Canning.

For his part, George dumped Lady Jersey and crawled back to his "real and true love" Mrs Fitzherbert. She received him coldly. In an attempt to worm his way back into her affections, George lost some of his considerable girth and began spending freely on his London home Carlton House and his Pavilion in Brighton, even though the Napoleonic Wars were putting a considerable strain on the public purse. Mrs Fitzherbert eventually took him back into her bed when the Pope sent confirmation that, in the eyes of the Church, she was the true wife of the Prince of Wales.

Of course, it was too much to expect him to be faithful. He sired a string of illegitimate children and slept with a number of French women, even though Britain and France were at war at the time. Mrs Fitzherbert, who was now in her middle age, accepted that he chased after pretty young women, but she was more than a little distressed when he sought out a series of grandmothers. When Napoleon heard that George was in love with the old and overweight Lady Hertford, he laughed uproariously.

In November 1810, George III became permanently insane and the Prince of Wales took over as prince regent. A king in all but name, he dismissed Mrs Fitzherbert coldly with the words: "Madam, you have no place."

This was no indication that he was taking his new responsibilities seriously. Mrs Fitzherbert and Lady Hertford had been dumped in favour of the portly Lady Bessborough, whom he begged to "live with him publicly". Her husband was made Lord Chamberlain and their son was also found a position in the royal household.

By this time the public were so used to George's excesses that such scandalous behaviour ceased to shock. However, new scandal was about to arrive from an unexpected quarter.

After the breakdown of the royal marriage, Caroline of Brunswick had moved to Blackheath. There, according to Lady Hester Stanhope, she had become "a downright whore". She was frequently "closeted with young men". In her front room, she had a Chinese clockwork figure that, when you wound it up, made gross sexual movements and she liked to dance around showing off a good deal of her body.

Her partner in crime was Lady Douglas, who had been shunned by polite society for having an affair with her husband's commanding officer, Sir Sidney Smith. Not only did Lady Douglas take lovers whenever she felt like it, she also slept with Caroline.

When the two of them fell out, Caroline sent Lady Douglas's husband, Sir John Douglas, an obscene drawing showing his wife making love to Sir Sidney Smith. Rumours flew that a four-year-old boy in their circle named William Austin was Caroline's illegitimate son by Prince Louis Ferdinand of Prussia. This caused such a scandal that parliament set up a Royal Commission to investigate the Princess of Wales's behaviour. It was called the "Delicate Investigation".

The commission investigated every sordid detail of the goings-on in Blackheath. Of particular public interest was her relationship with Captain Manby, a naval officer who was a frequent visitor. However, on the substantive charge, that she had an illegitimate child, Caroline was exonerated and Lady Douglas, who had started the rumour, was found guilty of perjury.

While the Delicate Investigation was supposed to be held in secret, it proved impossible to prevent the details leaking to the press who printed up every sordid detail.

In 1814, Caroline left England and started a scandalous progress across Europe. She began by dancing topless at a ball in Geneva given in her honour. In Naples, she had an affair with Napoleon's brother-in-law King Joachim. And in Milan, she took up with Bartolomeo Pergami, a former quartermaster in Napoleon's Italian Army. They travelled around Europe, North Africa and the Middle East together as man and wife, before setting up home in Como.

With her own reputation in tatters, Caroline tried to ruin her daughter's too. Charlotte had been strictly brought up by her maiden aunts in Windsor, but when she visited her mother, Caroline locked the young virgin in a room with Captain Hesse, who was said to be the illegitimate son of the Duke of York and one of Caroline's own lovers.

George III eventually died in 1820 and the Prince Regent came to the throne as George IV. He offered Caroline £50,000 a year if she promised to remain abroad. But Caroline saw herself queen of England and was determined to be crowned in Westminster Abbey alongside her husband.

She returned to England and was immediately arrested and arraigned before the House of Lords for "a most unbecoming and degrading intimacy with a foreigner of low station" – Pergami. A Bill of Pains and Penalties was drawn up which, George hoped, would strip Caroline of her title of queen consort and dissolve their marriage on the grounds of adultery.

The debate in the House of Lords went into the most lascivious detail. Witnesses were called, including servants from Caroline's own household, who said they had seen Caroline and Pergami naked together. Pergami had been seen caressing Caroline's breasts and her inner thigh. They slept together. He was frequently seen naked, or semi-naked in her bedroom and was present when she took a bath. It seemed an open-and-shut case.

The public lapped up every juicy detail. But people also knew what the king had been up to. What was sauce for the goose was sauce for the gander, was the consensus. When the Duke of Wellington was stopped by a mob, which shouted, "God Save the Queen", he replied, "Well, gentlemen, since you will have it so. God Save the Queen – and may all your wives be like her."

Caroline herself found that she was cheered by crowds when she travelled from her new home in Hammersmith to parliament to listen to the proceedings. The crowds of her supporters grew so huge that a stout timber fence had to be built around the House of Lords. The proceedings reached a climax when she was called to testify. Asked whether she had ever committed adultery, she said only when she slept with "Mrs Fitzherbert's husband".

The hearings went on for fifty-two days and the Bill was passed with a majority of just nine. But the matter had become a cause célèbre. To save the government any further embarrassment the Bill was discreetly dropped, rather than take it forward to the House of Commons, as there was little prospect of them passing it. Summing up the situation, one contemporary satirist wrote:

> Most gracious Queen we thee implore
> To go away and sin no more;
> Or if that effort be too great
> Go away at any rate.

But she was not about to. She was looking forward to the coronation, which was scheduled for 19 July 1821. Caroline wrote to the prime minister, Lord Liverpool, asking what she should wear. He wrote back saying that she could "form no part of the ceremony".

She turned up anyway, dressed in a sheer muslin slip and accompanied by a large contingent of supporters. Arriving at the doors of Westminster Abbey, she shouted, "Open for the queen. I am the queen of England."

The pages did as they were bid, but a courtier bellowed to the guards: "Do your duty. Shut the door." And the doors were slammed in Caroline's face. Undaunted, she sent the king a note asking for her coronation to be organized for the following Monday.

When news reached England of Napoleon's death on 5 May, George was told simply that his greatest enemy was dead. He replied, "Is she, by God."

Caroline did die, just three weeks after the king was crowned. It was so convenient that a popular conspiracy theory of the time was that she had been poisoned. The king, it was noted, was "gayer than might be proper to tell". When her body was being taken to the dock, to be shipped back to Brunswick, there was a riot along the way in Kensington. Bricks were thrown and two protesters were shot by Life Guards. Caroline was buried in Brunswick Cathedral and the inscription on her coffin reads: "The Injured Queen of England".

A free man once more, George IV continued in his scandalous ways. He exchanged Lady Hertford for Lady Conyngham, who was the same age as Lady Hertford but considerably fatter. Rumours soon circulated that they were deeply in love and he was seen nodding, winking and making eyes at Lady Conyngham in Westminster Abbey while the Archbishop of York was giving a sermon on the sovereign's duty to protect his people from "the contagion of vice".

He continued to be one of the most unpopular monarchs ever to sit on the throne of England. He had little influence with the Tory and coalition governments during his reign and the prominent Whig Lord Holland said that they encouraged "every species of satire against him and his mistresses".

When George IV died in 1830, his obituary in *The Times* said: "There never was an individual less regretted by his fellow creatures than this deceased king."

When he was buried, he had left instruction that a picture of Mrs Fitzherbert should be tied on a ribbon around his neck and placed on his heart. Although she had been estranged from him for many years, Mrs Fitzherbert wept when she heard of the king's instructions.

## Queen Christina of Sweden

In the seventeenth century, Sweden produced the brilliant and vivacious Queen Christina who wore men's clothes, refused to marry and gave up the throne to gallivant around Europe getting into all manner of scandals.

When she was born on 8 December 1626, she was so hairy and cried with such a deep voice that her father King Gustavus Adolphus was told that she was a much-hoped-for boy. Gustavus was killed in battle in 1632 when she was six. Her mother withdrew to a room hung in black and slept with Gustavus's shroud and a gold casket containing his heart. She also ordered that he should not be buried until she was buried with him and had the coffin lid left open so she could view him every day, despite the putrefaction.

Christina was left in the hands of five regents and surrounded by male courtiers who supervised her education. She had little opportunity to develop an interest in feminine pursuits and, when she was not indulging her amazing ability to learn languages, she loved to hunt reindeer on horseback in the snow. However, when she was thirteen, a French ballet master was brought to court to teach her to move more gracefully.

At the age of eighteen, she took the oath as queen of Sweden. Like all monarchs she was expected to produce an heir. In her autobiography, she said she felt "an insurmountable distaste for marriage" and "an insurmountable distaste for all the things that females talked about and did". She slept for three or four hours a night, rarely combed her hair, threw on any clothes that came to hand and wore men's shoes for the sake of convenience. Christina developed a passionate relationship with her beautiful Ebba Sparre, whom she called Belle. Most of her spare time was spent with "*la belle comtesse*" – and she often called attention to her beauty. She introduced her to the English envoy Bulstrode Whitelocke as her 'bed-fellow', assuring him that Sparre's mind was as beautiful as her body. Curiously,

Whitelocke had been sent by Cromwell's government to teach the ladies of the court "the English mode of salutation" which was sweeping the continent – kissing.

Christina hosted Ebba Sparre's marriage to Count Jakob Kasimir de la Gardie despite her jealousy. But just when everyone had concluded that she was a lesbian, Christina fell in love with the count's brother, Magnus Gabriel de la Gardie. She heaped honours on him and everyone assumed they were lovers. However, towards the end of her reign, he fell out of favour and she sent him away.

Christina fell out with her government over her refusal to marry. "Marriage would entail many things to which I cannot become accustomed," she told them. "I really cannot say when I will overcome this inhibition."

To make things worse she planned to convert to Catholicism. The French, she had concluded, had much more fun than dour Scandinavian Protestants. Her French doctor had brought Pietro Aretino's sixteen *Lewd Sonnets*, which were usually illustrated with pornographic engravings by Giulio Romano, to Sweden with him. She also learnt Ovid's erotic elegy *Ar Amatoria* by heart and read the scandalous works of Martial. Then she lost much of her popularity by executing the royal historian for calling her a Jezebel.

To that end, she abdicated in favour of her cousin Charles Gustavus who reigned as Charles X. During the abdication ceremony, she was stripped of her coronation robe and royal insignia, then she lifted the crown from her own head.

Christina had already stripped the palace in Stockholm of its furniture, which she had sent to Rome where she intended to settle. She set off via Denmark dressed as a man and calling herself Count Dohna. In tow was the lovely Ebba Sparre, who was now a widow. In Brussels, Christina declared herself a Catholic and threw herself into a round of parties. The scandal sheets happily chronicled her sexual misadventures, which grew so outrageous she was dubbed the "Queen of

Sodom" and the Swedish government threatened to cut off her pension.

In 1655, Christina arrived in Rome accompanied by two handsome brothers – Count Francisco Maria Santinelli, a poet and alchemist, and Ludovico Santinelli, an acrobat and dancer. She was welcomed in Rome by Pope Alexander VII as a prize convert and she was housed in a wing inside the Vatican. Soon graffiti appeared, saying: "*Omne malum ab Aquilone*" – "All evil comes from the North". The Pope had it painted over.

But Christina soon became an embarrassment. She had converted for fun, not piety. Making fun of the Church's holy relics, she spoke to her friends in a loud voice during Mass.

Settling in the Palazzo Farnese, she hung the walls with extremely indelicate pictures and had the fig leaves removed from all the statues. In the evenings, Christina would change out of men's clothing and into more alluring attire to entertain leading churchmen. Cardinal Colonna fell in love with her and the Pope had to send him away from Rome to avoid a public scandal.

Christina herself was in love with Cardinal Azzolino, though the two of them managed to be more discreet. However, some of their letters have survived. In one, she says that, although she does not want to give offence, this "does not prevent me from loving you until death, and since piety relieves you from being my lover, then I relieve you from being my servant, for I shall live and die as your slave". Her passion was evident. When he did not turn up for an assignation at the Villa Medici near Monte Pincio, she went to the Castel Sant'Angelo and fired one of the cannons. The mark on the bronze gate in front of Villa Medici is still visible.

She quit Rome for France, where she received a royal welcome. However, the ladies of the court were shocked by her masculine appearance and demeanour, and the frankness of her conversation. Anne Marie Louise d'Orléans, France's most wealthy heiress, who took her to the ballet, remarked that

Christina "surprised me very much – applauding the parts which pleased her, taking God to witness, throwing herself back in her chair, crossing her legs, resting them on the arms of her chair, and assuming other postures, such as I had never seen taken but by Travelin and Jodelet, two famous buffoons . . . She was in all respects a most extraordinary creature."

She stayed at Fontainebleau with her Italian courtiers, the Marquis Monaldeschi, her chief equerry, and the Santinelli brothers. Monaldeschi and Francisco Maria Santinelli loathed each other and vied for her favour. Christina suspected that Monaldeschi had swindled her over a property deal in Rome. To cover his tracks, he forged a series of letters blaming the swindle on Santinelli. They also made references to Christina's affair with Cardinal Azzolino and her intention of taking the throne of Naples.

However, Christina recognized his handwriting and summoned Monaldeschi. She asked him what he thought the punishment for treachery should be. Thinking that she had been convinced by the forgeries and that the forfeit would be paid by Santinelli, he said, "Death."

She agreed. On 10 November 1657, Monaldeschi was summoned to the Galerie de Cerfs in Fontainebleau and asked to read the letters. As he did so, he found the door barred behind him. Francisco and two guards entered with daggers in their hands.

Realizing he had been rumbled, Monaldeschi threw himself to his knees and begged Christina for mercy. She turned to Father Lebel, a prior who had been summoned from the nearby Mathurin Monastery, and asked him to prepare Monaldeschi for his death. Lebel also begged her to show mercy. So did Francisco. He said that the case should be taken before the Royal Courts of France. Christina refused, telling him to make haste and do his duty while she strode from the gallery. For the next fifteen minutes, she overheard Monaldeschi's screams as they hacked him to death.

The French were appalled at what they saw as an act of barbarity. Christina's host, Cardinal Mazarin, advised her to make herself scarce and she fled back to Rome. She was little more popular there and the Pope asked her to live outside the Papal See. As a sweetener, he offered her an annuity and an adviser to oversee her financial affairs – one Cardinal Azzolino.

When Charles X died in 1660, Christina thought it was time to return to Sweden. When she reached Hamburg, she received a letter making it plain that she was not welcome in her homeland. She took no notice. In Stockholm, the government had no option but to greet her with due respect and house her in the royal apartments. They even allowed her to use one of the royal estates. But when the locals complained that she was celebrating Mass there, the government had to ask her to leave.

She spent the rest of her life wandering aimlessly around Europe, growing fat, unpleasant and eccentric. As her health began to fail, she returned to Rome where she continued to put on plays with women on stage wearing décolleté dresses, despite a papal injunction. After all, the new pope, Innocent XI, had once been a guest in the royal box, along with other cardinals. She died on 19 April 1689, with the faithful Cardinal Azzolino by her side.

# 10

## Artistic Licence

### Tracey Emin

Leading Brit artist Tracey Emin has made a career out of sex scandal. It began with her tent *Everyone I Have Ever Slept With 1963–1995*. On the canvas she had appliquéd the names of her sexual partners, lovers and drinking partners, along with those of relatives she slept with as a child, her twin brother and the names she would have given to her two aborted children. It also included names of "some I'd had a shag with . . . against a wall". She described it, without irony, as a "seminal work".

Originally sold for £12,000, Charles Saatchi bought it later for £40,000 and it was thought to have been worth £300,000 in 2004, when it was destroyed in a warehouse fire in East London. Tracey was upset when everyone laughed, so the *Daily Mail* made another one for £67.50. This did not improve her humour.

Then came *My Bed*, an unmade bed littered with condoms and a pair of knickers with menstrual blood in them. It was shortlisted for the Turner Prize and Charles Saatchi bought it for £150,000. She took it in good heart when two Japanese performance artists, stripped to the waist, jumped on it. However, when a cleaner at the Tate tried to tidy it up, she had to be restrained.

In New York she exhibited an appliquéd blanket entitled *Psycho Slut* and, in a neon sculpture called *Very Happy Girl*, she announced the dimensions of her current boyfriend's penis.

In 2002, she produced a series of monoprints called *Something's Wrong* which included female torsos, legs splayed and with odd, spidery flows gushing from their vaginas. Her own naked body, sometimes doing weird things to herself, was another subject.

At the opening of her 2005 exhibition *When I Think About Sex*, she said, "I don't have sex, I make art. That's what I do. I think about sex when I make art."

In the exhibition, she displayed blankets embroidered with the slogans: "Feel Me", "Right Up Inside Of Me" and "People Like You Need To Fuck People Like Me".

She also produced that slogan in neon, along with "Is Legal Sex Anal" and "My Cunt Is Wet With Fear".

Brad Pitt and Jennifer Aniston, when they were still together, were seen eyeing up the "Anal Sex" piece in a London gallery, but were taken aback when they learnt that it was expected to fetch anywhere from £10,000 to £50,000. They must have figured they could make it themselves at home a whole lot cheaper. Other fans include George Michael, his boyfriend Kenny Goss and Elton John.

## Eric Gill

Tracey must have been jealous when the sex life of artist Eric Gill caused scandal nearly sixty years after his death. In 1998, the Catholic Archbishop of Westminster, Cardinal Hume, made a public apology for the harm done to children by priests after the first of a number of child abuse scandals involving the Christian Brothers erupted. However, Margaret Kennedy, founder of an organization called Christian Survivors of Sexual Abuse, noted that in his TV broadcast Cardinal Hume was standing in front of Eric Gill's *Stations of the Cross*, fourteen relief panels that decorate Westminster Cathedral. This, she said, caused her "a great deal of distress".

Writing to the *Catholic Herald*, she said, "These *Stations* do no honour to the Lord's house. Incest is inscribed into each carving. Should honour be given to a man whose hands carved sculptures and also carved into shame the small bodies of his sisters and children?" The panels should be removed, she insisted.

Soon daily papers were carrying headlines such as INCEST IN THE CATHEDRAL, UNHOLY ROW OVER ARTIST WITH A SHADY FAMILY LIFE, CATHEDRAL SHUNS PLEA ON PAEDOPHILE'S ART and DON'T RIP OUT THIS SEX FIEND'S ART OF STONE!

Eric Gill's reliefs adorn a number of public buildings in London, including Broadcasting House, home of the BBC. He also designed a number of typefaces, the most famous being Gill Sans and Perpetua that are in use worldwide. And, until 1989, he was considered a respectable, upstanding member of the Arts and Crafts movement and a noted Catholic convert. Then a new biography was published that drew heavily on his diaries. It revealed that Gill sexually abused his own children, had an incestuous relationship with his sister and performed sexual acts on his dog.

Gill was fascinated with sex from an early age. Of his first erection, he wrote: "How shall I ever forget the strange, inexplicable rapture of my first experience? What marvellous thing was this that suddenly transformed a mere water tap into a pillar of fire – and water into an elixir of life?"

In his adolescence, he picked up prostitutes. For him, a matter of burning curiosity was what their pubic hair was going to look like. These encounters were not always satisfactory. He complained boastfully that his cock was too big for one petite prostitute he picked up in Bond Street. It made the poor girl's eyes water. And there was a girl in a house in Fulham whom he did not like, but still he went there. His diary also recounts a bizarre encounter on Clapham Common with an elderly lady.

He told his fiancée Ethel about his experiences and his need for regular masturbation. To save him from this infernal practice, he said she must sleep with him and sent her a diagram explaining the principles of contraception. Inflamed by seeing naked women in the life class, he took Ethel to a hotel in Fleet Street and insisted that she strip off.

"Then for the first time I saw that she was a woman," he recorded. "I saw the dark full growth of hair on her belly. I touched it and kissed her. By now she was naked. Her breasts – her little tender nipples were against me – her hair down and covering my face – our lips kissing. So we lay together for the first time."

Ethel was the perfect sexual partner, he said. "The roundness and largeness of her legs and thighs and hips, the sudden smallness of her waist and the splendid fatness and softness of her buttocks, the thick hair on her belly are beautiful and very exciting."

Meanwhile she enthused about his "dear body" and "dear penis". This continued throughout their married life. Gill's diaries are full of remarks such as "great time in bed" and even "discovered a new *façon de faire*". According to his diaries they had a shag almost every day.

But for Gill that was not enough. He visited brothels and had casual encounters with prostitutes. One night, after leaving leading Bloomsburyite Lady Ottoline Morrell – the wife of an MP who counted among her lovers philosopher Bertrand Russell, writer Dorothy Bussy, painters Augustus John and Henry Lamb and the art historian Roger Fry – he picked up a girl in Guilford Street and went home with her. Then, after hearing a lecture by the writer Hilaire Belloc, he gave a woman two shillings to feel between her legs while she wanked him.

"No connection," he wrote. "No orgasm. Am I mad!"

Even on holiday, he would leave Ethel back at their hotel while he went out picking up women. And when Ethel fell pregnant, Gill asked their housemaid Lizzie to lend a hand.

"I said to her would she let me lie with her as Ethel was with child," he noted. "She agreed."

The following year he did what all self-respecting artists do. He took a prominent mistress. Lillian Meacham was a member of the Fabian Society and a "New Woman". He seduced her over readings of Nietzsche and at meetings of the Theosophical Society. Then he whisked her off to Chartres, where she became his "apprentice". His plan was to set up a ménage à trois as a rebellion against the moral order.

Gill also enjoyed casual sex in Turkish baths. Once he took Ethel and her brother-in-law Ernest along. Another time Ethel allowed Ernest to "play with her body" in bed, to Gill's evident delectation. Troilism was very much up Eric's street.

Gill did not mind being the other corner of the triangle in a ménage à trois. He liked to get naked with his patron Robert Gibbs and Gibbs's wife Moira while they kissed and fondled.

"Bath after supper and dancing (nude)," Gill confided to his diary. "R. and M. fucked one another after, M. holding me the while."

One thing led to another.

"A man's penis and balls are very beautiful things and the power to see this beauty is not confined to the opposite sex," he wrote. "The shape of the head of a man's erect penis is very excellent in the mouth. There is no doubt about this. I have often wondered – now I know."

Nevertheless, in accord with the teachings of the Church, he considered homosexuality to be "the ultimate disrespect both to the human body and to human love". But it was not an abiding passion. Usually he would move on to the wives and girlfriends of friends, considering all women to be essentially his. His secretary, Mrs Colette Yardley, was also fair game.

In 1907, he moved out to Ditchling in East Sussex, where he became fascinated with the sexual organs of animals. He would examine animal semen under the microscope, comparing it with his own. One day when the bull failed to mount a cow and service it, the vet prescribed a medicine. Instead of giving it to the bull, Gill gulped it down himself and proclaimed the following morning it was no good.

His animal experimentation did not end there.

"Expt with dog in eve," ran his diary entry for 8 December 1929. Five days later, he wrote: "Continued experiment with dog after and discovered that dog will join with man."

In his work, he often depicted couples copulating. One drawing shows two men penetrating one woman. And he did not like using professional models for his work, preferring to get people he knew to strip off. It was also a way of recruiting new lovers. He seduced Mrs Beatrice Wade, a lady friend of fellow typographer Stanley Morison, after she modelled nude for him. It was the beginning of an enduring affair.

When Joseph Cribb, Gill's apprentice, announced his engagement to sixteen-year-old farm girl Agnes Weller, Gill exercised his *droit de seigneur*. Sixteen-year-old Daisy Hawkins was also ensnared by fifty-year-old Gill. He had known her from childhood. Then when she came to the Gills as a servant, he persuaded her to model for his *Twenty-Five Nudes* and made her his mistress. Their affair continued for two years.

But what most outraged the Christian Survivors of Sexual Abuse, of course, was Gill having sex with his three daughters. Once they were pubescent, he loved to portray them nude. Moving on to sex was a matter of experimentation. For example, when his daughter Betty was sixteen, he recorded that he had made her come one afternoon. Then she had performed the same service for him. While they did it, he instructed her to watch the effects of orgasm on the anus. It raised important questions. Why should the sphincter contract during orgasm? he asked. And why should a man's anus behave the same way as a woman's?

More dastardly things happened at night when he visited his younger daughters' bedrooms at night.

"Stayed half an hour – put p. in her a/hole," he wrote in his diary. And he knew it was wrong. "This must stop," he added.

Received into the Catholic Church in 1913, Gill confessed to Father John O'Connor. But the priest knew so little about sex that Gill ended up doing a series of "fucking drawing and diagrams for Fr. O'C.". According to Gill's biographer Fiona MacCarthy, Father O'Connor was also a connoisseur of the nude. Gill even produced a wood engraving called *Nuptials of God*, showing Christ fucking on the Cross. Gill's brother, also a Catholic convert, went one better and seduced a nun.

When Eric Gill's daughters grew up and began to take lovers of their own, he was jealous. Nevertheless, they were surprisingly well adjusted and went on to lead contented married lives. But then incest was commonplace in the Gill family. Even though his father was a priest, nudity was de rigueur when Gill was young. One day, while out walking on the Downs with his sisters, they suddenly threw off their clothes and continued naked, shocking a passing shepherd. As a youth, he had sex with his older sister Cicely and her friend "Bunny" Browne.

Sex with his sister Gladys continued throughout their lives. He even liked to watch her at it with other men. Gladys and her husband Ernest Laughton were the models for a relief Gill called *Fucking*. Now in the Tate Gallery, it has been renamed tamely *Ecstasy*.

As to the *Stations of the Cross*, Westminster Cathedral stood firm. After all, if the Church began to remove the work of artists whose sex lives it disapproved of, it would have to close down the Sistine Chapel.

## Amedeo Modigliani

The painter Amedeo Modigliani had one exhibition of his work in his lifetime. It was immediately closed down by the chief of the Paris police, who was scandalized by Modigliani's nudes.

Even more scandalized were Monsieur and Madame Hébuterne. The naked form of their nineteen-year-old daughter – with a very prominent triangle of pubic hair – adorned the cover of the catalogue. They were good, respectable middle-class Catholics and she had shacked up with a penniless, thirty-four-year-old, drunken, drug-taking Jewish bohemian.

Modigliani was an Italian from Livorno who could never get enough nudes. Even in his religious paintings, the women had to strip off. And his nudes were extraordinarily seductive because he took the precaution of fucking the model first and then, some say, fucking them again afterwards.

At the age of eighteen, he enrolled in Giovanni Fattori's Scuola de Nudo – the School of Nude Studies – in Florence. A handsome man, there was no shortage of volunteers to help him with his home study and he was always seen about town with a beautiful young woman on his arm.

After further studies of a similar nature in Venice, he moved to Paris where he joined the life class at the Académie Colarossi. Picasso advised him to move to Montmartre. This was more to his tastes as the can-can dancers taking a break on the street corners were happy to show him that they wore no underwear under their dresses.

He got washerwomen and street girls, as well as well-bred virgins, to pose for him. He even took over one of Picasso's cast-offs and made love to her relentlessly in the hope that some of the master's genius would rub off. In homage to Picasso's blue period, he got women with syphilis to model nude for him.

His passion for nudity extended beyond his professional life. A Parisian lady recalled seeing Modigliani with his mistress Elvira, a ravishing courtesan who worked under the name La Quique, dancing naked in a garden. He took up with the artist and model Nina Hamnett, a woman who found it difficult to keep her clothes on in a public place. So he stripped off too and chased her up the street.

Modigliani shunned the Italian Futurists because they condemned the painting of nudes and remarked that "women of a beauty worth painting or sculpting often seem encumbered by their clothes" – which must have seemed like a pretty good chat-up line. He also smoked hash, which he found put his models in the mood, and was a fan of pornography.

He even found working girls who would pose nude for him for free, as well as wash, cook and clean. A prominent businessman foolishly commissioned him to paint a portrait of his wife. When he came home to find his wife nude, he tried to throw Modigliani out of the house. The painter resisted stoutly and the businessman fled. Later, when Modigliani returned to see his new mistress, she had disappeared along with his painting of her. It is said she died in an insane asylum, addicted to the drugs he introduced her to.

The art dealer Paul Chéron almost made the same mistake. He sent his wife to sit for Modigliani. But she was not to his taste, so he took Chéron's pretty young maid instead.

When he bedded Gaby, the thirty-year-old *maîtresse en titre* of a prominent lawyer, her boyfriend summoned Modigliani to the Café Panthéon on the Boulevard Saint-Michel. Before they could come to blows, Modigliani raved about Gaby's beauty, then produced a picture he had painted of her nude. United in their love for the beauty of this one woman, the two of them got drunk together and ended the evening swearing eternal friendship.

The feminist Beatrice Hastings came from London to meet Modigliani and filled her column in *The New Age* with stories about him. He painted her nude and as a courtesan and made no attempt to be faithful. They fought. One night, there was a commotion in her apartment. The concierge came to find out what was going on and knocked on the door. Modigliani answered it and said, "I am merely chopping firewood and beating my mistress like a gentleman."

Apparently Beatrice had bitten his balls.

One night at a party, he got so angry with her that he threw her out of a window. On another occasion, she complained that she had nothing to wear to a ball. He grabbed an old black silk dress of hers, painted a floral pattern on it and cut a new daring décolletage. The dress was a sensation. But then Modigliani became exasperated by her flirting and tore the dress to pieces.

He refused to allow her to pose for the painter Moïse Kisling. When asked why, Modigliani said, "As far as I am concerned, if a woman poses for you, she gives herself to you."

She was already having an affair with the Italian sculptor Alfredo Pina, then left Modigliani for Raymond Radiguet, the teenage author of the steamy bestseller *Le Diable au Corps*. She was forty. The pretty French Canadian model Simone Thiroux took over. She found him drunk one night in La Rotonde, took him home, put him to bed and got in with him.

Modigliani's new dealer Leopold Zborowski returned from the South of France to find that Modigliani had painted three portraits of his wife in the nude. To stop this happening again, Zborowski set up a studio for Modigliani and hired models for him. Naturally, he had to drop by occasionally to see that the artist and his model were hard at work.

In 1917, at the height of the slaughter of World War I, Modigliani painted a series of nudes. The models were shop girls, waitresses, seamstresses, prostitutes – openly sexual women in the flower of their youth. These suddenly found a buyer. Until then Modigliani had given away most of his work. Simone Thiroux then fell pregnant. Now he was selling, it was said, she wanted a Modigliani of her own. He refused to acknowledge the child, who was probably not his anyway, and the affair ended.

It was then that he met Jeanne Hébuterne. Although the Japanese artist Tsuguharu Foujita claimed to have had an affair with her, friends said she was a virgin when she met Modigliani. He painted her twenty-five times. She too became a celebrity thanks to his one and only show.

Numerous celebrities turned up for the opening. One of Modigliani's most inviting nudes hung in the window of the gallery. It drew a crowd. It also drew the police. When they entered the gallery and asked for it to be taken down, they found the walls crammed with more of the same. The commissioner was called and he ordered the gallery to be closed because – sin of sins – the female nudes had pubic hair.

Despite the success of the show in PR terms, he only sold two drawings for thirty francs each and was soon back in the study struggling with more nudes.

At the beginning of 1918, there were air raids on Paris and the city was now in range of the German long-range "Paris Gun". The art dealers fled south and Modigliani followed his market. He was joined by Jeanne, who was pregnant. As a statement of purpose to her parents, he acknowledged the child and promised to marry her when they returned. This can have been little consolation when they heard that Modigliani and their precious daughter had been accompanied by Foujita and his wife, the former prostitute Fernande Barrey.

Modigliani continued painting Jeanne and any other woman who would pose for him. He was also drinking heavily. When his daughter was born, he set off for the town hall to register the birth, but went on the piss instead. Then they were thrown out of the hotel after an altercation with a local pimp, whose girls were posing for him for free.

While in the South of France, he took time to visit Jean Renoir who said famously, "Before I paint, I caress the buttocks for hours . . ."

Modigliani said, "I don't like buttocks" and walked out.

True, Modigliani always did full frontals.

When they returned to Paris, Modigliani went out on the piss with the painter Maurice Utrillo. Finding they could not pay the bill at the famous artists' haunt Rosalie's, they decided to paint a mural. Rosalie was not amused and ordered them to clean it off. Today it would have been worth millions.

Jeanne found herself being edged out of Modigliani's life when fourteen-year-old Paulette Jourdain began posing for him. There was little she could do about it. Then he began painting two young Swedish girls. All she could do was look on.

By this time he was drinking so much, his health was failing. He died on 20 January 1920 of tubercular meningitis. On his deathbed it is thought that he suggested that Jeanne join him in death "so that I can have my favourite model in Paradise and with her enjoy eternal happiness". The day after his death, the heavily pregnant Jeanne jumped from a fifth-floor window and killed herself, mutilating the beautiful body that he had immortalized.

Modigliani was buried in Père Lachaise Cemetery. Jeanne Hébuterne was buried in the Cimetière de Bagneux outside Paris. It was not until 1930 that her grieving family allowed her body to be moved to rest beside Modigliani with a single tombstone that honours them both. His epitaph reads: "Struck down by Death at the moment of glory." Hers reads: "Devoted companion to the extreme sacrifice."

After his death, his work began to fetch high prices. But they retained their power to scandalize. In 1949, when *Life* magazine ran a feature showing Modigliani's nudes, readers from all over America cancelled their subscriptions.

## Leonardo da Vinci

In 1476, the twenty-four-year-old Leonardo da Vinci appeared in court in Florence charged with sodomy. This has been presented as incontrovertible proof that he was gay.

However, the accusation was made anonymously. On street corners in Renaissance Florence, there were drums or *tamburi* where you could leave unsigned notes denouncing your fellow citizens. One such faceless accuser alleged that Leonardo and three friends had sodomized seventeen-year-old prostitute

Jacopo Saltarelli. Sodomy was a serious charge, punishable by burning at the stake.

The accusation was registered and an investigation began. The first hearing was scheduled for 9 April 1476. But for the trial to proceed, statements from witnesses were required. There were none. The trial was postponed until 7 June. But again the prosecution turned up empty handed and the case was dropped. And that was the end of the scandal. It seems that one of Leonardo's co-defendants was a member of the ruling Medici family, who were becoming increasingly unpopular and the accusation was a political smear.

Sodomy was a common charge to throw at Renaissance artists and few could afford to marry. They also surrounded themselves with male models. Renaissance artists were emulating classical Greece and Rome where the male nude was the central icon. Leonardo, as an apprentice in the studio of Andrea del Verrocchio, would have posed nude. He is thought to have been the model for Verrocchio's bronze *David*. It is also thought that Leonardo's own *Vitruvian Man* – the naked man with his arms outstretched, framed by a circle and a square – is a self-portrait.

Benvenuto Cellini, no shrinking violet when it came to women, was convicted of sodomy twice. The first time he got off with paying just twelve measures of flour. Later, when he discovered his model for the *Nymph of Fontainebleau*, a young French woman named Caterina, was two-timing him with his friend Pagolo Micceri, he kicked her out. She then accused him of having "used her in the Italian fashion" – that is, sodomized her – though she was prepared to settle out of court for a few hundred ducats. In court, he denied everything, saying as she plainly knew what she was doing it must be the French fashion too. Then he got her to spell out, in detail, what he was supposed to have done, several times. Then he told the judge: "I know that by the laws of his Most Christian Majesty such crimes are punished by burning at the stake. The woman confesses her guilt, while I admit nothing."

He also demanded that her mother, who had provided Caterina as a model, should be burnt too, as a procurer. They dropped the case.

A third accusation came in February 1557. It was alleged that "for about five years he had kept as his apprentice a youth named Fernando di Giovanni de Montepulciano, with whom he had carnal intercourse very many times and committed the crime of sodomy, sleeping in the same bed with him as his wife". This was his model Dorotea. Though they were not married, Cellini had had their son legitimized.

Fernando had been his apprentice for five years. When he left his employ, Cellini had drawn up a will, leaving him thirty gold florins and thirty *staia* of grain. His family plainly wanted more. In the face of torture, Cellini pleaded guilty. He was fined fifty *scudi* and jailed, but he was soon released when his friend, the Bishop of Pavia, lodged an appeal on his behalf.

The rapacious Pietro Aretino was also accused of sodomy, though his literary output makes it clear where his proclivities lay. So was Botticelli, but his name alone invites suspicion.

Then there was Leonardo's pupil Giovanni Antonio Bazzi, a.k.a. Il Sodoma. But Raphael studied with Sodoma and he simply adored women. While he was betrothed to Maria Bibbiena, Cardinal Medici Bibbiena's niece, he had a number of other lovers. But the permanent fixture in his life was his model and mistress Margherita Luiti, whom he often depicts nude or semi-nude. The daughter of a baker from Sienna, she was known as La Fornarina, which means the "little baker", though it is just one syllable away from "little fornicator", which would be a more accurate description of her role. He grew so jealous that he would break off work from the fresco in the Farnesina palace to spend time with her. Eager to see the fresco completed, Raphael's patron Agostino Chigi persuaded La Fornarina to come and live in the palace so that the painter could get on with his work. There were unintended consequences. Giorgio Vasari, author of *Lives of the Most Eminent Painters, Sculptors and Architects*, put Raphael's death at the age of just thirty-seven down to the fact that he "continued with his amorous pleasures to an inordinate degree".

In his anatomical studies, Leonardo made detailed drawings of women's sexual organs, even depicting the vagina open as if the woman had just had sex, or was just about to. His drawings of the sexual act, which are part of Queen Elizabeth II's collection in Windsor Castle, certainly show that he knew what went where. He also knew how to seduce a woman – or thought he did.

"A man wishes to learn whether the woman will consent to the demands of his lust," he said, "and when he sees that this is so and she desires him, he asks her and puts his desire into action. But he cannot discover this unless he confesses, and when he confesses he fucks."

The phrase Leonardo used was "*e confessando fotte*", which really cannot be translated in any other way.

Leonardo was also the man who discovered that the penis becomes erect because of the retention of blood. Before Leonardo, it was thought that a hard-on was pumped up with air. He even wrote a famous essay called "*Della Vergha*" – "Concerning the Rod" – detailing what a troublesome thing a penis is.

## Concerning the Rod

It holds conference with the human intelligence and sometimes has intelligence itself. When the human will desires to stimulate it, it remains obstinate and follows its own way, sometimes moving by itself without the permission of the man or any mental impetus. Whether he is awake or asleep, it does as it desires. Often the man is asleep and it is awake, and often the man is awake while it sleeps, and often when the man wishes to use it, it desires otherwise, and often it wishes to be used and the man forbids it.

Therefore it appears that this creature possesses a life and intelligence alien from the man, and it seems that men are wrong to be ashamed of giving it a name or of showing it, always covering and concealing what deserves to be adorned and displayed with ceremony as a ministrant.

It is true that the penis does have a life of its own.

Alessandro Vezzoisi, the director of the Leonardo da Vinci museum in Vinci, unearthed evidence that Leonardo was particularly fond of one of the girls in a brothel he frequented in Milan in 1490, when he was thirty-eight. In his writings, Leonardo complained about the toll you had to pay to enter the city of Modesta, though he consoled himself with the fact that it cost less for your whole body to enter Modesta, than for just your prick to enter a prostitute in Florence.

Leonardo's painting *Leda and the Swan* would have been scandalous at the time. It was shockingly full frontal. Until that time, women were depicted in the *pudica* pose – the pose of shame – with one arm across the breasts and a hand over the pubic area. In *Leda and the Swan*, Leonardo breaks all the rules in his Leda. No arm coyly covers the breasts. No bashful hand, errant vegetation, stray tress, or flimsy fabric hides the female pubic area. For the first time in the Western canon, a woman is shown stark, bollock naked.

Worse. She has pubic hair. There is no depiction of female pubic hair in classical art. Look down behind the hand of a classical statue and you will see a smooth, hairless dome. Pubic hair was seen as a symbol of women's wild untamed sexual nature. This, in classical eyes, had to be restrained, if not eradicated.

Worse still. She is standing next to a swan that has its wing cupping her buttocks and she is holding it by its long phallic neck. At her feet are eggs that are hatching. There are babies inside, so there is no mistaking what they have been up to.

Then there is another, more controversial painting. It is called the *Mona Lisa Nude*. It shows a woman sitting in the same pose as the Mona Lisa, only she is naked. The model is the same woman as in *Leda and the Swan*. From her braided hair, we know that she was a prostitute – that was the fashion for prostitutes at the time. Respectable women kept their hair covered. Her name was La Cremona, which probably meant that she came from Cremona in the Duchy of Milan, though it was under Venetian control at the time. However, like Raphael, Leonardo was a punster. La Cremona is very nearly *Lacrimosa*, which means "tearful" or the "tearful woman". The *Mona Lisa* in Italy is known as *La Gioconda*; leading historians believe that the sitter was the wife of the Florentine merchant Francesco di Bartolomeo del Giocondo. But *La Gioconda* also means the jocund or joyful woman, drawing another parallel between the two paintings.

From Leonardo's domestic accounts, it is clear that La Cremona was part of his household for ten years. She also travelled with him. It is very probable that she was his mistress. He called himself the "disciple of experience". He studied the biology and mechanics of sexual intercourse and said that the only way to understand how the world worked was through *esperimento e esperienza* – experiment and experience. With La Cremona on staff there was always an opportunity to experience what he was studying first hand.

When Leonardo died in France in 1519, he left a very expensive fur coat to his housekeeper whom he called La Maturina. This is an affectionate diminutive that means "the little mature woman". La Cremona would then have been ten years older than she was when she is first mentioned as part of Leonardo's entourage. And La Maturina is exactly what you would call a prostitute ten years after her sell-by date.

Curiously Leonardo da Vinci did not give the *Mona Lisa* to whoever had commissioned it. It was with him and his model and mistress in Cloux when he died. Perhaps we can now see why she is smiling. It is the smile of a woman who has just been fucked, or is just about to be. It seems to say, come on Leonardo, put the brushes down . . .

## Michelangelo Buonarroti

Leonardo's great rival, Michelangelo, was gay. He could not stand to look at naked women. When he had to depict a female nude, he would get a man to pose for him, then make the appropriate adjustments. That is why the breasts of his women have been stuck on. He can do a pert-arsed *David*, but take a look at the figure *Night* on the tomb of Giulinao de' Medici. And if it was not bad enough being a sodomite in Renaissance Italy, Michelangelo was into some serious kinky stuff. Living in fear of discovery, he was regularly blackmailed. But, thanks to his talent, he managed to keep the lid on his scandalous sex life – while he was alive, at least.

Michelangelo was one of the Neoplatonic school who sought to re-establish the ideals of classical Greece and actively embraced homosexuality. This did not go down well in Florence where he was brought up. In 1502, the sodomy laws were tightened, outlawing any sort of homosexual practice. Four years later, amputation of the hand became the punishment for procuring. Houses where homosexual acts took place were burned down and fathers who allowed their sons to fiddle around with other boys were punished. So for Michelangelo to follow his natural impulses would be dangerous, possibly fatal. For much of his life he kept his urges under control and sublimated them into his art.

He also spent much of his life in Rome where attitudes were much more liberal, only returning to Florence in 1513 at the request of the Medici pope Leo X (see page 374) who shared his proclivities. But when Leo died in 1521, there was another clamp down. The new pope Hadrian VI complained: "For many years, abominable things have taken place in the

Chair of Peter, abuses in spiritual matters, transgressions of the commandments, so that everything here has been wickedly perverted."

But in 1522, at the age of forty-seven, Michelangelo could no longer contain himself. He was already writing to his model Gherardo Perini and giving him drawings. In February 1522, he sent a note to Perini begging him to come over. In the corner of the letter, he drew a small boy holding his penis. It was an image he would use again in *The Children's Bacchanal*. He also bought Perini expensive perfume, writing in a poem:

> I have bought you, at no small cost,
> A little something that smells sweet,
> Since by a scent one often knows a street,
> Wherever I am, where you may be,
> I can be clear and certain, free of doubt.
> If you hide from me, I'll pardon you,
> For, carrying this, always, as you pass,
> Even if I were blind, I would find you.

When Perini turned his back on Michelangelo, he was distraught, writing: "For myself I wept here, and with infinite sorrow" and "He who stole myself from me and never turned back."

Sixteen-year-old Antonio Mini moved into Michelangelo's house. They lived together for nine years until Mini left for France in 1531. As a parting gift, Michelangelo gave him his version of *Leda and the Swan*. The painting shows a naked Leda with the swan between her legs. She is clearly in ecstasy as the swan's phallic neck nestles between her breasts and its beak enters her mouth. And the swan is not having a bad time either. This is by far the most erotic image Michelangelo ever created.

By the time Mini left, Michelangelo had already meet Andrea Quaratesi. The son of a Florentine banking family, he sat for Michelangelo – the only portrait he ever finished. In a note, Michelangelo called Quaratesi his "great consolation" and begs him to "love me".

Another depiction of Quaratesi exists. It is on an exercise sheet and he appears to be about fourteen. Next to him are a screaming satyr and a man shitting. Draw your own conclusions. Cellini also said that Michelangelo was enamoured of the poet Luigi Pulci who was later beheaded for committing incest with his daughters.

Now all this could have been entirely innocent. But in 1533 Michelangelo was forced to leave Florence for ever because of his model Febo di Poggio, whom he called "that little blackmailer". Febo even sent a letter to Rome, telling Michelangelo to send a money order to Florence by messenger.

"Do not fail to answer," he threatened. "I will not write more . . . praying to God to keep you from harm." Is that a threat?

Michelangelo left clues to why he was being blackmailed in his poetry, where he alluded to Febo as Phoebus. He wrote:

> I truly should, so happy was my lot,
> While Phoebus was inflaming all the hill,
> Have risen from the earth while I was able,
> Using his feathers and thus make my dying sweet.

*Poggio* means hill, so is Phoebus inflaming his own hill or Michelangelo's? The feathers come up again in a later verse:

> His feathers were my wings, his hill my steps,
> Phoebus was a lamp for my feet. To die then
> Would have been my salvation and pleasure.

Feathers were important to Michelangelo. Indeed, *Leda and the Swan* is not the only place that Michelangelo depicts sex with birds. In *The Rape of Ganymede*, he shows the naked Ganymede being sexually assaulted from behind by Zeus in the form of an eagle. The boy is clearly in ecstasy while the eagle's clawed feet spread his legs. Ganymede goes on to be Zeus's willing catamite

In *The Punishment of Tityus*, Michelangelo shows a naked man being overpowered by a big bird. In Renaissance Florence, the word "bird" – *uccello* – was slang for the male genitals, just as it was in the United States in the late nineteenth century. And "bird" or "young thrush", in Florentine slang, was also a boy who might be bagged and plucked.

In the louche environs of Rome, the fifty-seven-year-old Michelangelo met a handsome twenty-three-year-old aristocrat named Tommaso de' Cavalieri. It was for him that Michelangelo drew *The Rape of Ganymede*, *The Punishment of Tityus* and *The Children's Bacchanal*. The latter shows an orgy of drunken boys with just two adult figures – an old hag with wizened breasts and a sleeping man.

Although Michelangelo claimed, at first, that his love for Tommaso was "chaste", he plied the young man with compliments – he had "not only incomparable physical beauty, but so much elegance in manners, such excellent intelligence, and such graceful behaviour, that he well deserved, and still deserves, to win more love the better he is known".

Tommaso responded: "I swear to return your love. Never have I loved a man more than I love you, never have I wished for a friendship more than I wish for yours."

Soon, Michelangelo's poems to Tommaso were full of words like "burning" and the "fire that consumes me".

> If the hope you have given me is true,
> And true the good desire that's granted me,
> Let the wall set between us fall away,
> And there is double power in secret woe.

Michelangelo is plainly on a promise. Then later:

> If capture and defeat must be my joy,
> It is no wonder that, alone and naked,
> I remain prisoner of a knight-at-arms.

Now he has got what he wanted. A knight-at-arms in late medieval Italian is *un cavalier armato*, clearly a pun on Tommaso de' Cavalieri's name. They lived together for six months, but their relationship endured, even after Tommaso was married. Ten years later, Michelangelo wrote to Tommaso:

> The love for what I speak of reaches higher;
> Woman's too much unlike, no heart by rights
> Ought to grow hot for her, if wise and male.
>
> One draws to Heaven and to earth the other,
> One in the soul, one living in the sense
> Drawing its bow on what is base and vile.

It may not be base and vile, but as the poem goes on, Michelangelo regurgitates images of birds descending to pluck up mortal men, hearts melting and things being pierced.

By then, Michelangelo had a new love – Cecchino de' Bracci, the nephew and "adopted son" of Michelangelo's close friend Luigi del Riccio. When he died at the age of fifteen in 1544, the sixty-nine-year-old Michelangelo wrote forty-eight epitaphs, a sonnet and a madrigal, raving about the beautiful youth. From his writing one can discern that, if they did not have a physical relationship, Michelangelo wanted one.

His love for the dead boy also found visual expression in his drawing *The Dream* which shows a winged boy blowing a horn into the ear of a naked man as if awakening him to higher things. The dreamscape behind him is full of naked figures copulating.

While he raves about male beauty, women are "pigs and prostitutes". He wrote poems vilifying them on the back of sketches and letters. In one, he talks of an ugly, tormenting old woman, with teeth like turnips, hair like leeks, a mouth that resembles a bog filled with beans and breasts like two watermelons in a bag. He gives us one clue of the disgusting things they get up to. On the ceiling of the Sistine Chapel, in the panel depicting the temptation scene in the Garden of Eden, Adam's penis is suspiciously near the mouth of the kneeling Eve. If that is not scandalous, I don't know what is.

# 11

## Literary Lapses

### Oscar Wilde

The trial of Oscar Wilde was one of the great sex scandals of the Victorian era. He was found guilty of "gross indecency" and sent to jail for two years' hard labour. He is now seen as a gay martyr – a man destroyed by society's prejudice against homosexuality. However, he was not interested in having sex with other men, but rather underage boys. These days he would have gone to prison for much longer and would have spent the rest of his life on the Sex Offender Register.

Wilde would not have considered himself "gay". In his day, the word was used for a prostitute of either sex. Its current meaning comes from slang of the twenties. He would not have been too keen on being called homosexual either. The word had come into the language with the publication of *Psychopathia Sexualis* by Richard von Krafft-Ebing in English in 1892, when Wilde was thirty-eight. In that tome, it was considered an aberrant condition requiring the attention of a doctor, not a harmless proclivity or a lifestyle choice. No, Wilde would have called himself a uranist, which gave Wilde the delightful pun in the title of his most famous play *The Importance of Being Earnest*. It comes from a reference made by Plato in his *Symposiums* to the Greek goddess of love Aphrodite – also known as Urania. A uranian is another nineteenth-century word for homosexual.

Sadly it also means an inhabitant of Uranus – though there is no evidence that Oscar was a science-fiction fan.

Oscar Wilde's father, Sir William Wilde, was a womanizer whose personal hygiene repelled his fastidious son. He was embroiled in a sex scandal when Oscar was a boy. A woman named Miss Mary Josephine Travers claimed that Sir William, a prominent surgeon, had given her a whiff of chloroform so that he could have his way with her. The trial in Dublin was the sensation of the 1860s. Sir William lost, but Miss Travers was awarded just one farthing, the smallest coin of the realm. Her chastity, it seems, was worth just over a tenth of a penny.

Oscar's mother, Lady Jane Wilde, wanted a daughter and dressed her son in girl's clothes until he went to school. A boarder at Portora Royal School, Enniskillen, he reported no sexual adventures. However, the day he left school another boy came up and kissed him. Tears ran down his face.

Uranism may already have been stirring.

"I was nearly sixteen when the wonder and beauty of the old Greek life began to dawn upon me," said Oscar.

At the time, John Pentland Mahaffy, a noted classic scholar at Trinity College Dublin and close friend of the Archbishop, was writing a book called *Social Life in Greece* and he encouraged Oscar to lend a hand. This was the first book to contain a frank discussion of "Greek love" – that is, the romantic affections between an older man and a beautiful young boy. Oscar called Mahaffy "my first and best teacher . . . the scholar who showed me how to love Greek things". They sampled the pleasures of Greece together, taking a holiday there one summer.

At Oxford, Wilde wrote poetry celebrating male lovers in Greek history. He and fellow undergraduate Cresswell Augustus "Gussy" Cresswell had "long chats and walks". Oscar used the word "spooning" to describe other activities undertaken with choirboys. According to the *Oxford English Dictionary*, by that time spooning already meant "to lie close together, to fit into each other, in the manner of spoons".

Surely that's forking. Oscar also wrote a poem called "Choir Boy" which spelt out what he wanted to do in the stalls. When asked what he wanted to do in life, Oscar said that he "would like nothing better in after life than to be the hero of such a *cause célèbre* and to go down to posterity as the first defendant in such a case as *Regina* versus *Wilde*". Well, he got his wish.

Wilde mixed with other uranists who believed, like the Greeks, that you pretty much gave up same-sex love when you reached marriageable age. As an adult under the law, it was best to avoid sodomy. In 1828, the penalty for sodomy had been increased from imprisonment to death. Understandably, like his friends, Oscar began to show an interest in girls. After a number of flirtations, he fell in love with Florence Balcombe. However, he delayed his proposal because he had caught syphilis. Florrie had a lucky escape when she married Bram Stoker, author of *Dracula*.

Wilde was not too put out by this as he was having an affair with a portrait painter named Frank Miles, whom he slept with while still at Oxford. Through Miles he met the sculptor Lord Ronald Gower, who introduced him to London's sexual underworld and the delights of "rough trade" with soldiers, sailors and labourers. Gower was the model for Lord Henry Wotton, the corrupting influence in *The Picture of Dorian Gray*. He soon tossed aside Miles for a younger artist named Arthur May.

In 1877, Oscar reviewed an exhibition at the Grosvenor Galley where he drools over the images of beautiful young boys and the "bloom and vitality and the radiance of this adolescent beauty". It is stuffed with references to Greek mythology and Ganymede, the beautiful shepherd boy raped by Zeus in the shape of an eagle. This attracted the attention of the art critic Walter Pater, leader of the Aesthetic movement who had already courted scandal through his relationship with the "Balliol Bugger" William Money Hardinge. It was said that

Oscar's "intimacy" with Pater turned him, by his own account, into an "extreme aesthete".

He told Pater of his ambition, saying, "Somehow or other I'll be famous, and if not famous, I'll be notorious." Steaming straight down that track, he began to publish homoerotic poetry.

Coming down from Oxford, Wilde lived with like-minded young men in Salisbury Street off the Strand. When Lillie Langtry came for tea, he was smitten. He threw himself at a number of actresses but, after growing his hair long, dressing in a flowing velvet jacket and knee breeches and being seen holding a single lily as he walked down Piccadilly, he was lampooned in *Punch* magazine for being a tad fey. Gilbert and Sullivan satirized him in their comic opera *Patience* as the effeminate "fleshly poet" Bunthorne – Bum-horn more like, sorry. But Oscar was to gain from the notoriety this parody gave him when the production opened to rave reviews in New York. The impresario Richard D'Oyly Carte sent for him. When he arrived in America, he certainly dressed the part. The *New York World* reported: "He wore patent-leather shoes, a smoking-cap or turban, and his shirt might be termed ultra-Byronic, or perhaps *décolleté*. A sky-blue cravat of the sailor style hung well down upon his chest. His hair flowed over his shoulders in dark-brown waves, curling slightly upwards at the ends."

On his tour of the US, he was widely mocked and scorned, while male followers painted their faces and rouged their cheeks. But Oscar did not care. He kissed Walt Whitman on the lips and praised his poetry as "Greek". People drew their own conclusions.

After having a couple more marriage proposals rejected, Oscar settled on twenty-three-year-old Constance Mary Lloyd, the sister of a friend at Oxford. He was plainly serious about the marriage as he immediately set about trying to "cure" his homosexuality by having sex with a number of prostitutes.

When he proposed to Constance, she accepted immediately, though she had already condemned some of his work for its lack of "morality". He was attracted to her slim, boyish figure. The problem was that he could not keep his hands off the real thing.

Once he was married, Oscar felt quite at liberty to go off with other men. This was because, after Constance gave birth to their two sons, she lost her boyish figure and became round and womanly, which repelled Wilde.

"When I married, my wife was a beautiful girl, white and slim as a lily, with dancing eyes and rippling laughter like music," he told Frank Harris. "Within a year or so the flower-like grace had all vanished; she became heavy, shapeless, deformed. She dragged herself about the house in uncouth misery with a drawn blotched face and hideous body, sick at heart because of our love. It was dreadful. I tried to be kind to her, forced myself to touch and kiss her; but she was sick always and – oh! I cannot recall it, it is all loathsome. I used to wash my mouth and open the window to cleanse my lips in the pure air."

Pregnancy he considered a deformity; menstruation an abomination.

"There is no comparison between a boy and a girl," he told Harris. "Think of the enormous, fat hips which every sculptor has to tone down, and make lighter, and the great udder breasts which the artist has to make small and round and firm." When it came to sex: "A woman's passion is degrading. She is continually tempting you. She wants your desire as a satisfaction for her vanity more than anything else, and her vanity is insatiable if her desire is weak, and so she continually tempts you to excess, and then blames you for the physical satiety and disgust which she herself created." And women only stopped shagging when they had "glutted their lust". Fortunately, he was away from home a lot.

Sodomy had long been against the law, but it was hard to prove unless there was evidence of the "emission of seed" up the rectum. However, in 1885, the Criminal Law Amendment Act outlawed other acts of "gross indecency" between men. The irony was that the act was not designed to persecute homosexuals. It was, it said: "An Act to make further provision for the Protection of Women and Girls, the suppression of brothels, and other purposes."

In July 1885, the crusading editor of the *Pall Mall Gazette* W. T. Stead caused a scandal when he published a series of articles called "The Maiden Tribute of Modern Babylon". He showed that in Victorian London underage girls were being sold into prostitution. To prove his case, he bought thirteen-year-old Eliza Armstrong from her alcoholic mother for £5. The newspaper sold out day after day, while Stead was jailed for three months for making the purchase.

England was in a moral panic about the sex trade and the 1885 Act was introduced to raise the age of consent for women from thirteen to sixteen and further tighten the curbs on prostitution. However, maverick Liberal MP Henry Labouchère seized the opportunity to introduce an amendment that read:

> Any male person who, in public or private, commits, or is party to the commission of, or procures or attempts to procure the commission by any male person of, any act of gross indecency with another male person, shall be guilty of a misdemeanour, and being convicted thereof shall be liable at the discretion of the court to be imprisoned for any term not exceeding two years, with or without hard labour.

Even though Wilde wrote for the *Pall Mall Gazette*, he seemed oblivious to the change in the law and continued picking up young men in public lavatories. He even brought some of his young conquests with him to the marital home in Tite Street in Chelsea. Others took him to pubs where he could pick up young boys. Wilde also had procurers supplying underage talent and was sleeping with Fred Atkins, a female impersonator, male prostitute and professional blackmailer. Wilde regularly paid off male prostitutes who blackmailed him.

And it was not as if Oscar was discreet. When he published *The Happy Prince and Other Tales* in 1888, he gave a copy to the young American playwright Clyde Fitch with, written on the flyleaf: "Clyde Fitch from his friend Oscar Wilde. Faëry-Stories for one who lives in Faëry-Land." Fairy was already New York slang for an effeminate gay man.

*The Picture of Dorian Gray*, published in 1890, is positively throbbing with homosexual innuendo. Even fellow uranists thought he had gone too far. The gay undertones were not lost on the press either. Dorian was compared to Ganymede. But, like all bad publicity, it didn't half help sales – especially in the wake of the Cleveland Street Scandal (see page 426). Meanwhile the public – and Henry Labouchère – were baying for the blood of "sodomites".

Wilde's play *Salomé* was banned in Britain and had to be staged in Paris where homosexuality was legal under the Napoleonic Code. Gay men in Paris had taken to wearing green cravats as green was the colour favoured by effeminate men in classical Rome. Then in 1891, they began sporting green carnations in their buttonholes. Oscar seized on the fashion. At the opening of *Lady Windermere's Fan* in London in 1892, a dozen young men, some wearing make-up, took their seats in the stalls wearing green carnations. Another young man wore one on stage.

At the end of the play, Oscar made a speech saying how much he had enjoyed it, then lit a cigarette – at a time when a gentleman did not smoke in the presence of a lady. He puffed on his cigarette deliberately as "puff" had just come in as slang for an effeminate man. The cartoonists had a field day.

The play and Wilde's performance were a deliberate affront to Constance who had to sit through the whole thing with his former lover Arthur Clifton. Wilde was there with his new beaux and ignored her throughout. She had to go home alone, while he entertained his friends in the Albemarle Hotel, where he bedded a seventeen-year-old boy whom he had seduced a few days before by plying him with whisky and champagne.

In 1891, he had met Lord Alfred Douglas, nicknamed "Bosie", who was still a student at Oxford. They had a brief affair.

"Wilde treated me as an older boy treats a younger one at school," Bosie told Frank Harris. "What was new to me and was not (as far as I know) known or practised among my contemporaries: he 'sucked' me."

Bosie's father, the Marquess of Queensberry, who famously lent his name to the rules of boxing, was right on the button when he later accused Oscar of being a "cock-sucker". Wilde said that it gave him "inspiration". He would pay delivery boys to let him suck them off.

"Love is a sacrament that should be taken kneeling," he said.

Two months after being bedded by Oscar, Bosie penned the poem "Two Loves" which contains the line "I am the love that dare not speak its name" – presumably because it has got its mouth full. He also published a poem on the joys of oral sex, described in a suitably veiled Victorian way.

Oscar and Bosie soon stopped having sex with each other. Instead, as they shared an interest in "Greek love", they took to swapping young partners. They took adjoining rooms in the Savoy Hotel and shared rent boys, some as young as fourteen. The chambermaids complained that the sheets and nightshirts were stained with Vaseline, semen and excrement. Eventually the laundry staff rebelled and they were kicked out, only to continue the action back at the Albemarle.

No one was under any illusion what was going on. Constance had turned up at the Savoy, begging Oscar to come home to see the children at least. He said he could not. It had been so long since he had been in Tite Street he could not remember the number of the house. The news even reached Paris, where his behaviour was the talk of the literary set. Henri de Régnier told Edmond de Goncourt: "He admits to being a pederast. He told me that he has been married three times: once to a woman and twice to men. Following the success of his play in London, he left his wife and three children and moved into a hotel where he lived conjugally with a young British lord."

Rumours that Constance was considering divorcing Oscar on the grounds of sodomy reached the ears of the Marquess of Queensberry, who questioned Bosie about it. After a brief and scandalous holiday in Paris, Bosie went back to Oxford where the two of them shared sixteen-year-old Walter Grainger. When Oscar and Bosie set up home together at "The Cottage" in Goring, Grainger was taken on as assistant butler with a room next to Oscar's. Grainger said Wilde would "work me up with his hand and then made me spend in his mouth". Again this was hardly a secret. The head butler caught Grainger naked in Wilde's room.

Oscar and Bosie would cavort naked around the garden. When the vicar turned up unexpectedly, he was told: "You have come just in time to enjoy a perfect Greek scene." The poor man fled. Constance and the boys also had to put up with this when they visited.

Back in London for the opening of *An Ideal Husband*, which also has a clearly homosexual subplot, Wilde boasted to his new friend Aubrey Beardsley that he was "having five love affairs and resultant copulations with telegraph and district messenger boys in one night. I kissed each one of them in every part of their bodies. They were all dirty and appealed to me for just that reason."

Despite all appearances, Beardsley was straight. He was shocked to the core when Oscar then proceeded to describe in mouth-watering detail the delights of rimming.

The circle surrounding Wilde grew more reckless. One of Oscar's old lovers, Robbie Ross, slept with a schoolboy who was supposed to be back in school the following day. When

Bosie heard about it, he went round, stole the boy off Ross and slept with him himself. The following day he passed him on to Oscar. The next night Bosie paid for the boy to have sex with a female prostitute. The boy arrived back at school three days late. His father was only dissuaded from going to the police when he was told by Wilde's solicitor that his son would almost certainly be prosecuted as well.

Fearing that this might not be the end of the matter, Bosie took off to Egypt and Oscar tried to dump him. Bosie threatened suicide. There was a passionate reunion in Paris. They then returned to London where the Marquess of Queensberry joined them for lunch at the Café Royal. Everything passed off peacefully. But then Queensberry was standing by the window in Carter's Hotel, when he saw Oscar and Bosie and saw Wilde "caress" his son in what he described as an "effeminate and indecent fashion".

Queensberry was particularly hot on this sort of thing. When he heard that his elder son, Viscount Drumlanrig, had been sodomized by Lord Rosebery, the Foreign Secretary, he set off to Bad Homburg, where Rosebery was at the time, to administer a sound thrashing. Rosebery was only saved by the personal intervention of the Prince of Wales, who was also taking the waters in Bad Homburg.

Bosie mocked his father, calling him a "funny little man" and declining any further support from him. Queensberry had problems of his own. Having been divorced by Bosie's mother five years earlier for drinking and womanizing, Queensberry had married a younger woman who, after a disastrous wedding night, asked for an annulment on the grounds of "impotence" and "malformation of the parts of generation".

Queensberry turned up at Tite Street and accused Wilde of "posing as a sodomite". Bosie urged Oscar to sue his father for criminal libel, but others advised caution. Lord Rosebery was now prime minister and Bosie's older brother Viscount Drumlanrig was a junior minister in the Liberal administration.

Given the relationship between the two men, any scandal could bring the government down.

Wilde sent a solicitor's letter to Queensberry, asking him to retract his accusations and make an apology. The marquess refused. Bosie goaded his father, while he and Oscar were as promiscuous as ever. They even indulged on a family holiday with Constance and the boys in Worthing, where Bosie expressed a desire for Oscar's nine-year-old son Cyril. Back in London, Bosie's chum Robert Hichens published, anonymously, *The Green Carnation*, which was clearly based on the love affair between Oscar and Bosie, and painted a vicious portrait of the Marquess of Queensberry. The book confirmed everyone's worst suspicions and, by the end of the year, it had gone through four editions.

Short of cash, Oscar got to work on *The Importance of Being Earnest*. The play is chock-full of uranist references. The ploy the two young male protagonists use to escape the society of women is called "Bunburying". I rest my case. Meanwhile, on a uranian roll, Bosie began to publish more explicit material in the daring new magazine *Chameleon*.

*The Importance of Being Earnest* was an instant success, which meant Oscar could entertain his upper-class uranian friends lavishly in the best restaurants again, while entertaining himself with lower-class rent boys back at the Albemarle Hotel. Then he and Bosie took off for Algiers where thirteen-year-old Arab boys "fluted on our reeds for us".

Queensberry wanted the government to prosecute Wilde over his relationship with Bosie and threatened to expose Rosebery's relationship with Viscount Drumlanrig. To protect Rosebery, Drumlanrig planned to marry, but died in what was recorded as a shotgun accident. It is plain that he committed suicide. Queensberry believed that "Snob Queens like Rosebery" – and Wilde, presumably – were responsible for the corruption of his sons and the death of one of them.

With Drumlanrig was beyond saving, Queensberry went on the offensive. He had planned to disrupt the first night of *The*

*Importance of Being Earnest*, condemning Wilde as a sodomite from the stalls and pelting him with rotting vegetables. But Oscar got wind of it and the theatre was ringed by police.

Nevertheless, when he returned to the Albemarle Hotel, he found a note from Queensberry waiting for him. It read: "For Oscar Wilde ponce and somdomite [*sic*]". Without the funds to flee, Wilde was forced to sue.

However, Queensberry was way ahead of him. He had hired George Lewis, the solicitor Wilde used to pay off blackmailers and straighten out the other problems his irregular lifestyle invited. Instead, Wilde had to hire a new solicitor, Charles Humphreys, who asked him to swear that there was no truth in the libel. Wilde did so. But then, he had written an essay called "The Decay of Lying".

Queensberry was arrested. Under the Libel Act of 1843, Queensberry faced two years in jail and a heavy fine. To avoid prison, he would have to prove that what he had said was true. Wilde and Bosie were sure that Queensberry could not come up with enough evidence to convince a court. But George Lewis could. Even though Lewis then withdrew from the case, Queensberry told the press that the note he had sent to the Albemarle Hotel was a trap and Wilde had walked into it.

Detectives working for Queensberry scoured the West End. In the lodgings of Alfred Taylor, a friend of Wilde's who had skipped town, they found letters and cheques indicating that Taylor had pimped boys to Oscar and others. The boys were tracked and told they faced prosecution unless they made statements incriminating Wilde. Queensberry's investigators also questioned the staff of the Savoy, the Albemarle and other hotels Wilde had used. Queensberry was rich so could afford to pay informants well.

In an attempt to bluff it out, Oscar took Constance out on the town, accompanied by Bosie. They even appeared in a box, watching *The Importance of Being Earnest* together. If his wife saw nothing wrong with Wilde's friendship with Lord Alfred Douglas, who else could condemn it?

They were, it was to prove, a tad overconfident. Bosie arrived at the court in a coach with a liveried coachman and a footman wearing a cockade. Dressed in one of his more outré outfits, Oscar announced: "Have no fear. The working classes are with me, to a boy."

The preliminary hearing had to be adjourned as letters were entered into evidence that mentioned "exalted persons" – Lord Rosebery, perhaps – that were not to be read out in open court. Though Bosie already had some inkling of the evidence his father had amassed and they should have been working on their defence, Bosie persuaded Oscar to take him on holiday to Monte Carlo, where they were thrown out of their hotel when other guests complained.

Back in London, George Bernard Shaw and Frank Harris begged Wilde to drop his prosecution. Oscar refused, saying that he found it both his duty and pleasure to stand up for uranians everywhere. So Oscar hired the leading advocate of the day, Sir Edward Clarke, who said he would take on the case only if Oscar swore on his honour as an English gentleman that Queensberry's accusations were groundless. Wilde was, of course, Irish.

Three days before the trial was due to open, Queensberry filed a Plea of Justification. It cited *The Picture of Dorian Gray* and poems in the *Chameleon* that promoted "sodomitical" practices. But Oscar was on safe ground when it came to literature. However, the Plea went on to mention names, dates, places and details of what Wilde had been up to. These began to appear in the press. It soon became clear that the libel suit was unwinnable. But worse, Queensberry was not just accusing Wilde of "gross indecency" under the Labouchère amendment, he was alleging attempted sodomy in every case. Oscar was now facing life imprisonment. All Wilde could do was keep on lying.

As this was a case of criminal libel – sodomy being a crime – it was heard at the Old Bailey. The press and public galleries were packed. Opening the proceedings, Sir Edward Clarke claimed that the Marquess of Queensberry had hounded Mr Wilde over his entirely innocent relationship with Lord Alfred. They had been seen out together in the company of Mrs Wilde and dined with her in Tite Street. Wilde and Douglas had even dined with Queensberry in the Café Royal. Of course, Sir Edward would not distress the jury with a detailed blow-by-blow repost to the hideous sexual allegations the Marquess had made.

When cross-questioned by Sir Edward, Oscar discharged himself well and the jury warmed to him. But then Queensberry's defence counsel Edward Carson QC rose. He was a childhood friend of Wilde's and they had been up at Oxford together. His first question was an easy one. He simply asked Oscar how old he was.

Wilde said, "Thirty-nine."

With a flourish, Carson produced Wilde's birth certificate. He was forty-one. Wilde had been caught, lying under oath. For Carson, this was a gift. If Wilde had lied about his age, might he not lie about other things? If he posed as being younger than he was, might he not pose as a sodomite? When pressed, Wilde could hardly deny that he was a poser.

The questioning was relentless. It went on for a day and a half. Denied the opiate cigarettes he normally smoked, Oscar was not on the form he might have been, even when it came to literature. He was asked if he had read Bosie's poems. Did he approve of them? What about the other things in the *Chameleon*? Did he approve or did he condemn them?

Then there was *The Picture of Dorian Gray*. He was forced to admit that it could be read as a story about sodomy. Had he even adored a younger man, as Dorian Gray had in the book? He was forced to admit that there was one man he loved, but it was a sacred love, in no way base or sordid.

He was asked about his relations with the boys mentioned in the Plea of Justification. Why did he associate with young men from the lower classes? He recognized no social barriers, Wilde said, and enjoyed the society of young men. Why had he lavished expensive gifts on them? They were close friends, Wilde said. While the jury might be able to accept that he could find the company of Oxford undergraduates stimulating, what stimulation did he get out of the company of a fifteen-year-old boy he had picked up on the beach at Worthing, or the cockney scamps introduced to him by Alfred Taylor? The clear implication was that they were prostitutes.

It soon became clear to Wilde's own lawyers that their client was lying and they tried to persuade him to drop the case. But Bosie urged him to fight on.

The following day, Carson asked him about Alfred Taylor. What did he do for a living? Had he ever seen him in women's attire? How many young men had Taylor introduced him to? Why had he taken the female impersonator Fred Atkins to Paris with him?

Wilde was then asked whether he had ever kissed Walter Grainger. He replied, "Oh, dear no. He was a particularly plain boy – unfortunately ugly – I pitied him for it."

It got a laugh, but Carson pressed him on why the boy's ugliness was relevant. Wilde grew flustered.

"You sting me and insult me and try to unnerve me," he said, "and at times one says things flippantly when one ought to speak more seriously."

Carson opened the case for the defence with a roster of boys and young men who said they had had sex with Wilde. The following day there were queues to get into the courtroom. By then Oscar had decided to drop the case. Sir Edward Clarke conceded that Wilde had "posed as a sodomite" in his literary work. But this was not good enough for the judge. It was, after all, a criminal trial. Queensberry must be found guilty or not guilty. His Plea of Justification was either true or not true. If it was true it must be published in the public interest. The jury took a matter of minutes to find Queensberry not guilty. Wilde's goose was cooked.

He went to see George Lewis who said that, if Oscar had brought Queensberry's note to him in the first place, he would have torn it up. Wilde withdrew to the Cadogan Hotel where he awaited the inevitable.

Queensberry sent a note to the government. Either they prosecute Wilde or he would out a number of senior Liberal politicians. Despite Queensberry's allegations of sodomy, they decided to charge Wilde with "gross indecency". It was the least they could get away with. Bosie would not face prosecution. That might have alienated Queensberry – not a good thing to do with the reputations of so many government ministers at stake. Besides it could be argued that Bosie was one of Wilde's victims.

Five hours after Queensberry's acquittal, warrants were issued for the arrest of Wilde and Taylor. At 6.20 p.m., Oscar was arrested and taken to Bow Street where he was charged. Bosie arrived to stand surety, but there was no possibility of bail. Unable to get his friend out of jail, he started a vigorous campaign to change sexual attitudes, which, under the circumstances, hardly helped.

At the committal proceedings, a number of those mentioned in Queensberry's Plea of Justification testified, along with chambermaids, housekeepers and landladies who said what they knew about the state of the bedlinen.

At their trial at the Old Bailey, Wilde and Taylor were charged with twenty-five counts of gross indecency and conspiracy to commit gross indecency. Wilde made an eloquent speech in his own defence. When asked about "the love that dare not speak its name" – from Douglas's poem "Two Loves" – he talked of the love between an older, intellectual man and a joyful youth as a beautiful and noble thing.

The jury could not reach a verdict and Wilde was released, but the scandal did not die down. The newspapers demanded a retrial. Did the government have something to hide? At a second trial, Wilde was found guilty on seven counts of gross indecency and sentenced to two years hard labour. The judge rued that this was the maximum sentence he could give.

The Liberal government organized a special soft regime for him, but less than a month after Wilde was sent down it was voted out of office. Still owing a bill at the Savoy, he went bankrupt. Constance sought a divorce. At first Wilde fought it but, fearing that evidence of sodomy that might come up in divorce courts would provoke new criminal charges, he relented. Under the terms of the divorce, he would have to live abroad and renounce "any moral misconduct or notoriously consort with evil or disreputable companions" – Bosie – in return for a small allowance.

At the time, Bosie was having a high old time on the Continent. He was warned that if he were not a little more discreet about his activities with young boys the French authorities would deport him back to England, so he moved on to Italy.

In jail, while forswearing homosexuality, Wilde indulged himself with other inmates. At the end of his sentence, he sailed for France where he adopted the name Sebastian Melmouth. While having sex with any young boy he could lay his hands on, he begged Constance for a reconciliation. As a gesture, at Berneval-le-Grand, a town just outside Dieppe, under the sponsorship of the poet Ernest Dowson, he visited a local brothel in an effort to acquire "a more wholesome taste in sex". This was done in the presence of a cheering crowd.

After having a woman, he told the onlookers: "The first these ten years, and it will be the last. But tell it in England, for it will entirely restore my character."

Despite his agreement with Constance, he did see Bosie again. They moved to southern Italy and set up home in

Posillippo – where Lord Rosebery had a villa – with a maid and two boys to serve them. When Constance got wind of this, she threatened to cut him off without a penny.

They made a public show of splitting up, but continued seeing each other, while Wilde teamed up with a former soldier named Maurice Gilbert, who kept two boys – one fourteen, the other twelve. There were plenty of other boys to pass the time.

Oscar Wilde died of cerebral meningitis in Paris in 1900 after being baptized into the Catholic faith. Bosie went on to become engaged to the American lesbian poet Natalie Barney, known in Paris as l'Amazone. However, her strait-laced father did not want the family's name tainted by the Oscar Wilde scandal and broke it off.

## Charles Dickens

The works of Charles Dickens embody many of the stern Victorian values, especially those concerning the sanctity of family life. But scandal bubbled beneath the surface of his own complex private affairs.

He married in 1836 and his wife Catherine gave him ten children. When the growing family moved into a house in Doughty Street in London in 1839, Catherine's younger sister Mary moved in with them. Among his descendants there is a story that Dickens then had an affair with Mary. At the age of seventeen, she died in his arms. He wore her ring on his finger for the rest of his life. In his will, he insisted on being buried with her, though in the event he was interred in Westminster Abbey.

In 1846, his interest turned to fallen women. Well, if it was good enough for Gladstone. He set up a home for fallen women called Urania Cottage. At the time, homes for fallen women provided a stern, punishing regime. In contrast, Urania Cottage offered inmates a chance to learn to read and write, and taught them domestic skills so that they could find employment as servants. Dickens was involved in the day-to-day running of the home, setting the house rules and vetting prospective residents. He would scour prisons and workhouses for suitable candidates and friends, such as the magistrate John Hardwick, would bring them to his attention. They would be given a printed invitation written by Dickens called "An Appeal to Fallen Women", which he signed as "Your friend". If a woman accepted the invitation, Dickens would interview her personally.

In 1857, Dickens hired professional actresses for the play *The Frozen Deep*, which he and his protégé Wilkie Collins, who lived openly with two mistresses, had written. One of the actresses was Ellen Ternan, whose sister married Thomas Trollope, brother of the novelist Anthony. Dickens was forty-four; Ternan was eighteen. They began a passionate affair.

Dickens's wife had lost her figure, grew depressed and took to drink. They split in 1858. However, another of her sisters, Georgina, who had joined the household at the age of fifteen, stayed on with Dickens. This caused a scandal.

Meanwhile, Dickens had set up Ellen in a house in Slough and, later, Nunhead, under a false name. They had a child together that died in infancy. Often she would travel with him, though he abandoned plans to take her on a trip to America in 1867, fearing that the relationship would be revealed in the American press.

When he died in 1870, he left her £1,000, enough to ensure that she would never have to work again. But in 1876, she married George Robinson. He was twelve years her junior, but she shaved fourteen years off her age for the occasion.

## Mae West

Mae West is now remembered, if she is remembered at all, as a bosomy movie actress or a World War II inflatable life vest.

However, in the twenties, thanks to a series of scandalous plays and a notorious novel, she was hailed as America's answer to Oscar Wilde.

Born Mary Jane West in Brooklyn in 1893, she changed her name to Mae, she said, because she did not like the droopy tail on the "y" – or on anything else. She inherited her hourglass figure from her mother who had a brief career as a corset model. Her father was a boxer. In later life, she would cruise gyms looking for sexual partners, taking a special pleasure in having sex with boxers on the night of a bout.

She claimed to have had her first orgasm as a child with a teddy bear. At thirteen, she surrendered her virginity to a twenty-one-year-old actor. This led her to the stage where, as a novelty act, she sang risqué songs, loaded with innuendo, while wiggling her hips.

Mae was more open about sex at all-male parties, where "I'd play with their – umm, you know," she said.

Her father went wild, but her mother told him to leave Mae alone. "Mae's different. She's not like other girls," she said.

Through theatrical lovers, she became a chorus girl, with a sideline as a fan dancer. While dancing nude, she was supposed to cover herself coyly with two enormous fans. But Mae could not be bothered to titillate. She was determined to give her audiences their money's worth.

She started a double act with comedian William Hogan, then went on the road with dancer Frank Wallace. They did an uninhibited ragtime act copied from the African-Americans Mae lived among in Brooklyn. This was condemned both by the church and social reformers, always a good sign. Even *Variety* said their act was "close to the line". Mae's response was that it "may develop".

When Mae fell pregnant in 1911, she married Frank. She was just seventeen and lied about her age. She continued to sleep about, denying that she was married even to her own mother. Fearing that marriage would hurt her career, she would have carried her secret to the grave if an officious clerk in the Milwaukee County Register of Deeds had not unearthed the licence in 1935. Marriage simply did not suit her.

"I was born to be a solo act," she said, "on and off stage."

Back in New York, Mae stole the show at the Folies Bergère in red harem trousers and a bare midriff and came to the attention of Lorenz Ziegfeld, famous for his casting couch. Mae was sacked from her next show after causing a riot. So Mae went back on the road, this time with two well-built male dancers. Her suggestive lyrics and provocative songs were guaranteed to cause a disturbance. In New Haven, Connecticut, students from Yale trashed the theatre. But headlines such as HER WIGGLES COST MAE WEST HER JOB made her a name. New York was now at her feet, partly because she had taken the precaution of sleeping with her agent Frank Bohm.

Back on Broadway in the Ziegfeld show, Mae borrowed from the over-the-top female impersonators she had seen on the circuit. She also had her own drag act, playing the boyfriend to her sister Beverley. She became a gay icon and surrounded herself with excessively effeminate men. Soon her songs were falling foul of the censors and she picked up more raunchy dances from African-Americans – such as the bump, the jelly roll and the shimmy – which were censured by local morals commissions. But the audiences loved it, while, offstage, her lovers found her insatiable. As well as enjoying the sex, for her, men were stepping stones to further her career.

With America's entry into World War I, the 1917 Ziegfeld Follies' Kay Laurell tore open her blouse in front of the French and American flags, exposing one breast. Isadora Duncan did the same at the Metropolitan Opera House while dancing to the "Marseillaise", explaining later that she was paying homage to the figures on the Arc de Triomphe. Needless to say, Mae West was not to be outdone.

In *Sometime* on Broadway, she played a vamp – the voracious man-eating role recently made famous by Theda Bara on the silent screen. Her shimmy stopped the show. While judges were closing down shimmy clubs and shimmy acts in burlesque houses, Mae became the toast of Broadway, wearing a dress that was "not only décolleté to the waistline at the back but is cut at either side to display her bare hips".

She wrote her first play, *The Ruby Ring*, in 1921. In it, the protagonist Gloria says that her ideal man was a combination of heavyweight boxing champion Jack Dempsey, the tenor John McCormack and the legendary baseball player Babe Ruth. Dempsey had been seen coming out of Mae's dressing room after a gruelling bout, and she was a big fan of music and baseball.

She teamed up with pianist Harry Richman. Their act included a scene called "The Gladiator," where she played an empress who wants to hire a gladiator dressed in a squirrel pelt – she wants him to show some skin, she said. The audience howled its appreciation. But there were also howls of complaint. The manager of the theatre chain Edward F. Albee got her to run through her act in the front office. One of the lines that had been blue-pencilled was: "If you don't like my peaches, why do you shake my tree?" Mae performed it with such wide-eyed innocence, that Mr Albee declared that not even a priest could be offended by it. That night she performed the same line with a wiggle and brought the house down.

Her next show was called, brazenly, *The Ginger Box Revue*. It included a master-and-slave routine that hinted at sex across the colour line. This was taboo in America at that time, but Mae did not care. She was hanging out in Harlem at night.

Then Mae West geared up for the biggest scandal of her career. She wrote a play called *Sex*. In it, she played a prostitute who rises from a rundown brothel in Montreal to the poshest part of Westchester County. Mae claimed she got the idea after seeing a prostitute down by the docks who was servicing sailors for fifty cents a trick. She did not mind the woman selling herself, she said, but she did mind the woman selling herself so cheap.

Mae put on the play with her current boyfriend James A. Timony, who set up the Morals Production Company. The money came from British-born underworld boss Owney "The Killer" Madden, owner of the Cotton Club and one of Mae's other lovers.

Her formula for the play was simple: "People want dirt in plays, so I give 'em dirt."

It was guaranteed to offend and Mae flaunted her body.

"She undresses before the public, and appears to enjoy doing so," wrote the *New York Daily Mirror*, shocked.

In the brothel scene, she played on the piano "Honey Let Yo' Drawers Hang Low", "Sweet Man" and "Shake That Thing", all drawn from the underside of Harlem. Consequently, Mae was criticized for having "much more flavour of the turpentine quarters than of the white bawd".

In publicity pictures for the tabloids, she appeared in provocative poses, wearing next to nothing. In the newspapers ads in Chicago warned: "If you cannot stand the excitement – see your doctor before visiting Mae West in *Sex*." She also plastered the town with handbills saying simply: "SEX". Some papers would not even print the name of the play in the ad. But the scandal surrounding the play was soon so huge that all the notice would have to say was "Mae West in That Certain Play" to ensure a sell-out.

The critics were universally hostile. The play was "disgraceful", "nasty", "vicious", "disgusting" and "infantile". It was condemned for "depravity" and portraying "not sex but lust – stark, naked lust". "Fumigation needed," said the *Milwaukee Sentinel*. The *New York Daily Mirror* called it "an offensive play plucked from the garbage can, destined for the sewer". However, in Los Angeles, where it played without Mae West, it was referred to as "*Hamlet* without the Dane." Walter Winchell in the *New York Evening Graphic* – sometimes known as the *Pornographic* – called it a "bold and cheeky enterprise". However, he said he found it morally "unpardonable" and had to hold his nose to escape the "stench".

*Variety* said Mae West had now typecast herself as a tramp, "good enough to fool a travelling salesmen's convention". She was dubbed the "Babe Ruth of the stage prosties".

With reviews like this, the play was, naturally, a huge hit, while the Catholic Church and the Society for the Suppression of Vice petitioned to have it closed down.

As if this had not caused an outrage, Mae quickly followed up with a play called *The Drag*. While homosexuality had been hinted at in plays before – not least by Oscar Wilde – Mae's play would feature openly gay men and transvestites.

"I've got seventeen real live fairies on stage," she crowed.

It was banned in Stamford, but opened in Bridgeport, Connecticut. *Variety* condemned it as "a jazzed-up revel in a garbage heap". Nevertheless crowds flocked from Boston, Philadelphia and New York. Without naming the play, the New York *American* warned: "A disgusting theatrical challenge to decency at Bridgeport, where the foulest use of sex perversions for dirty dollars, is being polished for a metropolitan run." It was scheduled to go into Daly's 63rd Street Theater after *Sex* finished its run.

A week after *The Drag* opened in Bridgeport, New York's Mayor Jimmy Walker, a playboy who relished the company of good-looking young actresses and hoodlums such as Owney Madden, went off on a junket to Florida and the Acting Mayor Joseph V. "Holy Joe" McKee seized the chance to close down *Sex* as part of his long-promised campaign to clean up Broadway. Mae West, Jim Timony, the director C. William Morganstern and twenty-one members of the cast, still in their make-up and costumes, were arrested and charged with "corrupting the morals of youth, or others".

This played directly into Mae's hands. The play had been running for forty-one weeks. Some 325,000 people had seen it, including members of the police department and their wives, judges of the criminal courts and seven members of the district attorney's staff. But sales at the box office were beginning to flag. What it needed was a fresh infusion of publicity. Mae was bailed for $1,000, the rest of the cast for $500 each, but ticket sales soared and the run was extended.

McKee's move against the play had nothing to do with *Sex* itself. He feared that if *The Drag* appeared on Broadway there would be riots. But with Daly's still coining it in from *Sex*, *The Drag* was blocked from coming into town as no other theatre would take it.

The trial, which opened on 15 February 1927, quickly turned into a farce. A police inspector called on to read out the offending lines was so embarrassed that he bowdlerized them as he went. There was more laughter when, describing Mae's provocative belly dancing, an arresting officer said, "Something in her middle moved from east to west." Mae explained that she was doing a simple bodybuilding exercise her father had taught her in the gym.

The defence attorney pointed out that one judge had sat through the play six times, and the court had to be cleared when Mae made a monkey of the prosecution witness. By then the play had come off anyway, as the court case had pulled a bigger audience than the show.

After five hours' deliberation, the jury returned a verdict of guilty. Mae and Timony were sentenced to ten days in jail and fined $500, and the judge admonished Mae for both writing and acting in objectionable scenes, while going "to extremes in order to make the play as immoral as possible". On the steps of the courtroom, she told the press that she would spend her time in prison writing more plays.

Taken to the Welfare Island Women's Workhouse, she was told to strip.

"I thought this was a respectable place," she said.

After she complained about the coarse prison underwear, the warden, a man, allowed her to wear silk. She dined with him and he took her out for drives. In her spare time, she wrote articles, earning $1,000 for one for *Liberty* magazine. The other women in the workhouse did not mind that she was excused cooking, cleaning or washing – "never having had any experience," she explained. Instead, they reeled off lines they had learnt from *Sex*.

She got on well with the other women, especially the prostitutes, saying that, if she had not starting writing plays, she might have joined their profession. And she was given one day's remission because, as the warden explained, she was a "fine woman and a great character".

The *Sex* scandal and her brief imprisonment made Mae West a star. She even had her imitators. The *Grand Street Follies* featured a sketch called "Stars in Stripes" where a Mae West character in a prison uniform seduces every man in sight. Mae claimed that her time on Welfare Island gave her enough material for six plays. The first was *The Wicked Age* about the bathing beauty contests that were sweeping the country. It was just an excuse to put lots of pretty young women in bathing suits on stage.

Next came *Diamond Lil* about "one of the finest women ever to walk the streets". It was set in a bar in Bowery and, though it was the height of Prohibition, real beer flowed from the pumps on stage, thanks to Owney Madden. The play was a financial and critical success. The *New York Times* called it "almost Elizabethan", though she had one brush with the law in Detroit when she distributed a mock-up of the *Police Gazette* as a publicity handout, featuring her picture with a caption comparing her to Madame du Barry, the mistress of Louis XV.

Mae claimed the play was a classic: "Like *Hamlet*, sort of, but funnier."

It was studded with the one-line double entendres she made her trademark in the movies and she played Diamond Lil off stage as well as on, installing a gilded bed, shaped like a swan, in her dressing room.

She did not appear in *The Pleasure Man* where a man who is having an affair with a married woman dies after being castrated by a young man whose sister he had also seduced. At the time she was having an affair with a married man.

"We met any place we could – dressing rooms, elevators, the back seat of his car or my limousine," she said. "A kind of hit-and-run affair, you might say ... One Saturday night we were at it till four the next afternoon. A dozen rubber things. Twenty-two times. I was sorta tired."

She dropped him when his wife turned up. Besides, she had plenty more men on tap at the time, including gangster-turned-movie-star George Raft.

*The Pleasure Man* used several scenes recycled from *The Drag*. Mae did not appear because she did not want to upstage the trannies. *Variety* described the play as "filth". It "paraded and glorified sexual perversion". This was enough to ensure a huge audience on the first night, hoping to see an arrest. They were not disappointed. During a drag party in the third act, the police burst on stage and carted off the cast, some still in their frocks.

Mae was blamed. The *American Mercury* said: "Her sole purpose seems to be to make money out of out-and-out fornicatory and homosexual rodeos."

On the second night, the theatre was raided again. This time Mae managed to get herself arrested too. Once more she bailed out the cast and took on the entire cost of the defence. She explained in *Parade* magazine that her motive was "the education of the masses to certain sex truths" – though she somehow ended the piece saying, "Marriage, love, and home should be sacred."

In court, Mae West had to stuff a handkerchief in her mouth to stop herself laughing when the judge called on one of the transvestites to perform some of the songs that were alleged to be "indecent". These included "Officer, May I Pat Your Horse" and "I'm the Queen of the Beaches" – which he/

she pronounced "bitches". A team of German acrobats then had to perform their act, which the police maintained was "suggestive". But the unwitting star of the show was Police Captain James J. Coy who was asked to demonstrate a snake act that he found particularly objectionable. The defendants were acquitted amid gales of laughter.

The Wall Street Crash hit box-office takings, so Mae tried her hand at writing a novel with the working title *Black and White*. Set among the brothels, bars, peep shows and clip joints of Harlem, it was about mixed-race sex. Mae had had several affairs with black boxers, so she was writing from experience.

"They don't smoke, don't drink and understand the importance of keeping their bodies in top working order," she said.

It was first published under the title *Babe Gordon* after the main character, the wife of a white boxer named Bearcat Delaney. She takes a black lover, Money Johnson, a pimp and bookmaker with a magnificent body that both black and white women drool over. When Delaney quits the ring, Babe makes a living peddling morphine, heroin, and coke, while indulging herself in opium with Money Johnson. One night, wealthy aristocrat Wayne Baldwin sees Money Johnson caressing "her cream, white throat". He finds the thoughts of "Babe's white body and Johnson's black body . . . terrible, yet it gives him a sensual thrill".

Baldwin and Babe become lovers. Johnson goes to jail. When he is released, Babe and Johnson indulge in a drug-fuelled lovers' spree in a Harlem tenement. Baldwin bursts in, shoots Johnson, frames Babe's husband Bearcat Delaney, then hires him an expensive lawyer who gets him off by convincing the all-white jury that he "upheld the best traditions of the white race [and] the honour of its womanhood" by protecting her from assault by "a low, lustful, black beast". Babe then gives Bearcat, anonymously, the money to go back into training. Meanwhile, she heads off to Paris with Baldwin, with no intention of being faithful to him. "Even if she decided to marry Baldwin, that would not prevent her having a lover, or lovers, on the side. That is Babe Gordon." As for Baldwin: "He cannot avoid thinking of Babe's white body and Johnson's black body, darkness mating with dawn . . ."

It is hard to imagine a more deliciously scandalous tale in 1930 and it sold well. But to promote a second edition, *Publishers Weekly* ran a competition to give it a new title. The winning entry was *The Constant Sinner* – an ironic reference to Somerset Maugham's *The Constant Wife*.

The book went through five editions and sold 94,000 copies, so Mae put it on the stage with herself playing Babe, whom she called a *femme amoureuse*.

"Babe was the type that thrived on men," she wrote. "She needed them. She enjoyed them and had to have them. Without them she was cold and alone . . . There are women so formed in body and mind that they are predestined to be daughters of joy. These women whom the French call '*femmes amoureuse*' are found not alone among the women of the streets, but in every stratum of society. History's pages reveal the power of these women that thrive on love, whose lives are centred on men. Babe was a born '*femme amoureuse*.' Her idea was that if a man can have as many women as he wants, there is no reason why a woman should not do the same thing. She was one of those women who were put on this earth for men – not one man but many men . . . She was one of those rare type of women who uses her beauty and sexual allure as a soldier uses his weapons – without mercy or scruple."

Again this was guaranteed to cause a scandal. Seven years before, when Paul Robeson had played a black man married to a white woman in Eugene O'Neill's *All God's Chillun Got Wings* on Broadway, there was practically a riot. But in 1931, race tension was worse. The country was gripped by the Scottsboro case. Nine black youths had been convicted of raping two white prostitutes in Alabama, even though doctors had testified that no rape had taken place. An all-white jury had sentenced all except the youngest, who was twelve, to death. As a precaution, over Mae's objections, a Caucasian actor would play the part of Money Johnson in black face, then remove his wig and make-up at the curtain, revealing himself to be white. Nevertheless, he was given the usual privileges in the dressing room.

The first-night audience loved it, though the critics again dismissed it as "filth". However, they were quite taken with a scene where she crossed the dimly lit stage in sheer chiffon gown and changed into a robe.

"I wasn't really nude," she said, merely adding to the titillation.

With a black actor in the lead role, she tried to take it on the road. But in Washington, DC, then a segregated Southern city, it was closed after two performances when the district attorney threatened to jail the cast.

George Raft got her a part playing a prostitute in his latest movie *Night After Night* and she headed for the West Coast. She signed to Paramount for $5,000, but stayed at home until they gave her script approval. Then she wrote her own dialogue. In a scene in a nightclub, the hatcheck girl says: "Goodness, what lovely diamonds."

Mae snaps back: "Goodness had nothing to do with it."

She is asked: "Do you believe in love at first sight?"

"I don't know," she replies, "but it sure saves an awful lot of time."

Cinema audiences had never heard anything like this. There had been strict censorship since the Arbuckle scandal and the advent of talkies.

"There was a terrific explosion," said *Photoplay*. "A bomb had gone off in a cream-puff factory . . . Blonde, buxom, rowdy Mae – slithering across the screen in a spangled, sausage-skin gown! Yanking our eyes from George Raft and Connie Cummings—" nominally the stars of the movie "—I dare say that the theatre has never seen Hollywood a more fascinating, spectacular and useful figure than bounding Mae West, queen of the big-hearted, bad girls of show business."

"She stole everything but the camera," said Raft.

To celebrate, Mae commissioned a nude portrait of herself being ogled by a monkey. This hung in her living room. In the bedroom, she installed a mirrored ceiling above her huge bed. When asked what the mirror was for, she said, "I like to see how I am doing." Adding: "I do my best work in bed."

Audiences were soon clamouring for more Mae West movies. Filming her stage hit *Diamond Lil* was the obvious solution. But *Diamond Lil* was on the Hayes Office blacklist. So Paramount changed the title to *She Done Him Wrong* and watered down the plot. Mae responded by adding more suggestive one-liners. These included "When women go wrong, men go right after them," and "Haven't you ever met a man that can make you happy?" "Sure, lots of times." Nevertheless, the Hays Office passed the picture. The obvious sexual contents of the songs "Frankie and Johnny", "A Guy What Takes His Time" and "Easy Rider" – thirties African-American slang for a pimp – passed Will Hays right by. In the film she is seen handing out pictures of herself, said to be for use in the bedroom, which were "a little bit spicy, but not too raw". Although these photographs are never shown on camera, she insisted on using real soft-core shots, which she sold off afterwards. On screen, there was a nude painting of her hanging over the bar – was Hays blind? When a man comments on it, she says, "I do wish Gus hadn't hung it up over the free lunch." The Hays Office's only comment on the movie was that it was a "hearty, if somewhat rowdy amusement". Nevertheless, it was cut in several states, censored in Britain and banned outright in Austria, Latvia, Java and Australia.

The Great Depression had also hit the box office at the cinema. By the time it came out, Paramount had gone into receivership. But then *She Done Him Wrong* began breaking box-office records across the country. It grossed over $2 million in the first three months. One newspaper proclaimed that the movie and Mae's décolletage both hit THE BULLS'-EYE OF LUSTY ENTERTAINMENT, while *Variety* reminded readers that scandalous Miss West was "the *Sex* star".

"Her handling of lovers, past and present and prospective, comprises the whole movie," it said. Again priests and prudes railed against her.

But *She Done Him Wrong* saved Paramount from bankruptcy. It also helped out a number of old prizefighters and other former lovers she hired for bit parts and it was just the tonic that Depression-ridden America needed. It was nominated for an Oscar.

Paramount pumped up the scandal. With Prohibition about to be repealed, Mae posed in a brewery, saying, "Girls, drink beer. It'll give you those sexy curves." Then they put on a stage show where she played a "bad, bad lady who gets more applicants than a want ad". In a clinging black gown, she tells her maid not to call her madam, negotiates with a gigolo and fields numerous calls from lovers.

She answered her critics in an article entitled "Who Says I'm A Bad Woman".

"Virtue may have its own reward, but it isn't at the box office," she said. "Men like women with a past, because they hope history will repeat itself. Women like to see them too, because almost every woman (although she won't admit it) would like to be a scarlet adventuress – without any of the penalties, of course . . . Why should I be attacked as a menace to movie morals because I present sex on the screen as it really is? Is it not far less dangerous to do it that way than to give it a phonily romantic and mysterious label and a fancy foreign accent? Sex is not necessarily vulgar. I don't think it is any more so than eating. Sex is never vulgar except to vulgar people. Why is it necessary to weep or gnash teeth over the process of nature? . . . Love is a woman's stock-in-trade and she always ought to be overstocked."

Six months after the opening of *She Done Him Wrong*, the National Legion of Decency was founded and the Hays Office pulled its socks up. Mae's next movie, *I'm No Angel*, was the story of a girl who climbs the social ladder "wrong by wrong". It was a problem from the off. In the opening scene, Mae appears in a carnival sideshow doing a belly dance in a Salome costume with tassels on the nipples. Her barker announces that she is "the girl who discovered you don't have to have feet to be a dancer". But the lines "she's given the old biological urge to a Civil War veteran" and "the only girl who satisfied more patrons that Chesterfields" had to go. White musicians had to replace black ones and the line "that's all, boys, now you can go home and beat your wives" was cut. But she was allowed to say of a young male acrobat, "I'm not going to hurt him, I only want to feel his muscles." And the song "They Call Me Sister Honky-Tonk" also got by.

A fortune-teller says: "I see a man in your life."

"What, only one?" she replies. But she must have pleased the censor when she maintained that she was a one-man woman – "one at a time".

She even got away with lines that now grace dictionaries of quotations: "It's not the men in my life, it's the life in my men" and "When I'm good, I'm very, very good, but when I'm bad, I'm better", along with the entirely innocuous "Beulah, peel me a grape."

But the censor had no control over what happened off camera. Among the numerous visitors to her dressing room was the bisexual Marlene Dietrich. A bodyguard gave Mae the line: "Is that a gun in your pocket, or are you just pleased to see me?" and she claimed to own a part of heavyweight champion Joe Louis – the "Brown Bomber" – but she did not say which part.

The *Hollywood Confidential* eventually ran an exposé on "the Empress of Sex", taking her to task for her preference for "bronze boxers" and other "tan warriors". She defended herself against the charge of having loose morals with typical aplomb: "Loose morals? Why, after four years of Depression, you'd be lucky if you could find a loose nickel."

She was also accused of bringing sex into the movies.

"When were pictures ever without sex?" she said. "Have we forgotten the vampish writhings of Theda Bara and Valeska Suratt? Sex is considered the strongest instinct next to self-preservation. When will humans lose interest in it?"

Even Chaplin had "a lot of sex in his pictures," she said, "and he never made it obvious either. He kidded it, and that's exactly what I do."

The Catholic Church led the attack on Mae West, though privately she attended Mass every day.

"I have never done anything to harm the Catholic Church," she said. "Why does the Catholic Church start preaching against me?"

But there were people on her side

"Sex, unashamed and unabashed, has built her into her present international fame," said *Motion Picture*. "Prudery will slaughter her."

Other critics implored her to keep it "spicy, straight from the shoulder, without compromise or one eye on the Woman's Club". Who would want the "expurgated edition"?

Her sexual frankness was praised by Will Rogers, F. Scott Fitzgerald, D. W. Griffith and Hugh Walpole. But the studio tried to clean up her image, signing her up for a radio campaign for the local Community Chest. Mae could not help herself, though.

"Love your neighbour," she urged, "and by that I don't mean his wife."

Articles about her home showed she had two new nude statues – of herself. Comparing herself to the Venus de Milo, she said, "I've got it on her. I've got two arms and I know how to use them. Besides, I ain't marble."

Journalists were invited to interview her in bed and she boasted about her sexual activities. And she urged President

Roosevelt to introduce a New Deal for women. It should involve "jewellery, motor cars, flowers, furs and candy". And the NRA (Roosevelt's National Recovery Administration), she said, "stands for No Regrets After".

But the campaign to clean up Hollywood was gaining steam. FILM MORALS – OR ELSE ran a headline in *Variety* and film censors talked of the "Mae West Menace". According to the *Chicago Tribune*: "She really and truly doesn't give a damn."

There were even dissenters within Paramount. Studio boss, Adolf Zukor, a family man, reprimanded publicist Arthur Mayer for using such a "dirty word as 'lusty'" in a poster that showed Mae's swelling bosom above the line: "Hitting the High Spots of Lusty Entertainment".

Mayer insisted that the word lusty was innocent. It derived from the German *lustig* which meant merry or jolly.

"Look, Mr Mayer," said Zukor. "I don't need your Harvard education. When I look at that dame's tits, I know what lusty means."

One man who did approve was Italy's Fascist dictator Benito Mussolini who was trying to encourage Italians to have bigger families at the time. She had put sex on the world stage. For *Variety*: "She's as hot an issue as Hitler." Invited to England to celebrate the Silver Jubilee of George V, she declined with a cable, saying simply: "Sorry, George."

*I'm No Angel* was another box office smash, further reviving Paramount's coffers. But in Omaha there were sexually segregated shows. Mae countered by giving out copies of her "NRA code for bachelor girls".

Her next movie was originally called *It Ain't No Sin*. When the first posters went up on Broadway, priests marched up and down carrying signs saying: "It is." The name was changed to *Belle of the Nineties*, even though a Paramount publicist had already trained forty parrots to say "It ain't no sin," for a publicity stunt.

The man responsible for the change was Joseph Breen, a hitman the National Legion of Decency had sent to Hollywood to enforce the new Production Code. *Film Weekly* dubbed him the "Hitler of Hollywood". First he demanded that *She Done Him Wrong* and *I'm No Angel* be withdrawn. Then he got to work on the script of *It Ain't No Sin*. He demanded that all references to sex, prostitution, crime, drugs and gambling be removed. That did for the entire plot. Kissing and fondling were out, and bedrooms were for sleeping in. So there went the action too. Mindful of the New York protest, the title had to be changed as well.

Breen knew that Mae could make the most innocuous line suggestive by a wiggle of her hips, so dispatched a watchdog to the set. Mae sought to frustrate him at every turn. She invented a kidnap threat and insisted on hiring a bunch of bodybuilders to protect her. After each take, they would march into her dressing room with her and a sign would be hung on the door that read: DO NOT DISTURB – EXCEPT IN CASE OF FIRE.

Despite the close scrutiny, she got away with a few lines: "A man in the house is worth two in the street" and "It is better to be looked over than overlooked." Shown a portrait of a woman, said to be an Old Master, she says, "Looks more like an old mistress to me." And when a character complains that all she thinks about is having a good time, she says, "I don't just think about it."

Playing a burlesque queen, the statuesque Mae even gets away with wearing a skintight dress, then slowly transmogrifying into the Statue of Liberty, or the "Statue of Libido" as one critic remarked. Nevertheless, the censors won out and the movie ends with a wedding.

"Mae West has graciously permitted the New York censors to make an honest woman of her in her new picture," said the *New York Times*.

It was a "shotgun wedding", said *Literary Digest*.

But Mae had played a skilful game. She had deliberately peppered the script with lines that she knew they would cut, to distract them from other more subtle, more suggestive passages. Besides the sex was not in words, but in her personality.

"The censors could never beat that," she said.

And she was tougher than they were.

"I've never had a wishbone where my backbone should be," she said.

Mae continued battling with Breen – and besting him – throughout her Hollywood career. However, she made an enemy of William Randolph Hearst by an off-hand remark about the acting ability of his mistress Marion Davis. He banned ads for her movies from his newspapers and published an op-ed piece asking: "Is it not time Congress did something about Mae West?"

"The nearest Congress came to that," Mae said in her autobiography, "was almost naming twin lakes, round ones, after me."

But Hearst's opposition did little to hurt the success of her movies. Then she moved on to the radio with ventriloquist Edgar Bergen and his dummy Charlie McCarthy, whom Mae said she loved because he was "all wood and a yard long".

In a sketch where she plays Eve, she feeds Adam "forbidden applesauce" to get sex, then says, "I've just made a little more history. I'm the first woman to have her own way – and the snake'll take the rap for it."

Again this was guaranteed to offend. NBC was barraged with letters of complaint. The *Catholic Monitor* carried the headline: MAE WEST POLLUTES HOMES. And the comment of the professor of religion at the Catholic University – that Mae was "the very personification of sex in its lowest connotation" – was read into the Congressional record. Despite pulling an audience of forty million on her Sunday night spot, Mae was banned from the radio.

"Did they expect a sermon?" said Mae. "Why weren't they in church if they were so religious?"

Mae went back on the road with *Diamond Lil*. In Britain, where the theatre was still regulated by the Lord Chancellor's office, she had trouble with the scene where her breasts were fondled. Nevertheless she still had young actors rehearse the scene.

Back in the US, she toured with *Come On Up, Ring Twice* and *Catherine Was Great,* her take on the life of Catherine the Great of Russia. In one scene where she inspects her male courtiers at crotch level, one shows a prominent bulge in his trousers and she says, "You're new here." She adapted her old "gun-in-the-pocket" line. When her leading man's scabbard accidentally stabs her, she says, "Is that your sword, or are you just pleased to see me?" And in a curtain speech at the end of the performance, she told the audience: "Catherine was a great empress. She also had three thousand lovers. I did the best I could in a couple of hours."

She developed a nightclub act where she was surrounded by bodybuilders dressed in loincloths – though the young Kirk Douglas was rejected as substandard.

"Why marry a ball player, when you can have the whole team," she told the audience.

At one stage, she examines the troupe in bathrobes, as if they were naked underneath. Later they appeared in G-strings.

"Tonight I feel like a million," she said, "but one at a time."

This may have been an exaggeration, but the singer she engaged, Steve Rossi, told the *Globe*: "She insisted on having sex every day, otherwise she wouldn't feel right."

She was sixty-one at the time.

Stories about her relationship with "her boys" filtered into the press, especially when Jayne Mansfield ran off with one of them. Another moved into her Santa Monica beach house, which was decorated with erect penises.

Though she was still in demand by directors, she only took parts where she could flaunt her sexuality – such as the agent in Gore Vidal's X-rated *Myra Breckinridge* who beds all her clients and the movie star and sex symbol in *Sextette*, a film version of her own play, whose five ex-husbands try to stop her bedding her sixth. In it she is asked: "Do you get a lot of proposals from your male fans?"

"Yeah," she says, "and what they propose is nobody's business."

Her scandalous sex life lasted until the end of her life. She continued to audition the male parts and fans sent nude pictures of themselves. In 1979, the year before she died, a young African-American man, about seventeen years old, turned up at her apartment block. Mae, then eighty-seven, had him sent up. When he came down again ninety minutes later, he said to the receptionist, "I will never forget you and what you have done for me for the rest of my life."

## Jeffrey Archer

In 1998, bestselling author Jeffrey Archer published a novel, *The Eleventh Commandment – Thou Shalt Not Be Caught*. Within a year, he had broken his own fictional commandment.

A career politician, he had risen through the ranks of the Conservative Party, becoming deputy chairman. He was eventually ennobled as Baron Archer of Weston-Super-Mare, though the satirical magazine *Private Eye* always referred to him as Lord Archole.

Then in October 1986 the *News of the World* ran the headline TORY BOSS ARCHER PAYS VICE-GIRL on its front page, with a picture of Monica Coghlan, who was a streetwalker under the name "Debbie". Archer's aide Michael Stacpoole had met her on platform three at Victoria Station and offered an envelope stuffed with £2,000 in £50 notes. The story said Archer had told Coghlan to leave the country. The paper did not say that Archer had slept with her, but that was clearly the implication.

The *Daily Star* followed up the story, alleging that Archer had had sex with her on the night of 9 September, though they later changed the date of the alleged liaison to the eighth. It said that Archer and Coghlan had met in a central London area long renowned for its sex trade, and, after coming to an agreement, the pair repaired to room 6A on the second floor of the Albion Hotel. According to the *Star*, £70 changed hands. Archer resigned as deputy chairman of the Conservative Party and sued for libel.

Critical to his case was his alibi. On the night of Monday 8 September 1986, when the *Daily Star* alleged he was with Ms Coghlan, his literary agent Richard Cohen and his wife had dined with Archer at Le Caprice, a posh restaurant. They had left at 10.30 p.m. But Terence Baker, one of his film agents, testified that he had met Archer in the bar and Archer had given him a lift back to Camberwell in south London at around 12.45 a.m.

Archer's wife Mary also appeared at the trial, telling the jury that they had a "happy marriage" and enjoyed "a full life" together. The allegation was ludicrous.

"Anyone who knows him well," she said, "knows that far from Jeffrey accosting a prostitute, if one accosted him he would run several miles in the opposite direction, very fast."

It was revealed later that the Archers were living separate lives at the time.

Monica Coghlan – just four foot eleven, "a tiny but well-proportioned thirty-five-year-old" according to the *New York Press* – maintained that Archer had paid her £70 for sex, £50 up front and £20 afterwards.

"I had no difficulty seeing his face," she testified. "I was lying on top of him the whole time. He commented on how lovely I was. He was quite surprised by my nipples. It was over very quickly – about ten minutes, what with getting undressed and the actual sex. Because it was over so quickly, I suggested that he relax for a while and he could try again. I lit a cigarette and I lay down on the bed with him. I asked him what he did for a living. He said, 'I sell cars,' and he had no sooner said that than he jumped off the bed and said he should go and move his car."

Famously, she said she could identify Archer from his spotty back, much to the amusement of the nation.

Mrs Archer returned to the witness box to testify that: "Jeffrey has excellent skin, sir. He has no spots or blemishes anywhere."

"He had no spots on his back?" asked Mr Archer's QC.

Mrs Archer replied, "No, sir."

Through tears Ms Coghlan admitted that she had slept with "many thousands of men" while earning "hundreds and thousands of pounds". She also said that she had paid no income tax while still collecting government benefits and that the *News of the World* had paid her £6,000 for her story. While Archer's QC tried to undermine her credibility, she screamed through her tears: "You're a liar. He's a liar and he knows it. He's even putting his wife through it. I've got nothing; he's got money. I can't even go back to work."

And she was unapologetic about her "work". She told the court: "I enjoy my job. As long as the men are all right with me, I'm all right with them." When asked if some of those men were in search of kinky sex in anonymous hotel rooms, she said, "What's wrong with that? Half the time it keeps marriages together."

But the judge, Mr Justice Caulfield, was completely spellbound by Mrs Archer. He told the jury: "Remember Mary Archer in the witness box. Your vision of her probably will never disappear. Has she elegance? Has she fragrance? Would she have, without the strain of this trial, radiance? How would she appeal? Has she had a happy married life? Has she been able to enjoy, rather than endure, her husband Jeffrey?"

Of Archer, he said, "Is he in need of cold, unloving, rubber-insulated sex in a seedy hotel round about quarter to one on a Tuesday morning after an evening at the Caprice?"

"Did you at any time that evening pick up any girl or prostitute?" Archer was asked. "Did you go to the Albion Hotel?"

He denied it. So why had he given her £2,000?

Two weeks after the supposed sexual encounter, Archer said Coghlan had phoned him in apparent distress, claiming that one of her clients, a lawyer, had spotted them together that night at the Albion and was now urging her to go to the tabloids with her story. Archer reacted with "initial surprise and disbelief", but nevertheless consented to give her £2,000.

"I was worried obviously that anyone could be going round telling lies," he testified. "But I did not take that seriously. I knew it was not true."

He admitted that giving her the money was "clearly a very foolish thing to do". But it was not hush money. It was, rather, a humanitarian gesture, allowing Ms Coghlan to leave the country and escape the hounding of the press.

The jury believed him. Archer won £500,000 damages, a new British record, and the editor of the *Daily Star* was sacked.

After the trial Monica Coghlan cashed in on her notoriety by posing topless for a newspaper for £5,400. She died on 26 April 2001 after being hit by a getaway car and before she could relish the denouement of the scandal.

In 1999, Archer was standing as Conservative candidate for mayor of London when the *News of the World* struck again. A former friend of Archer's, TV producer Ted Francis told them that, before the libel trial, Archer had asked him to cook up an alibi and he had tapes of the conversation to prove it. Francis was to say that he was having dinner with Archer on the night of 9 September. That night, Archer was, in fact, having dinner with his mistress Andrina Colquhoun.

Archer had also got his secretary to compile a fake appointments book to show that he had arranged to have dinner with Francis that night. Neither the book nor Francis's alibi were used when the *Daily Star* changed the date of the alleged assignation with Coghlan to the eighth. However, Archer's bagman Michael Stacpoole then resurfaced. He told the *Mail on Sunday* that Archer had given him £40,000 to leave the country before the trial.

"In effect he was paying me to keep my mouth shut – perverting the course of justice is what it is," he said. "If I'd have been asked under oath if Archer was a faithful husband, I would have had to confirm he was not because of his affairs with other women."

The Conservative Party pulled the plug on Archer's campaign for mayor and he withdrew his candidacy. He was then expelled from the Conservative Party for five years.

TV producer Nick Elliott then said before Terence Baker had died in 1991 he had told him that he had committed perjury to protect Archer. The tale of Archer giving him a lift home from Le Caprice was a complete fabrication. Richard Cohen also said that Archer had asked him to change his testimony, saying that he had left the restaurant later than had been the case. He refused.

Scotland Yard swooped and Archer was charged with two counts of perverting the course of justice, two counts of perjury and one of preparing a "false instrument", the bogus appointment book.

Before the trial started, Archer appeared as the defendant in a production of his own play *The Accused*, though critics said that, had Agatha Christie been alive, he would be facing an additional charge of plagiarism. The audience acted as the jury in the piece and, at the end of each performance, was invited to vote on his guilt or innocence.

In the Old Bailey, he was found guilty of perjury and perverting the course of justice and was sentenced to four years in jail. He also repaid £500,000 to the *Daily Star* along with legal costs of £1.3 million.

Of course, Archer did not suffer as a result of the sex scandal. He wrote three books about his prison experiences. He was expelled from the MCC (Marylebone Cricket Club), but only for seven years. Released after serving half his sentence, he returned to the bosom of the establishment, being embraced by Mrs Thatcher at a memorial service.

This was in stark contrast to the fate of Monica Coghlan. Shortly before her death, she said: "Jeffrey Archer took everything away from me. I lost my home, my dignity, my self-respect, and any hope of a future. While I was scrimping and scraping, he was clawing his way back to power and lording it up in his manor house. It just wasn't fair, simple as that. I have never denied what I was. I was a prostitute."

# 12

## Raunchy Republicans

### Abraham Lincoln

There are have been a number of attempts to prove that Abraham Lincoln was gay, largely based on the fact that he slept with other men. But men often shared a bed in the nineteenth century, often simply to save money. On the other hand, William H. Herndale, Lincoln's partner in his law practice, said: "Lincoln had a strong, if not terrible, passion for women. He could hardly keep his hands off a woman; and yet, much to his credit, he lived a pure and virtuous life. His idea was that a woman has as much right to violate the marriage vow as a man – no more, no less."

The source of a scandal in his life was his wife Mary Todd. Taking him at his word, when they were engaged, she was seen out with Stephen A. Douglas, Lincoln's great rival in the debates over slavery. The engagement was broken off. Lincoln then declared his love for her best friend, while Mary took up with a widower, but decided that she could not take on his children.

They got back together again and married, but she continued flirting. When they arrived in the White House, she was much criticized for her daring décolletage. Once visitor wrote: "Mrs Lincoln had her bosom on exhibition."

During the Civil War she was known to have Confederate sympathies – she came from a slave-owning family in

Kentucky. Her extravagance brought accusations of treason and in ribald songs round the Union campfires her name was linked with that of Jefferson Davis. Rumours abounded about Mary and the men she planned to elope to the South with. Although there was no truth to this, she continued to flirt with any man in sight, including Charles Sumner who secured her a pension after her husband was assassinated.

Lincoln also took to flirting. When Mary was out of town, he would go to see dancing girls. One night in Ford's Theatre he took a private box and carried on "a hefty flirtation with the girls in the flies". After he died, Mary went to France. On the way back, on-board the *Amérique*, she became friendly with the notorious actress Sarah Bernhardt.

## Ulysses S. Grant

Attempts to stir up sex scandals during the political career of Ulysses S. Grant broadly failed. During the presidential campaign of 1868, it was alleged that he had sired an illegitimate daughter with an Indian squaw at Fort Vancouver in Oregon Territory. However, the child had been born less than nine months after he arrived there. It seems to have been a case of mistaken identity and the real father was one Richard Grant.

During the notorious Whiskey Ring that skimmed off the tax revenue from liquor into private hands, a telegram warning the conspirators of the investigation came to light. It was signed "Sylph". According to one of the conspirators, "'Sylph' was a lewd woman with whom the President of the United States had been in intimate association . . ." After he had broken off the extramarital affair, she had continued to pester him.

It was also said that she was "'unquestionably the handsomest woman in St Louis. Her form was petite, and yet withal, a plumpness and development which made her a being whose tempting, luscious deliciousness was irresistible".

No one believed that Grant could possibly have been involved with such a woman, which must have done wonders for his self-esteem.

## James Garfield

As a youth, James Garfield used to work on a canal near Ohio City where, in 1849, it was necessary to pass a law banning "lewd and lascivious behaviour in any of the streets, lanes, alleys or public places".

"At the time," he said, "I was ripe for ruin and an active and willing servant of sin. How fearfully I was rushing both soul and body to destruction."

It is not clear what the exact nature of this sin was. His diaries reveal that he was unsure of his own masculinity. He made several attempts to get married, but got cold feet and one writer has concluded that he had a homosexual infatuation with a young man named Oliver B. Stone.

He later fell for one of his students though, again, backed out at the prospect of marriage. Then he tried to break off his engagement to Lucretia Rudolph to marry Rebecca Selleck, but relented. After he married Lucretia, he continued seeing Rebecca. In 1862, he had a fling with Mrs Lucia Calhoun, an eighteen-year-old reporter for the *New York Times* – not something an aspiring politician would risk today. He confessed this to his wife, but went to see Mrs Calhoun again, ostensibly to pick up indiscreet letters he had written to her that might damage his political career. Fearing that the affair would rekindle, Lucretia prayed that "the fire of such a lawless passion would burn itself out unfed and unnoticed".

During the 1880 election, there were allegations that he had been with a prostitute in New Orleans. Months after taking office, he was assassinated, but talk of his womanizing continued. For the remaining thirty-six years of her life, Lucretia Garfield continued to deny all rumours of her husband's infidelity.

## Chester Arthur

Chester Arthur was a widower when he came to office. He left his daughter at home with a governess and sent his son to Princeton, where he majored in expensive clothes, wild parties and girls. The matrons of Washington paraded eligible women in front of him.

"No president since the war has been so popular," said one newspaper.

Gossip was rife, but he did not like people prying into his love life.

"I may be president of the United States," he told one persistent enquirer, "but my private life is nobody's damned business."

What a shame modern-day politicians do not take up such a robust position.

## Benjamin Harrison

When Benjamin Harrison was ousted by Grover Cleveland, he was free to have something of a sex scandal of his own. In 1892, while he had been president, his wife had died and her young niece, Mary Scott Lord Dimmick, a widow, took over as official hostess. After he left office, he married Mrs Dimmick, who was twenty-five years his junior. His children from his first marriage, who were both older than his new bride, did not approve and did not show up at the wedding. A year later, Harrison became a father again at the age of sixty-three.

## Theodore Roosevelt

Despite having a condom named after him, the "Rough Rider" Theodore Roosevelt managed to avoid getting personally involved in scandals. He was a virgin when he married his first wife. When she died in childbirth, he married a former girlfriend whom he had thrown over when he discovered that she had "had a romance".

However, his wayward cousin Cornelius married a French actress! Roosevelt wrote: "He has disgraced the family, the vulgar brute . . . She turned out to be a mere courtesan! A harlot!"

Then there was Theodore's brother Elliott, who was an alcoholic and a drug addict. A former maid named Katy Mann claimed that he was the father of her illegitimate child and demanded $10,000 for the child's upkeep. Elliott, who had been hooked on laudanum and morphine since an accident, vehemently denied her accusations. The family called in an "expert in likeness" who examined the child. He concluded that the maid was telling the truth and the family paid her off.

Roosevelt believed that marital infidelity reduced the perpetrator to the level of a "flagrant man-swine" and proposed that Elliott cease having sex with his wife Anne until he expunge his "hideous depravity" by several years of celibacy. Elliot promptly took a new mistress and resumed heavy drinking. His wife then moved to seize her husband's $170,000 estate before he blew it. Roosevelt, himself, applied for a writ to have his brother declared legally insane. The press got wind of it and went to town.

Theodore Roosevelt followed John Quincy Adams's habit of skinny-dipping in the Potomac. However, he risked scandal because, since Adams's time, photography had been invented. To prevent him being ambushed by the press while naked, he took with him his good friend, the French ambassador Jean Jules Jusserand. However, Jusserand would keep his gloves on "in case we meet a lady". Roosevelt dispensed with this nicety. A Rough Rider he may have been, but he was no gentleman.

## Warren Harding

The election of Warren Harding promised a "return to normalcy". In a way, it was. He was a tireless womanizer.

However, he died in office before it came out that he had an illegitimate child by a young campaign worker. If any of that sounds familiar, hold hard – Warren Harding was America's first black president. Or, at least, that was the allegation made at the time.

It had long been rumoured in Ohio that Harding's great-grandmother had been a black woman, that Harding's father's second wife had divorced him because he was "much too Negro for her to endure", and that Harding's father-in-law had denounced his daughter for "polluting the family line". This was at a time when the "one drop" rule applied in Southern states – that is, when one drop of black blood meant that you were considered black and, thus, ineligible to vote or hold office.

When Harding became president in 1922, historian William Estabrook Chancellor had toured Ohio, compiling these rumours and accusations. The resulting book can be seen as the partisan smear of a racial bigot. Nevertheless, there may be some truth to it. The dark-skinned Oliver Harding, said to be the president's great-uncle, appeared in *Abbott's Monthly*, a black-owned Chicago magazine, in 1932. As recently as 2005, a Michigan schoolteacher named Marsha Stewart made her own claim to Harding's ancestry. "While growing up," she wrote, "we were never allowed to talk about the relationship to a US president outside family gatherings because we were 'coloured' and Warren was 'passing'."

Harding himself appeared to believe it. His political allies hit back against Chancellor, driving him out of his job and destroying all but a handful of published copies of his book. The fact of his womanizing, though, is undoubtedly true. His attorney general Harry M. Daughtery said that no president had more "woman scrapes" than Harding. Fearing that he might be found out, he stunned a private party of reporters at the National Press Club by confessing his carnal desires.

"It's a good thing I am not a woman," the president said. "I would always be pregnant. I can't say no."

The truth is he never wanted to be president.

"I knew this job would be too much for me," he said when his administration was falling apart. "I am not fit for this office and never should have been here."

But one of his major backers said that he "looked like a president" and was forced into office by an ambitious and conniving wife. The daughter of a prominent banker in Marion, Ohio, Florence Kling ran off with drunken spendthrift Henry DeWolfe at the age of nineteen. After she gave birth to a son, he abandoned her and she returned to Marion shamefaced.

In 1884, Harding and two partners had bought the *Marion Daily Star* and to improve its profitability began to take advertising from the Republican Party. Two years later, he was appointed to the Republican County Committee.

Harding was more interested in drinking and playing cards than journalism. Florence turned up at the newspaper to help out and, despite the objections of her father, they married in 1891. She was thirty; he was twenty-five. While being a divorcee in those days was considered racy, she was cold and passionless. A plain woman, Harding called her "Duchess". She was considered to be the power behind the throne and, when he became president, a cartoon depicted the couple as "The Chief Executive and Mr Harding".

He began to look for passion elsewhere. First he turned to Florence's childhood friend, Susan Hodder, who is thought to have given birth to his child Marion Louise Hodder in Nebraska in 1895.

Then he began an affair with another of her friends, Mrs Carrie Phillips, the wife of a neighbour. This began in 1905 when Florence was in hospital having a kidney removed. Mrs Phillips had just lost a son and Harding comforted her. It was a passionate affair that continued for fifteen years. With all his mistresses, Harding was a passionate letter writer. In one of his missives to Mrs Phillips, he included a poem that read:

> I love your back, I love your breasts
> Darling to feel, where my face rests,
> I love your skin, so soft and white,
> So dear to feel and sweet to bite . . .
> I love your poise of perfect thighs,
> When they hold me in paradise . . .

At Florence's behest, Harding put his political career on a statewide footing. Though no politician, this suited him. Florence would have to stay in Marion running the paper, while he roamed Ohio. Carrie could then find some excuse to get away from her husband and meet up with him in an anonymous hotel room in some remote town in the boondocks.

No one suspected anything back in Marion, where the Phillipses and the Hardings would be seen socializing together. When Harding bought his first automobile, they would go out for an early evening drive together. They even took a holiday cruise together in 1909, with Warren and Carrie taking pleasure in having illicit sex in darkened corners of the deck, practically under the noses of their spouses. Rumours buzzed around Marion but, somehow, Florence, the managing editor of the local newspaper, did not get to hear about it. When she eventually found out in 1911, she considered filing for divorce, but then thought better of it when he agreed to end the affair.

Carrie begged him to leave his wife. But by then he was too embroiled in his political career. She fled to Germany, but the beginning of the First World War brought her scuttling home again and the affair resumed. Her husband, John, eventually found out about his wife's adultery in 1920. This brought the affair to an end, though John Phillips seems to have harboured no lasting resentment.

By this time, Harding was a United States senator and was having an affair with Grace Cross, member of his Senate staff. He had assorted other flings, including one with Augusta Cole, who said her pregnancy by Harding was terminated when he sent her to a Battle Creek Sanitarium, and one with Rosa Hoyle, who claimed to have given birth to his only illegitimate son and committed suicide when he would not leave Florence. He bedded an employee of the *Washington Post* known as Miss Allicott, and former chorus girls Maize Haywood and Blossom Jones – all procured by Harding's crony, Ned McLean, the owner and publisher of the *Washington Post*. Then there was the string of "New York women" – including one who committed suicide after Harding wouldn't marry her, and another who had a stash of incriminating love letters that had to be purchased by Harding loyalists.

But by far the most scandalous relationship was that with Nan Britton, a girl he had known since she was a child in Marion. At thirteen, she had become obsessed with him, filling her room with his campaign posters when he was running for the Senate. Her father, a friend of Harding's, told him of her infatuation and, when she went round to his house with her mother to have a chat with the candidate, he gave her a photograph of himself to add to her collection. Florence was as cold as ice.

In his book, *Warren Gamaliel Harding – An American Comedy*, Clement Wood claimed that Harding fell for her when she was a child and took her to his newspaper office where he bounced her on his lap, though it is generally accepted that the affair took a little longer to develop. However, while still in her early teens, according to her own account, she would hang around outside the newspaper office in the hope of bumping into him.

When Nan's father died, Harding found her mother a job as a substitute teacher and promised Nan that if there was anything he could do for her, she only had to ask. Taking him at his word, when she graduated from secretarial school in New York three years later, she wrote to him, asking whether he remembered her and whether he could find her a job in Washington. He wrote back saying that he did, indeed, remember her – "most agreeably too" – and that he would go personally to the War and Navy Departments to find her an appointment. He also said that he would probably be in New York the following week. He would like to phone her or look her up and would "take pleasure in doing it".

Their letters progress by innuendo. She wrote back saying "an hour's talk would be much more satisfactory", so that "I could give you a better idea of my ability . . . and you could judge for yourself as to the sort of position I could completely fill". This, she said "would please me immensely".

Early the next day, Harding was in New York. He phoned and asked her to meet him at his hotel. They walked through the foyer arm in arm. Then on a settee in reception, she blurted out her girlhood feelings for him. He suggested that they go up to his room where they would not be interrupted. But there was a convention in town, he said. All the rooms were taken. Except for one – the bridal suite.

"We had scarcely closed the door behind us when we shared our first kiss," she wrote later.

"Tell me it isn't hateful for you to have me kiss you," said the fifty-year-old senator, occasionally sighing "God! God! Nan," before going back for more.

Harding then admitted that he needed a woman and had come from Washington just to see her. She explained that she was still a virgin and was not ready to explore the "lovely mystery" of sex. To ease the situation, he tucked $30 into the top of her stocking.

Between feverish kisses, he explained that it would not be a good idea for her to come to Washington. The town was notorious for gossip. Instead, he would find her a good job in New York.

After lunch they took a taxi to the head office of US Steel. On the way, Harding decided to test her shorthand. He would dictate a letter. It began: "My darling Nan; I love you more than the world, and I want you to belong to me. Could you belong to me, dearie? I want you . . . and I need you so . . ."

But he could not finish because she began to smother him with kisses.

The head of US Steel gave her a job immediately, without question. When they got back to the hotel, Harding tripped when he got out of the taxi. "You see, dearie, I'm so crazy about you I don't know where I am stepping," he said.

Back in the bridal suite, she sat in his lap, though it is not recorded whether any bouncing took place.

"I'd like to make you my bride," he said. "We were made for each other" – ignoring the thirty-one-year age difference.

Before she started her new job, she went to visit her sister in Chicago. He sent her a picture of himself on the steps of the Capitol – another one for her collection – and one of his lengthy love letters. In reply, she made her first casual request for money. He sent $42. He always sent odd sums, as in the accounts, it would appear that she had run up some expenses on his behalf as a campaign volunteer.

Harding had a speaking tour of the Midwest lined up. He wrote, asking her to meet him in Indianapolis. When she arrived, he met her at the station. At the Claypool Hotel, they checked into separate rooms, though they spent most of the night together. She was, ostensibly, his niece and withheld what she called "love's sweetest intimacy".

The next day they travelled to a speaking engagement in Connersville, Indiana. There she checked in under the name of his secretary Elizabeth N. Christian. Then they travelled back to Chicago by Pullman. On the way to the station, he asked: "Dearie, are you going to sleep with me?"

He booked a berth, which they shared, but Nan was still a little naive about sex, according to her account, at least.

"I had earlier reached this conclusion," she wrote. "People got married and undressed and slept together, therefore, one must be undressed in order for any harm to come to them. I remember that this belief was so strong in my mind that when, during our ride together from Connersville to Chicago,

I experienced sweet thrills from just having Mr Harding's hands upon the outside of my nightdress, I became panic-stricken. I enquired tearfully whether he really thought I would have a child right away. Of course, this absurdity amused him greatly, but the fact that I was so ignorant seemed to add to his cherishment of me for some reason. And I loved him so dearly."

Back in Chicago, they tried to book into a hotel as man and wife. A disbelieving desk clerk said that, if they could prove they were married, he would give them the room for free.

The moment of "climactic intimacy" had to wait until they got back to New York. On a hot day in July 1917, he took her to the Imperial Hotel, an out-of-the-way establishment on lower Broadway that friends recommended for "unconventional activities".

"I remember so well, I wore a pink linen dress which was rather short and enhanced the little-girl look which was often my despair," she admitted. "There were no words going up in the elevator. The day was exceedingly warm and we were glad to see that the room which had been assigned to us had two large windows. The boy threw them open for us and left. The room faced Broadway, but we were high enough not to be bothered by street noises."

It was there, that torrid afternoon, that "I became Mr Harding's bride – as he called me – on that day."

They were lying in bed together in post-coital rapture when the phone rang.

"You have the wrong party," Harding said, answering it.

Then there was a knock on the door. A key turned in the lock and two detectives burst in. They demanded to know her name and address.

"Tell them the truth," he said to Nan, adding disconsolately, "they've got us."

As the detectives wrote down her details, Harding begged them to let her go. The scandal would ruin his career. "We've hurt no one," he said.

"Tell that to the judge," they replied, telling him that a paddy wagon was on its way.

But then one of the detectives picked up his hat and noticed the name W. G. Harding in the sweatband. Realizing that they had just arrested a US senator, they became deferential – obsequious, even – and left the room while the couple dressed. Then they led them to a side exit. At the door, Harding slipped them $20. Afterwards, in the taxi, Harding said, "Gee, Nan, I thought I wouldn't get out of that for under a thousand dollars."

But this brush with scandal did not put him off. He would come up from Washington once a week to sleep with her. And they were hardly discreet. She would meet him at Penn Station. They would go to see Al Jolson at the Wintergarden or a musical comedy on Broadway, then have a romantic dinner for two in a nearby restaurant.

"We were so sweetly intimate and it was a joy just to sit and look at him," she said. "The way he used his hands, the adorable way he used to put choice bits of meat from his own plate onto mine, the way he would say with a sort of tense nervousness, 'That's a very becoming hat, Nan,' or 'God, Nan, you're pretty!' used to go to my head like wine and made food seem for the moment the least needful thing in the world."

They would talk about what they would do if Mrs Harding died. He said he would give up politics and move to a farm if he could where Nan would be his "darling wife". Nan was less than charmed by the bucolic vision. She liked the way that he was an important man whom people recognized and, she said, she knew that one day he would be president. After dinner they would check into some anonymous hotel in downtown Manhattan to spend the night.

Otherwise, when he was out on a tour of speaking engagements, she would take a train ride out to meet him. They would sleep together in provincial hotels and make love out in the countryside. They even made out in a secluded corner of Central Park.

Sometimes, they borrowed a friend's apartment – Harding would get out of the elevator on the floor below to allay suspicion. Then Nan moved into an apartment on West 136th Street where they set up home together. They were like two newlyweds.

"His pangs seemed almost virginal in their intensity and surpassed any longings he had experienced in his life," she wrote.

However, they were far from virginal as he was still carrying on his affairs with Carrie Phillips and Grace Cross. And there was always his wife. During debates in the Senate he would crank out lengthy love letters, sometimes sixty pages long. He would send money and ply her with presents.

Sometimes she would go down to Washington to visit him. Her boss at US Steel was understanding when she needed to take time off. Everyone in the office knew that she had a lover in an exalted position. As Florence Harding suffered from a kidney infection that kept her indoors, Warren and Nan could stroll carelessly down Pennsylvania Avenue.

They made love in his office. Harding liked to see her naked there, so that he could fantasize about her when he was working. But, as she recalled, his workspace lacked the "usual paraphernalia which we always took to the hotels . . . and of course, the Senate Offices do not provide preventive facilities for use in such emergencies". On one of these occasions, she got pregnant.

Nan was thrilled by the news. Harding less so. He bought a bottle of Dr Humphrey's Number 11 pills. When Nan refused to take them, he suggested an abortion. She wanted to have his child. When she would not be shaken, he bought her a sapphire ring and he "performed a sweet ceremony . . . and declared that I could not belong to him more utterly had we been joined together by fifty ministers".

When the pregnancy began to show, Nan moved out to New Jersey, where she pretended that her husband was away at the war and that she was all alone because her mother did not approve of the match. On 22 October 1919, she gave birth to a daughter, Elizabeth Ann. Afterwards, he thought it best if they did not see each other any more as he was in line for the presidency. However, when he won the nomination, he could not help phoning her to tell her the news. She then appeared in the gallery at the convention to hear his acceptance speech.

Now it was time to clean up his act. His affair with Carrie Phillips had to end. Her husband was told about his wife's infidelity and, during the election, the couple were sent off on a world cruise paid for by the Republican Party. Carrie was also given $25,000 and a monthly stipend of $2,000 a month through a secret bank account to keep quiet about their affair while he was in office.

Harding gave Nan's sister and her husband $500 a month to adopt their child. Grace Cross proved more troublesome. They had already had one close scrape with scandal. While Harding was a senator they had had a row and she cut his back. The police were called, but the matter was hushed up. So, after a late-night assignation in the Willard Hotel on the eve of his inauguration, Grace Cross was told to pack her bags and leave town.

After a phony affidavit claiming that she was a liar and a blackmailer failed to shut Cross up, Jess Smith, the bootlegger who provided booze for White House parties during prohibition, dragooned Cross's friend Bertha Martin to purloin the love letters Harding had sent to Cross in return for being made society editor of the *Washington Post*. When Ned McLean sanctioned the deal, Martin took Cross to lunch, asked Cross to show her Harding's letters, then grabbed them and ran from the restaurant. Nevertheless, the two stayed friends and took a European vacation together, courtesy of Harding's secret blackmail fund. Martin was later found dressed in her fur coat, pearls and white gloves with her head in the oven, another alleged suicide.

Other mistresses were tracked down and were paid to sign affidavits denying their affairs. These found their way to the First Lady. Nan Britton was more of a problem. Once he was in office, her letters, which were marked "personal" and "private and confidential", were opened in the mailroom of the White House. They contained pictures of a child who bore a suspicious likeness to the president and asked for money. White House staffers dutifully destroyed them.

But Harding could not give her up. He sent for Nan. A White House aide met her at the station and brought her to him in the Oval Office. However, with its large windows overlooking the White House lawn, it was hardly discreet. But there was a solution.

"He introduced me to the one place where, he said, he thought we might share kisses in safety," Nan recounted. "This was a small closet in the anteroom, evidently a place for hats and coats, but entirely empty most of the times we used it, for we repaired there many times in the course of my visits to the White House, and in the darkness of a space not more than five feet square the president of the United States and his adoring sweetheart made love."

After their first encounter there, they worked out a way for her letters to get through to him. She was to address them to his valet, who would pass them on. After he had read them, he would destroy them. She was to destroy his letters too. She was also warned not to spend the money he gave her on expensive jewellery or fur coats. That would attract attention and they needed to avoid scandal at all costs.

Harding already had a heart condition. It was not helped when Elizabeth Ann got locked in a bathroom in Chicago and he saw in the papers pictures of firemen rescuing her.

The assignations in the closet were facilitated by Secret Service agents James Sloan and Walter Ferguson.

"Harding hated to have them around, for he despised being watched," said the chief usher.

Proceedings came to an abrupt end when another agent, Harry Barker, tipped Florence off, and she ran down for a confrontation. But Sloan and Ferguson barred her way. When she demanded that they stand aside, they told her that it was a rule among the Secret Service that no one was to see the president when he told them that he was not to be disturbed. Florence headed around to another door that gave access to the Oval Office through his secretary's office. This gave the couple enough time to put their clothes on and for Harding to bundle Nan out of a side door.

Harding often complained of his wife's inconsiderate behaviour. "She makes my life hell for me," he told Nan.

If this was not bad enough, another sex scandal loomed on the horizon. Harding's father had taken a new mistress who was five years younger than Harding himself. This threatened to draw attention to Harding's own peccadilloes.

Florence was also on the warpath. She employed a shady sleuth named Gaston Means to deal with Nan Britton.

"Warren Harding has had a very ugly affair with a girl named Nan Britton from Marion," Florence told him. "It goes back to the actual childhood of this girl. When she was but a child, she was greatly over-developed and wore extremely short dresses above the knees. It was not considered quite decent. And she was always doing everything on earth that she could do to attract Warren's attention. This over-development tended to attract men on the street and, together with her unusually short dresses, she attracted the attention of course and in not a very nice way. Why, I have watched men watch her even before she was in her early teens."

She also explained that Nan had a child and claimed that Harding was the father, though she did not believe it. Florence hired Means to investigate Nan. His job, he realized, was to prove that Harding and Nan were not lovers and that he was not the father of her child. It was an impossible task. Means soon concluded that, not only was Nan Britton Warren Harding's lover, but that she was also faithful to him. He even claimed to have broken into Nan's sister's apartment in Chicago and purloined love letters that Harding had written. Florence insisted that he hand them over, but he refused at first, saying that he had been hired to supply information, not stolen goods.

Eventually he handed over a bundle tied up in pink silk corset ribbon. When Florence read them she went white and moaned, "Could you believe it?"

Nevertheless, she refused to believe that Harding was the father of Nan's child. She believed that he was sterile. After all, he had never got her pregnant. Means then produced pictures of the child, showing that Warren Harding was not only willing but capable.

Florence then summoned her husband and confronted him with the evidence. He turned on Means.

"By what authority do you put the president of the United States under surveillance?" he insisted to know.

Means said that he had not put the president under surveillance, only his mistress. It mattered little. Within twenty-four hours, Means was indicted and, in due course, went to jail.

Harding then had bitter words for Florence. "You have ruined me with your contemptible detectives," he said, shaking his fist at her.

"Warren, Warren," she begged. "Think of our young love . . ."

"Our young love?" he yelled. "Love? I never loved you. You want the truth. Now you've got the truth. Young love? You ran me down."

Despite this confrontation, he did not stop seeing Nan. Nor did he stop seeing other women. Warren Harding "could no more resist a pretty girl or woman than he could resist food when hungry," a friend said. The public were all too well aware of this when he was caught ogling Margaret Gooding, the first Miss America, days after her crowning in Atlantic City.

Bootlegger Jess Smith and Attorney General Harry M. Daughtery laid on parties in a house they called the "Love Nest" on H Street, complete with a pink taffeta bedroom. One night some New York chorus girls were brought down to entertain a stag party. In attendance was the president. When glasses and bottles were being flung off the table so the dancing girls could perform, one Washington prostitute, identified only as a Miss Walsh, was knocked unconscious. Harding was hustled out. The woman died and was buried in a field.

Women who took Harding's fancy – and there were many of them – were given lucrative government jobs. Others, who turned up with incriminating letters, were paid off. The Justice Department was used to intimidate anyone who threatened to make a scandal. They even managed to seize and destroy a small, privately printed book, *The Illustrated Life of Warren Gamaliel Harding*, that revealed Harding's affair with Carrie Phillips, the blackmail pay-off and Florence's out-of-wedlock child by a common-law first husband. It was the only book in the history of the United States to be suppressed by the government in peacetime.

The action was entirely illegal. The books were not even impounded on government property. Rather they were taken to Ned McLean's estate where they were burnt. However, one escaped the conflagration. It can now be found among the papers of McLean's wife Evelyn in the Library of Congress, along with a letter from Harding to Grace Cross. It seems that Ned McLean had been made a special agent, who sought to thwart any threats to Harding he heard about as publisher of the *Washington Post*. In the privacy of his editorial office, he even ripped the blouse of Nan Britton trying to snatch letters she claimed to be carrying.

Warren Harding's sexual misdemeanours were overlooked because his administration was so deeply mired in other scandals. Daughtery's relationship with Jess Smith was investigated by the Senate. When he was brought to trial, the jury could not agree a verdict after sixty-six hours' deliberation and he was acquitted. However, Harding's secretary of the interior Albert B. Fall was found guilty of accepting $100,000 to lease the US Navy oil reserves at Tea Pot Dome to private interest. He was the first Cabinet member to be sent to prison. There were also scandals in the Veterans' Bureau, the Shipping Board, the Office of Alien Property, the Prohibition Bureau and the Bureau of Investigation – the forerunner of the FBI. Jess Smith was found with a bullet in his head. Rumours were spread that he was homosexual.

"I have no trouble with my enemies," President Harding said. "But my damned friends, they're the ones that keep me walking the floor at night."

Warren Harding died suddenly of a heart attack or stroke in San Francisco while returning from a visit to Alaska, after being given purgatives by Florence's homeopath Charles "Doc" Sawyer whose mistress was the First Lady's housekeeper. Florence then rushed back to Washington to burn his papers. There were rumours that Harding had committed suicide or been killed by his wife to avoid impeachment. In his book *The Strange Death of Warren Harding*, Gaston Means claimed that Florence poisoned him in revenge for his affair with Nan Britton. The book was a runaway bestseller.

Florence Harding was a believer in astrology and consulted the capital's society psychic Madame Marcia. Her diary, which surfaced in a barn auction in 1997, shows that she consulted Madame Marcia on February 1920. Curiously, the seer predicted that if Harding ran for president that year, he would be nominated – but that if he won the election, he would not live through his full term and instead die of "sudden, peculiar, violent . . . death by poison".

Nan Britton rekindled the scandal surrounding Warren Harding's sex life with her own kiss-and-tell book *The President's Daughter*. The Society for the Suppression of Vice wanted to ban it. They went to the printing plant and seized the plates, but they were ordered by a court to give them back. Bookshops refused to carry the book, but Nan managed to sell 90,000 copies under the counter at $5 a time. The campaigning journalist H. L. Mencken – who loved a good sex scandal – then took up the story in the *Baltimore Sun* to smear the Republican administration of Harding's successor Calvin Coolidge.

When Carrie Phillips died in Willets Home for the Elderly in Marion in 1960, her possessions were sold off. Among them was a box that contained ninety-eight handwritten letters from Harding. In one, dated 1911, he said: "I love you garbed, but naked more . . ." The word "naked" was underlined twice. In another there was a poem that began: "Carrie, take me panting to your heaving breast." They bore a striking similarity to the letters Nan Britton said that Harding wrote to her.

## Dwight D. Eisenhower

During World War II, Eisenhower was posted to London to prepare for the D-Day landings. His wife Mamie stayed at home. But Ike did not want for female company. The British assigned him a driver from the Women's Royal Army Corps. Her name was Kay Summersby. Born in County Cork, she had been a model and movie actress.

"She is also very pretty," Eisenhower wrote tactlessly in a letter home to Mamie. "Irish and slender and I think in the process of getting a divorce, which is all that worries me."

Luckily, Eisenhower's aide Harry Butcher forgot to post this letter. However, he recorded in his own diary a much more frank assessment of the situation: "Ike defines this member of the WAC as 'a double-breasted GI with a built-in foxhole'."

After his first letter had gone astray, Eisenhower omitted any further reference to Kay in his letters home. But Mamie would have had to have been blind not to see what was going on. In the press coverage of Eisenhower, he was always pictured with

Kay by his side. Asked about the rumour that Eisenhower was having an affair with a woman twenty years his junior, John Thompson of the *Chicago Tribune* said, "Well, I have never before seen a chauffeur get out of a car and kiss the General good morning when he comes from his office."

Not only was she his driver, he also employed her as a secretary at AFHQ and they were constant companions. She even accompanied him to meetings with Churchill, George VI and President Roosevelt. Then there were the trips abroad to Algiers, Egypt and Palestine.

Brigadier General Everett Hughes, Eisenhower's deputy, wrote in his diary: "Kay is helping Ike win the war." But he feared a scandal.

Mamie kicked up a fuss when she read in *Life* magazine that Ike's "London driver" was with him during his stay in North Africa.

"She is terribly in love with a young American colonel and is to be married to him come June, assuming both are alive," Eisenhower wrote back. "I doubt that *Life* told you that."

He also told Mamie that she could not come and stay with him in London because of the bombing.

On the eve of Kay's wedding, her fiancé was killed by a landmine. Ike told Mamie that Kay "cannot long continue to drive – she is too sunk". But he did not sack her. Instead he consoled her – and began a passionate affair.

"It was like an explosion," Kay wrote in her memoirs *Past Forgetting: My Love Affair with Dwight D. Eisenhower*. "We were suddenly in each other's arms. His kisses absolutely unravelled me. Hungry, strong, demanding. And I responded every bit as passionately. He stopped, took my face between his hands. 'Goddamn it,' he said. 'I love you.'

"We were breathing as if we had run up a dozen flights of stairs. God must have been watching over us, because no one came bursting into the office. It was lovers' luck, but we both came to our senses, remembering how Tex [his aide Colonel Ernest R. 'Tex' Lee] had walked in earlier that day. Ike had lipstick smudges on his face. I started scrubbing at them frantically with my handkerchief."

With the largest amphibious landing in history to plan they were seldom alone. But one evening they were having a nightcap when everyone else had mysteriously disappeared.

"Ike refilled our glasses several times," she recalled, "and then, I suppose inevitably, we found ourselves in each other's embrace. Our ties came off. Our jackets came off. Buttons were unbuttoned. It was as if we were frantic. And we were.

"But it was not what I expected. Wearily, we slowly calmed down. He snuggled his face into the hollow between my neck and shoulder and said: 'Oh, God, Kay. I'm sorry. I'm not going to be any good for you.'"

Ike could not get it up. Kay made excuses for him. It was pressure of work. He had a lot on his mind. There was his wife waiting for him at home and his innate sense of morality.

So here was another – worse – scandal. A general having a bit on the side is one thing. It was wartime. There were air raids. Everyone was living for today. Who knew whether there would be a tomorrow? But for the Allies' leading general to be found wanting in the sexual department. What would German propaganda make out of that if they got to know of it? Dr Goebbels would have a field day. How could an impotent old man like Eisenhower hope to defeat a frothing stud like Hitler? Or, at least, that was how it could be made to look.

But Ike had not given up. Maybe things would work out in more relaxed circumstances. So he fixed up a rural retreat called Telegraph Cottage on Kingston Hill in Surrey and bought her a puppy they called Telek – the "Tele" from Telegraph Cottage and the "k" from Kay. They tried to make love again at Telegraph Cottage. Again they failed.

Nevertheless Eisenhower asked the Chief of Staff, General George Marshall, for permission to divorce Mamie and marry Kay. Marshall threatened to bust Eisenhower down to private if he tried.

With the end of the war in Europe, Eisenhower returned to the US. The American people gave him a hero's welcome. Mamie's welcome was a little more restrained. Ike was then posted to Germany as military governor of the US zone of occupation. The war was over. There was no more bombing, but Mamie did not go with him. Kay did.

He arranged for her to become a US citizen so that she could continue working for him, telling her that she was going to be on his personal staff in the Pentagon. When he told her the news, she kissed him.

"We sat there on the sofa making daydreamy plans for the future, kissing, holding hands being quite indiscreet for the rest of the afternoon," she wrote. "Never in all the time I had known him had I had to hold Ike back. He had always been circumspect, but this afternoon he was an eager lover."

The door was closed and she knew that nobody from the household would be walking in.

"The fire was warm. The sofa soft. We held each other close, closer. Excitedly, I remember thinking, the way one thinks odd thoughts at significant moments, wouldn't it be wonderful if this were the day I was to conceive a baby – our very first time. Ike was tender, careful, loving. But it didn't work.

"'Wait,' I said. 'You're too excited. It will be all right.'

"'No,' he said flatly. 'It won't. It's too late. I can't.' He was bitter. We dressed slowly. Kissing occasionally. Smiling a bit sadly.

"'Comb your hair,' he said. 'I'm going to ask them to serve supper in here.'"

When she came back from the bathroom, there was a small table in front of the fire with a bottle of wine in a cooler, some chicken and salad. They drank and talked. The door was closed again.

"It seemed as if Ike had decided that he no longer cared what anyone thought or said."

They ate and drank and talked about "what had happened. Or had not happened."

She said: "It's not important, not the least bit important. It just takes time. That's all. And I'm very stubborn. You've said so yourself."

"I know you are," said Ike, "but I'm not sure that you are right."

She did not get the opportunity to find out whether she was right or wrong. When Eisenhower returned to Washington, she found that she had been dropped from the roster of people going with him. Instead she was given a job in Berlin working for the Deputy Military Governor of Germany, General Lucius Clay.

When she eventually turned up in Washington, she was something of an embarrassment. Men she had known in Europe during the war now shunned her. After visiting Eisenhower in the Pentagon with Telek, she found herself posted to a small public relations unit in California.

After she was discharged from the army, she began stalking Eisenhower, who was then president of Columbia University in New York City. Bumping into him on campus one day, she said she was visiting a friend who was a student there. He did not believe her.

"Kay, it's impossible," he said. "There's nothing I can do."

A few months later, she discovered that he was going to speak at the Fellowship of United States–British Comrades at the Seventh Regiment Armoury on Park Avenue. She went to the meeting, sitting far back not to draw attention to herself. There was a reception afterwards. She did not go.

"I still did not trust myself to go up, shake his hand and say the conventional empty words," she said.

Her appearance there sparked a conflagration of gossip. Even the *New York Times* reported that she had been at the meeting but had left without talking to him.

She published her first volume of memoirs, *Eisenhower Was My Boss* which mentions nothing of their affair. He returned to Europe as supreme commander of NATO. Then he was on the campaign trail. Only in 1972, three years after Eisenhower's death, did she publish *Past Forgetting*.

## Richard Nixon

Nixon's career was dogged by scandal. In 1952, when he first ran for vice-president alongside Eisenhower, allegations were made about the funding of his campaign. He responded with a televised speech where he refused to return one gift – a black-and-white dog named Checkers. Then as president he was brought down by the Watergate scandal. However, there was little hint of any sex scandal. Indeed, despite being married with two daughters, Nixon always appeared rather asexual.

The famous journalist Adela Rogers St John once saw Nixon at a Republican rally where he was surrounded by some of Hollywood's most beautiful movie stars.

"You never saw such beautiful flesh," she said. "And he acted like a man utterly unsexed. It was as if he did not know they were there."

Nixon's closest friend was Cuban-exile Bebe Rebozo. They were friends for forty-four years. After losing the 1962 gubernatorial race in California, he told the press: "You won't have Nixon to kick around anymore because, gentlemen, this is my last press conference." Then he said he was going to go home to spend some time getting to know his family again. Instead, he spent three weeks alone with Rebozo on Paradise Island in the Bahamas.

White House Chief of Staff General Alexander Haig joked about the two men having a homosexual affair, even aping Nixon's limp-wristed manner. But there is no evidence that they were gay. They were both fiercely anti-homosexual in an old-fashioned way. Indeed, it was a smear Nixon liked to use against political opponents.

But as a young man, Nixon was interested in female flesh. He was an avid fan of striptease, even taking his fiancée Pat to seen the "blonde bombshell" Betty Roland at Topsy's in East Los Angeles before they were married.

However, there was a scandal lurking in the FBI's files that allowed J. Egar Hoover to stay on in office long after retirement age. Every time Nixon tried to fire Hoover he emerged from the meeting ashen-faced.

In 1958, forty-five-year-old Nixon, who was then vice-president, met a twenty-three-year-old tour guide in Hong Kong named Marianna Liu. Naturally Hoover had pictures of them together. They met again when he was a private citizen in 1964, 1965 and 1966. Then she was working as a cocktail waitress. Marianna and another waitress visited Nixon in Rebozo's suite in the Mandarin Hotel. Later, he sent flowers, a bottle of her favourite perfume and a note giving her his New York address.

The FBI took a particular interest in her because she was suspected of being a Communist spy. She had already been seen fraternizing with US Navy officers. British intelligence was also watching her. At the request of the CIA, Hong Kong Special Branch photographed Nixon and Liu through a hotel bedroom window using an infrared camera.

Then she turned up at the inaugural ball in 1969 and went to live in Nixon's hometown, Whittier in California. It was only after he fell from power over Watergate that the *National Equirer* ran a story about their "hot and heavy" romance. She threatened to sue, but admitted to *People* magazine that she had met Nixon when she was a "hostess" in the cocktail lounge of the Hong Kong Hilton, that she went to see him in Rebozo's suite in the Mandarin Hotel, that he had sent her flowers and a note when she was ill, and that he had given her legal advice on emigrating to the US.

Liu's lawyer said Nixon was so angry about the accusations that he had volunteered to take the stand on Marianna's behalf. The editor of the *Enquirer* said: "We hope he does."

Nixon had already been caught in enough lies.

## Ronald Reagan

When it came to scandals, President Gerald Ford was rather overshadowed by his wife Betty. She admitted in her autobiography that she was addicted to booze and pills, and started the Betty Ford Center for other lushes. Then there was Jimmy Carter who caused a frisson when he told *Playboy* magazine: "I've committed adultery in my heart many times." Must try harder.

But then with Ronald Reagan things went back to normal. He was, after all, a movie star before he became president. A well-known ladies' man back in Illinois, his first publicity shots in Hollywood show him bare-chested and surrounded by a bevy of bathing beauties. He was seen out with a number of stunning actresses, including "sweater girl" Lana Turner. He married his first wife, actress Jane Wyman, in 1938, but she famously complained that he was "about as good in bed as he was on screen". They divorced in 1949. But by the eighties, being a divorcee was no longer a bar to the presidency.

A free man again, he was out on the pull – a town that was full of starlets and other hopefuls. However, fellow actor Eddie Bracken said, "He was never looking for sexpots. He was never the guy looking for bed. He was a guy looking for companionship more than anything else."

In 1952, he married actress Nancy Davis, a woman with a history of her own. Her mother Edith Luckett was an actress and her godmother was famous silent-era lesbian movie star Alla Nazimova. According to Kitty Kelley's scurrilous biography *Nancy Reagan: The Unauthorized Biography*, she had a lesbian affair with a classmate when she was majoring in theatre at Smith College in Massachusetts. Then she fell in love with a young man who committed suicide. This had left her scarred.

During World War II, she was engaged to a US Navy officer who had a particularly feminine nature. She broke it off and indulged in a period of sexual experimentation, becoming what men at the time called "accessible". She even hit on married men who were friends of her parents.

In New York, she hung out with gay men, taking a bisexual as her lover. On Broadway in *Lute Song* in 1946, she had an affair with a dancer who had only been to bed with a woman twice before. She had three dates with Clark Gable and her phone number was passed around, guaranteeing a regular supply of dates.

Spencer Tracey, a notorious womanizer, drunk and friend of her mother's, organized a screen test. In Hollywood, she advanced her career by becoming the lover of MGM casting director Benjamin Thau. Just before he died in 1983, Thau gave an interview where he said that Nancy orally obliged men who furthered her career in the MGM offices. Her abilities were legendary.

In *The Peter Lawford Story: Life With the Kennedys, Monroe and the Rat Pack*, Lawford's widow Patricia said:

> Peter was watching the news right after Reagan was elected. He went over to the set, laughing and calling Mrs Reagan a vulgar name. I was shocked and wanted to know what was bothering him. He laughed again and said that when she was single, Nancy Davis was known for giving the best head in Hollywood. Then Peter told of driving to the Phoenix area with Nancy and Bob Walker [the actor who Lawford claims was Nancy's lover at the time]. Nancy would visit her parents, Dr and Mrs Loyal Davis, while Peter and Walker picked up girls at Arizona State University in Tempe, a Phoenix suburb. He claimed that she entertained them orally on those trips, apparently playing with whichever man was not driving at the moment. I have no idea if Peter was telling the truth, though I have to assume he was because Peter was not one to gossip.

Nancy's mouth must have worked its magic. Betty Powers, one of the bevy of models and starlets Reagan was running around with at the time, said that Reagan was so obsessed with his ex Jane Wyman that he could not get it up. Nancy must have given him oral encouragement.

Doris Lilly, author of *How to Marry a Millionaire* and *How to Make Love in Five Languages*, and thought to be the inspiration for Holly Golightly in Truman Capote's *Breakfast at Tiffany's*, complained that he was "passive . . . very gentle, very square" and, seemingly, more interested in drinking than sex.

Starlet Jacqueline Park, later the mistress of Warner Bros studio boss Jack Warner, told a similar story. When the two began dating, Reagan "couldn't perform sexually," she said. "I think he was still suffering withdrawal pains from Jane Wyman."

Throughout their liaison, Park said, "He never took me out in public, never gave me a present and never ever paid for a cab for me."

But then Park mysteriously became pregnant. Presumably she was not visited by the Holy Ghost.

"When I told him I was pregnant, he said he didn't want to have anything to do with me any more," she said. Who can blame him, if he could not deliver the old love juice? "He just ran out on me. He was a swinger in those days. He went out with this girl and that girl. But the moment he married Nancy and became a Republican, he was reformed, and there's nothing more boring than a reformed swinger."

According to Reagan's own account, he was tiring of the never-ending round of beauties he was bedding. "I woke up one morning and I couldn't remember the name of the gal I was in bed with," he told a friend – hey, it's happened to us all. "And I said get a grip here."

He proposed to glamour girl Christine Larson. Plainly, she did not get a grip and turned him down. Soon after, Nancy told him she was pregnant. She must have swallowed awfully hard.

But before the nuptials, Reagan encountered nineteen-year-old blonde Selene Walters. They met at a Hollywood nightclub.

"Although I was on a date," Walters said, "Ronnie kept whispering in my ear, 'I'd like to call you. How can I get in touch with you?'"

Reagan was then president of the Screen Actors Guild and she hoped that he could give her a leg up in her career, so she gave him her address and was surprised when he came calling at 3 a.m.

According to Kitty Kelley, Walters told her: "He pushed his way inside and said he just had to see me. He forced me on the couch ... and said, 'Let's just get to know each other.' It was the most pitched battle I've ever had, and suddenly in a matter of seconds I lost ... They call it date rape today."

Selene Walters later confirmed Kelley's account of what happened, except she said that Reagan did not force his way in.

"I opened the door," she told *People* magazine. "Then it was the battle of the couch. I was fighting him. I didn't want him to make love to me. He's a very big man, and he just had his way. Date rape? No, God, no, that's her [Kelley's] phrase. I didn't have a chance to have a date with him."

Walters said she bore Reagan no ill will, and even voted for him. "I don't think he meant to harm me," she said.

A week later, he announced his engagement to Nancy. They married in March 1952. Seven months later, she gave birth to their daughter Patti. Reagan was not present at the birth. He was with Christine Larson. The affair ended soon afterwards when he dropped around one afternoon to be greeted by a French actor dressed in nothing but a bath towel. Apart from a brief affair in 1968, he seems to have remained faithful.

Once married Nancy also became a good Republican wife. She quit work and dedicated herself to being a housewife.

"A woman's real happiness and real fulfilment come from within the home with her husband and children," she said.

According to Kitty Kelley, Nancy did not get on with her children. While Reagan was governor of California, Nancy began an affair with Frank Sinatra that "continued for years". As First Lady, Kelley writes, Nancy entertained Sinatra at the White House, which he entered "in the back way", for three-or four-hour "private 'luncheons'" in the family quarters. When Nancy was with him, Kelley quotes a staffer as saying, "She was not to be disturbed. For anything. And that included a call from the president himself."

At White House parties she would dance dreamily with her "Francis Albert" and got annoyed when Reagan tried to cut in. Even Sinatra's wife Barbara complained that Nancy was hogging him.

Ironically, Sinatra, a lifelong Democrat, hated Reagan, considering him a turncoat for switching parties. When Reagan was governor of California, he changed the lyrics of "The Lady is a Tramp" to "She hates California, it's Reagan and damp . . . that's why the lady is a tramp."

Reagan had already left office when Kitty Kelley's hatchet job on Nancy came out. Mercifully he was probably already too gaga to take it all in.

## George Bush

As unlikely as it may seem, George Herbert Walker Bush was in the centre of a sex scandal in the run-up to the 1992 election. But then when he was a congressman he had been nicknamed "Rubbers" because of his insistence on using a condom, unfashionable in the sixties, and it was said that he had set up an Italian woman in an apartment in New York. Then, on the eve of the Republican convention in Houston, Susan B. Trento published her book *The Power House*, which named British-born diplomat Jennifer Fitzgerald as First Mistress. She first met Bush during the Watergate scandal in 1974 and quit her job in the White House to become his secretary when he was appointed ambassador to China. She went on to work with him at the CIA and on his vice-presidential staff.

According to the book, US Ambassador Louis Fields arranged for then Vice President George Bush and his former appointments secretary Jennifer Fitzgerald to share a private cottage during an official visit to Geneva in 1984.

"It became clear that the vice president and Mrs Fitzgerald were romantically involved and this was not a business visit," said Fields. The couple had adjoining bedrooms but the rendezvous was "so heavy handed" that it made him feel "very uncomfortable". At the time, the First Lady Barbara Bush was in the US promoting her book about the family dog, *C. Fred's Story: A Dog's Life*.

The scandal broke when the story made the front page of the *New York Post*, which cited two other sources – a lawyer and a former reporter – who had also heard versions of the story.

When CNN reporter Mary Tillotson broached the topic at a joint news conference Bush was holding with Israeli Prime Minister Yitzhak Rabin at the family estate at Kennebunkport, Maine, Bush declared himself to be outraged.

"I'm not going to take any sleazy questions like that from CNN," said Bush. "I am very disappointed that you would ask such a question of me, and I will not respond to it. I haven't responded in the past. Nevertheless, in this kind of screwy climate we're in, why, I expect it. But I don't like it, and I'm not going to respond other than to say it's a lie."

Barbara Bush looked on with evident disgust.

Later in the day, when Bush returned to Washington, he was interviewed in the Oval Office by Stone Phillips, who asked him straight out: "Have you ever had an affair?"

"I'm not going to take any sleaze questions," Bush replied. "You're perpetuating the sleaze by even asking the question, to say nothing of asking it in the Oval Office. And I don't think you ought to do that, and I'm not going to answer the question."

Ironically, the interview went out on *Dateline NBC*.

Not wishing to take advantage of the situation, the Democratic presidential nominee Bill Clinton condemned the injection of allegations of marital infidelity into the presidential campaign. After all he was a gentleman. No hint of self-interest there.

Referring to rumours of adultery that had dogged his campaign earlier that year, Clinton said, "I didn't like it when it was done to me, and I don't like it when it's done to him."

After all Slick Willie was so much better at it.

Besides in May, when Hillary Clinton was fuming over stories about her husband's alleged affair with Gennifer Flowers, she complained in *Vanity Fair* that everyone knew there was also a "Jennifer", in Bush's life, but that no one was reporting it.

Ms Fitzgerald was then deputy chief of protocol in the State Department, an appointment arranged by Bush when he entered the White House. She was said to be out of the country on business, but her mother, eighty-six-year-old Frances Patteson-Knight, responding with evident distaste, said Jennifer was "devastated".

"She had a very unhappy marriage, and she can't stand men," she said, and she recalled her daughter once telling her, "I've been through so much. I couldn't have sex with anybody."

In 1955, Jennifer Patteson-Knight, the daughter of a British officer, had married a US Army private, Gerald FitzGerald. They divorced in 1959. However, she kept his surname, though made the G lower case, presumably making it harder to find.

This was not the first time the affair between Bush and Jennifer Fitzgerald surfaced. During the 1988 campaign, *LA Weekly* ran a story naming Fitzgerald as Bush's long-time mistress and quoting an unnamed source that Fitzgerald had spoken openly of the affair. But since then Gary Hart had declared open season.

## George W. Bush

In many ways George W. Bush could have been expected to rival Clinton. During his roistering days, a classmate from Yale said, "He flew jets, drove fast cars and screwed more women than Hugh Hefner."

One of them was Tina Cassini, daughter of movie actress Gene Tierney and fashion designer Oleg Cassini.

"She was a real show pony," said a friend. "They paraded for the summer. Tina was spectacular . . . It was a good fling."

He was a great drinker too. When he was at Moody Air Force Base with the Texas National Guard, he would get drunk, strip off and dance naked on the bar. He worked on a campaign for a friend of his father's in Alabama, where he was remembered as a "party boy who couldn't keep his hands off the girls".

At Harvard Business School, a classmate said, "We all had steady girlfriends, one week at a time. Drinking and womanizing – what else is there to do in your spare time? George was no different to anyone else."

Back in Texas, Julia Reed, later a writer on *Vogue* magazine said: "All the ladies were going crazy over him. When coupled with the young George's bad-boy good looks, the total package was enough to send the many eligible twenty-somethings into a collective swoon."

Friends noted that he dated good-looking women that gave him phone numbers. Otherwise he would find his own in the sweaty honky-tonks of Odessa.

All this seems very promising, but then he met Laura at a backyard barbecue in 1977. He sobered up, became a born-again Christian and got married. And that was that.

However, during the 2000 election, Tammy Phillips, a thirty-five-year-old stripper, came forward, claiming she just ended an eighteen-month affair with one George W. Bush. According to the *National Enquirer*, the *New York Post*, and Tony Snow on FOX TV, the affair had lasted from late 1966 until June 1999 when he decided to run for president. She told the *Enquirer* that she met Dubya at a hotel in Texas. She was wearing a micro-miniskirt. He "combusted" and became a born-again womanizer. But, rather than turning into a sex scandal, this was passed off as a smear.

Then in 2002, when he was securely in the White House, a thirty-eight-year-old African-American woman named Margie Denise Schoedinger from Missouri City, Texas, filed suit, claiming that he had raped her in October 2000. In her suit, she alleged "race-based harassment and individual sex crimes committed against her and her husband".

A seven-page document was filed at Ford Bend County Court Texas, which claimed that Bush drugged, raped and beat her. She also suggested that she "dated George W. Bush as a minor", and that the president may have been the father of the child she miscarried as a result of the alleged rape. She was asking for $1 million actual damages and $49 million punitive damages, due to her emotional distress and being deprived of her liberty.

Most commentators dismissed her as a nutcase. But then it was reported that Schoedinger died on 22 September 2003, of a gunshot wound to the head, nine months after filing the suit. The Harris County, TX, Medical Examiner's office ruled the death a suicide. Surely this has all the makings of a conspiracy theory. But if that is the best George W. Bush can do by way of a sex scandal we must all pray that Barack Obama can try a little harder.

## Clarence Thomas

In 1991, Clarence Thomas was nominated for the Supreme Court. The hearings turned into a scandal when a former colleague of Thomas's, University of Oklahoma law school professor Anita Hill, accused him of making unwelcome sexual comments to her when they worked together ten years earlier at the Department of Education and the Equal Employment Opportunity Commission in 1982.

Hill told the Senate Hearing that, in his office, instead of discussing work, Thomas would talk about "pornographic material".

> Question: What was the content of what he said?
> Answer: This was a reference to an individual who had a very large penis. And he used the name that he had been referred to in the pornographic material.
> Q: Do you recall what it was?
> A: Yes, I do. The name that was referred to was Long Dong Silver.

And she had gone into his office merely to "report on memos". Hill alleged that Thomas had already taken "more than a professional interest" in her.

"He said to me, very casually, you ought to go out with me sometime," she said. She declined.

On other occasions, he referred to the size of his own penis as being larger than normal, and he also spoke on some occasions of the pleasures he had given to women with oral sex. One time, she said he talked about "acts that he had seen in pornographic films involving such matters as women having sex with animals and films showing group sex or rape scenes. He talked about pornographic materials depicting individuals with large penises or large breasts involved in various sex acts." Pressed for the details, she said: "I really cannot quote him verbatim. I can remember something like, you really ought to see these films that I've seen, or this material that I've seen. This woman has this kind of breast, or breasts that measure this size. And they've got her in there with all kinds of things, she's doing all kinds of different sex acts, and you know, that kind of – those were the kind of words, where he expressed his enjoyment of it, and seemed to try to encourage me to enjoy that kind of material as well."

Hill thought that Thomas wanted to have sex with her, or at least wanted them to watch porn movies together – though he never actually asked her straight out, she admitted. However, she complained that the conversations were "very dirty, they were disgusting".

"On several occasions, Thomas told me graphically of his own sexual prowess," she said.

He also made references to "his own physical attributes". Naturally, the senators wanted to hear more.

Q: Can you tell us what he said?
A: Well, I can tell you that he compared his penis size – he measured his penis size in terms of length . . .

Senator Arlen Specter of Pennsylvania was not particularly disgusted by this. He pointed out that she had told Roger Tuttle, former dean of the Oral Roberts Law School that Thomas was a fine man and she had never made any derogatory comments about him. However, she had complained to the FBI about him, though she made "no reference to any mention of Judge Thomas's private parts or sexual prowess or size, etc.".

Q: Why didn't you tell the FBI about that?
A: Senator, in paragraph two on page two of the report, it says that he liked to discuss specific sex acts and frequency of sex . . .
Q: Now, are you saying, in response to my question as to why you didn't tell the FBI about the size of his private parts and his sexual prowess and Long Dong Silver that that information was comprehended within the statement, quote, Thomas liked to discuss specific acts and frequency of sex?
A: I am not saying that that information was included in that . . .

> Q: Professor Hill, you said that you took it to mean that Judge Thomas wanted to have sex with you, but, in fact, he never did ask you to have sex, correct?
>
> A: No, he did not ask me to have sex . . .
>
> Q: So that when you said you took it to mean, we ought to have sex, that that was an inference.
>
> A. Yes.

Sometimes it got a little bizarre.

"One of the oddest episodes I remember was an occasion in which Thomas was drinking a Coke in his office," she said. "He got up from the table at which we were working, went over to his desk to get the Coke, looked at the can and asked, 'Who has put pubic hair on my Coke?'"

Sadly, the Senate never got to the bottom of this. Who did put the pubic hair on Clarence's Coke can? I think we should be told.

Thomas denied everything and got on his high horse.

"How would any member on this committee, any person in this room, or any person in this country like sleaze said about him or her in this fashion?" he asked. "Or this dirt dredged up and this gossip and these lies displayed in this manner, how would any person like it? The Supreme Court is not worth it. No job is worth it. I am not here for that. I am here for my name, my family, my life and my integrity. I think something is dreadfully wrong with this country when any person, any person in this free country would be subjected to this."

Then he really got into his stride.

"This is a circus," he said. "It's a national disgrace."

The Senate Committee was determined to prove him right. Senator Orrin Hatch said: "People hearing yesterday's testimony are probably wondering how could this quiet, you know, retired woman know about something like Long Dong Silver. Did you tell her that?'

"No, I don't know how she knows," Thomas replied.

Q: Is that a black stereotype, something like "Long Dong
   Silver"?

A: To the extent, Senator, that it is a reference to one's
   sexual organs and the size of one's sexual organs, I think
   it is.

You can't get anything past Clarence. He's obviously the man
for the Supreme Court.

Hatch went on to suggest that someone who talked about
pornographic films featuring men with large penises and
women with large breasts – is there any other kind? – was a
psychopathic sex fiend or pervert. Instead of saying that a
pervert would surely be watching a porn film involving men
with large breasts and women with large penises, Thomas
simply said no.

He complained that the hearing was a racial witch-hunt.

"From my standpoint, as a black American," he said, "it is
a high-tech lynching for uppity blacks who in anyway deign
to think for themselves, to do for themselves, to have different
ideas, and it is a message that unless you kowtow to an old
order, this is what will happen to you. You will be lynched,
destroyed, caricatured by a committee of the US Senate rather
than hung from a tree."

Thomas, a literary man, compared himself to Josef K., the
protagonist in Franz Kafka's novel *The Trial* which begins:
"Someone must have been telling lies about Josef K. for
without having done anything wrong he was arrested one fine
morning."

Hold on Clarence, you didn't get arrested. You were up for
the Supreme Court. In the end, Josef K. is executed. You got
the job.

He also compared himself to the eponymous hero of Ralph
Ellison's novel *Invisible Man*. Invisible? The hearings were on
TV, night after night. And as the hero of Richard Wright's
*Native Son*, where a young black man is falsely accused of

raping and murdering a white girl and ends up in jail. Anita Hill was black and Clarence ended up on the Supreme Court. The protagonist's name is Bigger Thomas. Let's not go there.

But Senator Hatch was a literary man too. He plainly thought the hearing was a witch-hunt too and tracked the stray pubic hair down to *The Exorcist*. On page seventy, it read:

> "Oh, Burke," sighed Sharon. In a guarded tone she described an encounter between the senator and the director. Dennings had remarked to him in passing, said Sharon, that there appeared to be, quote, "an alien pubic hair floating around in my gin."

What did Judge Thomas think of that? Thomas said: "Senator, I think this whole affair is sick." Hatch had to agree with him, but then, he asked the question.

Clarence Thomas got to sit on the Supreme Court. Anita Hill went on to have a distinguished career in the media and academia. And Senator Hatch, a Mormon, got to write "Eight Days of Hanukkah", described by Jeffery Goldberg of *The Atlantic* magazine as "a hip hop Hanukkah song by the senior senator from Utah".

## Arnold Schwarzenegger

Muscleman turned movie star Arnold Schwarzenegger married John F. Kennedy's niece Maria Shriver in 1986. He said her parents, Eunice and Sargent Shriver, inspired him to get into politics. But instead of becoming a Democrat, he ran for election as governor of California in 2003 as a Republican.

Five days before the election, Schwarzenegger was hit with allegations of sexual harassment that went back over twenty-five years. Three women told the *Los Angeles Times* that he had grabbed their breasts. A fourth said he had reached under her skirt and gripped her buttocks. A fifth said that he had groped her and tried to remove her bathing suit in a hotel elevator. And a sixth said that he had pulled her onto his lap and asked whether certain sexual acts had ever been performed on her. They worked in Hollywood and four of the six would not let their names be used, lest it hurt their careers.

Assistant director Linnea Harwell told the *LA Times* that Schwarzenegger often displayed himself naked when she went to fetch him from his trailer and once pulled her onto a bed while he was wearing only his underwear.

"He was laughing like it was all a big joke," she said. "Well, it wasn't. It was scary."

She could easily have been terminated.

In another only-in-Hollywood story, Carla Baron, a stand-in for *Twins* female lead Kelly Preston, said Schwarzenegger and his own stand-in once crowded her from the front and back, and suggested "a Carla sandwich" as the Austrian star stuck his tongue in her mouth.

Most of the allegations were not true, Schwarzenegger said, though he could not remember what had happened twenty years earlier. However, he admitted that he had "behaved badly" in the past and apologized to anyone he had offended. According to an interview in *Oui* magazine in 1977, he had attended orgies and had girls on hand to give head before he went on stage as a bodybuilder. The London *Daily Mail* also said that he had a long extramarital affair with flight attendant Tammy Tousignant and fathered a love child by her, both things Tammy denies. At the same time, he was defending himself against allegations in the seventies that he had admired Adolf Hitler. A good Kennedy woman, it was said that Maria Shriver had been taught to look the other way. She stood by him, kissed him on the stump and he was elected governor.

A further allegation of groping came up when he was running for re-election and, according to the *Daily Mail*, rumours of his rampant womanizing continued to circulate. The *LA Times* also reported that former child actress Gigi Goyette had been paid $20,000 to keep quiet about their long-term affair. But the bombshell did not go off until he had stepped down as governor.

In May 2011, Schwarzenegger and his wife separated after twenty-five years of marriage, when she discovered that he had a fourteen-year-old child by their housekeeper, Guatemalan-born Mildred Patricia "Patty" Baena. In a statement on 17 May, the ex-governor said: "After leaving the governor's office I told my wife about this event, which occurred over a decade ago."

Ms Baena had worked for the Schwarzenegger-Shriver household for twenty years, until she retired that January. He bought her a four-bedroom house with a double garage and swimming pool in Bakersfield, around a hundred miles from his Brentwood home.

It seems that Maria got wind of the ancient affair between the maid and the muscleman and confronted Patty. She broke down and admitted that her son had been fathered by Arnie. Maria then had words with her horny husband, who also confessed.

TMZ reported that in the late nineties Patty began to "pursue Arnold". She told friends that they would have unprotected sex during the day at the house. Their randy romps even took place in the marital bed. The *Sun* also reported that he romped with the mother and sister of his love child's mom while they were working for him.

"He would touch all their backsides while they were doing the housework," the paper said. "He flirted with all of them, even the mother."

Patty never slept overnight at the house and was not caught on the job. Patty's son Joseph was born just six days after Maria's third child in 1997, six years before he ran for office.

Schwarzenegger accepted financial responsibility for the child. He also spent time with him and showered him with gifts. The star of *True Lies* took Maria and two of their kids to Joseph's christening. Family photos also show the Kindergarten Cop teaching the boy to play golf. In another shot, Schwarzenegger is seen hugging Rogelio Baena, the man who brought up the child as his own. He and Patty divorced in 2008. The boy did not know who his real father was until reports surfaced in the press.

"He kept this hidden for over a decade," said Jay Leno, "which is pretty shocking. I had no idea he was that good an actor."

While Conan O'Brien said: "Arnold Schwarzenegger secretly fathered a child outside of his marriage ten years ago. He told his wife at the time, but it took ten years for her to figure out what he was saying."

Not one to stay off a bandwagon, blonde-bombshell Brigitte Nielsen then admitted she was having an affair with him 1985, when they co-starred in *Red Sonja*.

"We both knew that it wouldn't last beyond the movie, we didn't hold back," she told the *Herald Sun*. "We wanted to try everything and so we did. There were no restrictions, no promises, nothing, and it was a great time in my life."

Arnold was already seeing Maria at the time.

"Maybe I wouldn't have got into it if he said 'I'm going to marry Maria' and this is dead serious, but he didn't, and our affair carried on," Nielsen said.

She went on to marry Sylvester Stallone, whom she called "the sexiest, most delicious man", while Arnie was "the sexiest actor I've known in real life". She also had a brief fling with Sean Penn.

"I haven't had many one-night stands, but he was one and oooh . . . he was amazing!" she said.

Nielson had no intention of marrying Schwarzenegger. She did not feel that she was political-wife material.

Far from being a boorish, sexual predator he was, she said, very romantic. Her kiss off was "a beautiful over-the-top present". He was, of course, in love with her. But "you don't just have a baby with someone else". And her heart went out to Maria.

It was just lucky that, at the time, she had a new book out, *You Only Get One Life*, $29.95.

## Mike Sanford

In June 2009, the governor of South Carolina Mark Sanford, tipped as a possible president by conservative Republicans, disappeared for six days. Neither his bodyguards nor his wife Jenny knew where he was, but she said she was not concerned as he needed time away from her and their children to write. However, she indicated that she was unaware of his travel plans over the Father's Day weekend.

When he finally got in touch, his staff said he had been hiking down the Appalachian Trail. But then he arrived at Atlanta's Hartsfield-Jackson International Airport on a flight from Buenos Aires.

"It's a great city," said Sanford.

Snared by lone reporter Gina Smith, Sanford said he had planned to go hiking, then decided: "I want to do something more exotic." He had got the ticket at the last moment by redeeming points on his frequent-flier scheme and had returned early when his staff informed him that his disappearance was attracting media attention.

Republican State Senator Jake Knotts dismissed this as "lies" and said he wanted to know: "Why all the big cover-up?"

Sanford was alone in Argentina and took a drive down the coast. However, in Buenos Aires, the Avenida Costanera is the only coastal road, and it's less than two miles long. Reaching coastal resorts to the south requires a drive of nearly four hours on an inland highway with views of endless cattle ranches. To the north is a river delta of islands reached only by boat.

Only hours after returning to the United States, Sanford called a press conference and admitted that he was having an extramarital affair with a woman in Argentina and had lied to cover up his tryst. Then his wife said that she had asked him to move out of the governor's mansion two weeks before.

Emails written the previous summer hit the press. They were addressed to "Maria" and Sanford characterized their relationship as a "hopelessly impossible situation of love".

Just after midnight on 10 July 2008, he wrote: "You have the ability to give magnificently gentle kisses . . . I love your tan lines . . . the curves of your hips, the erotic beauty of you holding yourself . . . in the faded glow of night's light."

On 4 July, she had written: "I wasn't aware till we met last week, the strong feelings I had for you. I haven't felt this since I was in my teen ages. I do love you."

He said he had met the woman concerned eight years before and, at one point, counselled her not to leave her husband for the sake of their sons. He admitted that there was a certain irony to this as he and his wife had four sons.

"It began very innocently . . . in just a casual email back and forth," Sanford said. Despite the distance between them, "It developed into something much more than that."

Sanford said he had seen the woman three times since their relationship became sexual. Then, when his wife had found a letter he had written to his Argentinian mistress, they had gone into counselling together. It obviously had not done him any good.

"I spent the last five days of my life crying in Argentina," he said. Some therapy.

During the press conference, he repeatedly quoted Scripture. He was a religious man, he said, and this was the first and only time he had been unfaithful during his nineteen-year marriage. Maybe he should have spent more time on his knees.

He stepped down as chairman of the Republican Governors' Association, a position he had taken to fight President Obama's economic stimulus package, which would have given $700 million in aid for a poor state racked by one of the country's highest unemployment rates. I am sure the people of South Carolina were very grateful.

Later, while saying that he wanted to reconcile with his wife and save what was left of his political career, Sanford admitted that he "crossed lines" with a handful of other women since he had been married. That would do it then.

He had met other women when he had gone abroad to "blow off steam". He met his Argentine amour Maria Belen Chapur at an open-air dance spot in Uruguay eight years before. They met again during the 2004 Republican convention in New York, when she was working as a correspondent for an Argentine TV station there. But the relationship only became physical, he said, during a government trip to Brazil and Argentina in June 2008. It was the government's fault then. No, that's unfair. After he was caught, he wrote a cheque for nearly $3,000 to reimburse the state for a state-funded trip to Argentina in 2008.

Over the previous year, he had met her five times. There were two romantic stays of several nights – one in Manhattan, one in the Hamptons. Both paid for in cash to cover his tracks. After his wife found out, he asked her permission several times to meet his mistress, but she said no. There's a surprise. However, when he agreed to break up, he got her permission to meet Chapur in New York again with a "trusted spiritual adviser" serving as chaperone. The threesome went to church and dinner together and parted ways the same night, he insisted.

But sex was not the only thing between them. He said that he could go to his grave "knowing that I had met my soul mate".

"This was a whole lot more than a simple affair, this was a love story," Sanford said. "A forbidden one, a tragic one, but a love story at the end of the day."

He drew a moral from the whole sorry story. "If you're a married guy at the end of the day you shouldn't be dancing with somebody else," Sanford said. No, maybe you shouldn't be fucking with somebody else.

I wonder whether that was what the controversial religious organization The Fellowship told him when he sought counselling there. It was there that he met Senator John Ensign, who resigned after having an affair with the wife of one of his top aides, and Congressman Chip Pickering, whose wife launched a lawsuit for alienation of affection against his mistress, who instead of praying with him was preying on him there.

Although they threatened to impeach Sanford, the state legislature censured him instead. He served out his governorship and divorced. In 2011, he was seen in Uruguay with Chapur. The *New York Times* asked if she was still his "soul mate", though the affair had torpedoed his promising political career.

"Out of fairness to my boys and to folks that I've hurt," he said, "I'm not going to say more than this: any of those seemingly goofy feelings that I described a couple years back have intensified, not dissipated, with time."

## Sarah Palin

Darling of the Tea Party, Sarah Palin was dropped into a sex scandal by the publication of Joe McGinniss's book *The Rogue: Searching for the Real Sarah Palin*. According to the book, in 1987, Palin, then a twenty-three-year-old sports reporter, had a one-night stand with college basketball stud Glen Rice. Obviously, it was an in-depth interview. Less than a year later, Palin married her husband Todd and became the hockey mom we all know.

Now normally, there would not be any problem with a little pre-marital hanky-panky. But, uh-oh, Palin has taken a stand on chastity. In 2006, when she was running to be governor of Alaska, she filled out a questionnaire supplied by the Eagle Forum, a conservative interest group. In it, she stated that she supported funding abstinence-until-marriage education programmes instead of teaching sex-education programmes.

The *Washington Post* published details of the dalliance under the headline: GLEN RICE AND SARAH PALIN: I DON'T WANT TO KNOW. But the *National Enquirer* seized eagerly on the story, reporting that "Sarah had a 'fetish' for black men at the time and ... had 'hauled [Rice's] ass down'," and that she also had an affair with her husband's former business partner, Brad Hanson. According to the news site Alaska Report, this may even prompt a divorce.

Thrust into the spotlight in 2008 when she became a Republican vice-presidential nominee, Palin was immediately caught with her pants down. The *National Enquirer* claimed that the First Lady of Alaska had been keeping a lover. Her presidential running partner, Senator John McCain, denied the rumour immediately on her behalf.

But following McGinniss's book, even the stuffy old *New York Times* could not help getting in on the act. Their reviewer Janet Maslin pulled a choice quote from *The Rogue*: "A friend says, 'Sarah and her sisters had a fetish for black guys for a while.'"

What a shame that she is not Barack Obama's type.

## Herman Cain

On 21 May 2011, the former CEO of Godfather's Pizza Herman Cain announced that he was running for president on the Republican ticket with his 999 tax plan. Plainly he had been practising for the position for some time.

On 30 October 2011, *Politico* reported that two female employees had complained about sexually suggestive behaviour by Cain when he was president of the National Restaurant Association. The women were said to have accepted financial settlements from the association, which barred them from discussing the matter any further. Cain initially refused to comment, glaring at a reporter who dared to ask him whether he had ever been accused of sexual harassment three times, while his campaign accused the "inside the Beltway" media of making unsubstantiated attacks on him and "dredging up thinly sourced allegations".

The following day, Cain told the National Press Club: "I have never sexually harassed anyone and those accusations are totally false."

He claimed that there was a "witch-hunt" against him and concluded proceedings by singing a few verses from "He Looked Beyond My Faults".

At first, he denied knowing anything about the financial settlement with his accusers, but later accepted that a payment had been made by the Restaurant Association. One of the allegations, he maintained, amounted to the fact that he had said that one of the women was the same height as his wife and made a gesture with the flat of his palm at about chin level. For that, the woman wanted a five-figure sum.

Joel Bennett, a lawyer representing one of the complainants, Karen Kraushaar, called Cain's version of events "goofy", saying, "My client would never have filed a complaint of sexual harassment on the basis that she was the same height as his wife. It is ridiculous."

At her next job, Kraushaar also made a complaint and demanded thousands of dollars to settle. She later dropped the matter. Then on 3 November 2011, a third woman told the Associated Press that Cain had commented on her attractiveness and invited her up to his corporate apartment. It made her feel very uncomfortable and others present asked him to stop, she said.

On 7 November, Sharon Bialek stepped forward. She told the packed press conference in New York that the incident had taken place in 1997. She had recently lost her job with an affiliate of the NRA and had come to Washington in the hope that he might be able to help her. He had upgraded her suite at the hotel and took her for dinner at an Italian restaurant. Then they drove over to the National Restaurant Association headquarters, but when he stopped the car outside, he made an advance.

"He suddenly reached over and put his hand on my leg under my skirt and reached for my genitals," said Bialek. "He also grabbed my head and pushed it toward his crotch."

He wanted to 999 her.

"I said, 'What are you doing?'" she continued. "'You know I have a boyfriend. This isn't what I came here for.' Mr Cain said, 'You want a job, right?' I asked him to stop and he did. I asked him to take me back to my hotel which he did, right away."

A member of the cast from the *Daily Show* was at the press conference, along with a heckler from the *Howard Stern Show*, but the best comedian on hand was Bialek's lawyer, celebrity attorney Gloria Allred. She said of her client, "Instead of receiving the help that she had hoped for, Mr Cain decided to provide her with his idea of a stimulus package."

But Bialek had some good lines of her own, urging Cain to "come clean". And Bennett said that he had heard from Bialek but she said she did not want to do anything because she had "too much on my plate".

Even Cain could not help getting in on the act, telling TV's *Jimmy Kimmel Live*: "We are taking this head on."

His initial response to Bialek's allegations was the suitably Clintonesque: "I have not acted inappropriately with anyone, period." And he claimed that he did not even recognize her. "I don't even know who this lady is," he said.

However, they had met just a month before at a Tea Party event, a witness said.

"I went up to him and asked him, 'Do you remember me?'" said Bialek. "He acknowledged that he remembered me from the foundation, but he kind of looked uncomfortable and he said nothing as he was whisked away for his speech by his handlers."

This annoyed her because she wanted to talk. He smiled at first, but after the words they had together, he was seen to be "stone-faced".

The Cain campaign hired attorney L. Lin Wood to head a team responding to the allegations. Wood warned that any other women coming forward with allegations would face intense scrutiny and might also be subject to legal action. So they are expecting some then.

And they weren't disappointed. On 28 November 2011, Georgia woman Ginger White told the local Fox affiliate in Atlanta that she had had a thirteen-year affair with Cain, which had ended eight months earlier, just before he announced he was running for the nomination. They met in Kentucky during the nineties when he was head of the National Restaurant Association. She was impressed by Cain and they had drinks, she said, before he invited her back to his hotel room. After that, he bought her airline tickets so that she could join him in different cities.

"It wasn't complicated," she said. "I was aware that he was married. And I was also aware I was involved in a very inappropriate situation, relationship."

She said that she had decided to speak out now about the affair before anyone else did.

In fact, Cain got in first on CNN, telling Wolf Blitzer: "This individual is going to accuse me of an affair for an extended period of time. It is someone that I know who is an acquaintance that I thought was a friend."

Again he claimed that it was not a sexual affair and he had done nothing wrong.

Lin Wood said: "If any candidate wants to publicly discuss his private sex life, that is his or her life. But I don't believe that there's an obligation on the part of any political candidate to do so."

No, but Mr Wood, you must admit it is more fun if they do.

**The Mammoth Book of Best New Erotica 10**
edited by Maxim Jakubowski

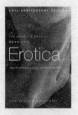

ISBN: 978-1-84901-365-9 (UK)
RRP: £7.99

ISBN: 978-0-7624-4097-9 (US)
RRP: $13.95

**The year's best erotica from the world's leading writers**

A collection of over 40 imaginative and intimately detailed
sexual adventures, *The Mammoth Book of Best New Erotica*
offers the very best new work of both well-known names and
up-and-coming talents. For the first time the collection features
the work of nearly as many male as female writers, offering a
wealth of perspectives from both sides of the gender divide.

Here you will find erotica of every kind, exploring the
full range of human sensual and sexual experience, from
voyeurism to swinging, from hotel rooms
to vampires, in ways both suggestive and explicit.

**'Honeymoon with Shannon', Thom Gautier**

**'In the Absence of Motion', Peter Baltensperger**

**'On My Knees in Barcelona', Kristina Lloyd**

**'Perfect Timing', Kristina Wright**

**'Double Take', Madeline Moore**

**'Careful What You Wish For', D. L. King**

## The Mammoth Book of Body Horror
edited by Marie O'Regan and Paul Kane

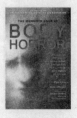

ISBN: 978-1-78033-039-6 (UK)
RRP: £7.99

ISBN: 978-0-7624-4432-8 (US)
RRP: $13.95

### 25 horrific tales of transformation, mutilation and contagion

This truly disturbing collection of 'body horror' ranges from Mary Shelley's revelatory 'Transformation' to H. P. Lovecraft's 'Herbert West – Reanimator', brought to a new audience by the success of Stuart Gordon's film *Re-Animator*, to George Langelaan's 'The Fly', filmed most recently by David Cronenberg, and a chilling story by Lovecraft's disciple, Robert Bloch, best known as the author of *Psycho*.

The term 'body horror' has long been used to describe films such as *The Thing*, based on John W. Campbell's 'Who Goes There?', which is reprinted here, and most recently *District 9*, but the subgenre did not begin with film.

Here you will find profoundly unsettling stories spanning the entire history of the subgenre by the very best writers of horror, such as Clive Barker, Ramsey Campbell, Nancy A. Collins, Neil Gaiman, James Herbert, Stephen King, Brian Lumley, Edgar Allan Poe and many more.